D1301186

Recent Results in Cancer Research

Fortschritte der Krebsforschung

Progrès dans les recherches sur le cancer

41

Edited by

Sponsored by the Swiss League against Cancer

Tumours in a Tropical Country

A Survey of Uganda 1964-1968

Edited by

A. C. Templeton

With 131 Figures

Springer-Verlag New York · Heidelberg · Berlin 1973

A. C. Templeton, M.R.C. Path. (U.K.), M.R.C.P. (Edin.), Professor of Pathology, University of Minnesota, Minneapolis, Minnesota, U.S.A.

Formerly Senior Lecturer in Pathology, Makerere University, Kampala, Uganda

Supported by a grant from the
Cancer Research Campaign, London

ISBN 0-387-06114-2   Springer-Verlag New York · Heidelberg · Berlin
ISBN 3-540-06114-2   Springer-Verlag Berlin · Heidelberg · New York

Foreword

The geography of medicine is a classical subject that can be studied wherever medicine is practised and the population counted. It has already contributed a great deal to knowledge of the causes of disease and it might be thought that the subject had little more to teach. This, however, is unlikely. First, there are many parts of the world that have only recently been provided with the full range of diagnostic services. Secondly, it is now realised that the observation that a disease occurs only very rarely under some conditions can be just as important as the observation that it occurs very often under others. Thirdly, the spread of industrialization has not yet eliminated the wide variety of conditions of life that has been produced by different cultures and different standards of living. We have still an opportunity to determine their effect on the incidence of disease, but not perhaps for long.

That an interest in the geography of cancer can pay dividends is shown by many examples ranging from the relationships between cancer of the buccal cavity and chewing habits and between cancer of the lung and smoking, to the current enquiries relating Burkitt's lymphoma to malaria, cancer of the oesophagus to the comsumption of maize beer, cancer of the liver to food contaminated with aflatoxin, and cancer of the large bowel to the dietary content of fibre and fat. Many of these observations have been made in Africa and particularly in Uganda, where Sir ALBERT COOK began to record clinical impressions of the incidence of cancer before the end of the last century. Now, in this book, Templeton and his colleagues add a mass of new data that will serve as a source of new ideas for many years to come.

The data refer to nearly 11,000 tumours registered in the Kampala Cancer Registry over the period 1964—68. With the exception of a few patients in whom cancer was diagnosed by clinical and radiological means in the immediate vicinity of Kampala, patients were registered only when specimens were received for pathological examination. It is obvious, therefore, that incidence rates must be grossly underestimated, particularly for those parts of Uganda that are remote from the capital. The value of the work lies, therefore, not so much in the provision of detailed incidence rates, but in the picture it provides of the distribution of cancer, subdivided by organ, site within an organ, and histological type and in the relationships that have been observed between these characteristics and the sex, age, tribe, and place of residence of the affected patients. With such data, bias due to incomplete registration may be unimportant and useful information can be obtained by comparing the relative proportions of different types of cancer recorded for different cultural groups in different parts of the country. It is, for example, unlikely that any sort of selective bias could have brought about the observation that cancers of the lower end of the oesophagus were reported relatively more often from the Eastern part of the country than cancers of the upper end of the oesophagus, while the reverse was true for cancers of the pyloric part of the stomach in comparison with cancers of the cardia. Similarly, it is difficult to see how bias could have brought about specific correlations between the tribal incidence of cancers of the penis and the vulva and, to a less extent, between cancers of the penis and the cervix uteri. Nor is there any reason to suppose that bias could have accounted for a high incidence of Hodgkin's disease of the mixed cellular type in childhood without any evidence of a peak incidence at older ages.

When, twenty five years ago, Sir AUSTIN BRADFORD HILL and I began to study the smoking histories of patients with and without lung cancer, we were immediately struck by the rarity with which patients with lung cancer were recorded as having been life-long non-smokers. For some time we had difficulty in persuading ourselves that the difference between the two groups of patients was not an artefact due, for example, to a difference in the intensity of questioning to which they had been subjected, or to exaggeration of their smoking habits by patients with respiratory symptoms. Gradually, however, as we reviewed the criteria on which the diagnoses were made, we became aware that the diagnosis of bronchial carcinoma had to be abandoned in a much higher proportion of the 'lung cancer' patients who had never smoked than of those who had. As one non-smoker after another was found to have had a fibrosarcoma of the chest wall, a hamartoma, or an alveolar cell carcinoma, the conviction grew that the difference we had observed was real; for the histological classifications had been made independently by many different pathologists and could not have been biassed by knowledge of our interest or of the patient's smoking history. Later, Court Brown and I had a similar experience when we were investigating the relationship between the use of radio-therapy for ankylosis spondylitis and the development of leukaemia. The more that radio-therapists wrote to report the occurence of leukaemia in an unirradiated patient, the fainter our doubts became; for the leukaemia that occurred in patients who had not been irradiated was most often chronic lymphatic in type, while that which occurred after irradiation was usually myeloid. These are two personal examples of the way in which statistics can be given life and meaning when symbiotic with pathology; the records of the Kampala Cancer Registry provide many more.

Oxford, April 1973

RICHARD DOLL

Preface

This monograph is based on material derived from the Kampala Cancer Registry of the Department of Pathology, Makerere University. The registry was founded by Prof. J. N. P. Davies and directed by him until 1962, and during the period of this survey was directed by Prof. M. S. R. Hutt. The collection analysed between 1964—1968 constitutes 10,945 tumours and at least eleven facts are known about each case. This whole activity has been generously financed by the British Empire Cancer Campaign (now the Cancer Research Campaign) but for which the Kampala Cancer Registry and this study could not exist.

The generation, classification and retrieval of these facts are obviously the work of many people. Details of individual cases have been submitted by doctors in all hospitals in Uganda. Many have spent a good deal of time ensuring that details of cases are accurately noted down and relayed to the Registry. Registration and coding has been the work of Mrs. Barbara Wright assisted at different times by Mrs. Claire D'Abreu, Mrs. Margaret Musoke, Mrs. Anne Huckstep, Mrs. Alexis Bianchi, Mrs. Elizabeth Buxton and Mrs. Carole Nickson. Computer programming and dealing with the numerous alterations caused by this study have been the work of Dr. Malcolm Pike and Mrs. Diana Bull of the Department of the Regius Professor of Medicine, Oxford University. Mr. Kenneth Hill advised on matters of population determination. Mr. Matt Findlay took, developed, and printed many of the illustrations. Messrs. Robertson, Serumaga and Busulwa of the Department of Medical Illustration, Makerere University, gave help with other illustrations, maps and charts. The secretarial work entailed has been patiently borne by Mrs. Jenny Whitehead. Advice on different aspects of this publication has been given by Professor Sir Richard Doll, Dr. Robert Harris, Mr. Dennis Burkitt and Dr. Robert Scully. Helpful discussions on various aspects of tumours in Uganda were held with Prof. Sir Ian McAdam, Prof. S. K. Kyalwazi, Dr. Rolf Schmauz, Dr. John Thomas and Dr. John Ziegler. Prof. R. R. Trussel, Dr. Pet Leighton and Mr. O. Zeigler kindly allowed access to the records of the cytology department. To all these and many others who helped in so many ways grateful thanks are given.

Minneapolis, January 1973   A. C. Templeton

Contents

Contributors

Dr. P. P. ANTHONY, M.R.C. Path., Senior Lecturer in Pathology, Middlesex Hospital Medical School, London, W. 1./ Great Britain. Formerly Senior Lecturer in Pathology, Makerere University, Kampala.

Liver, p. 57
Urinary Tract, p. 145

Professor J. N. P. DAVIES, M.D. (Bristol), F.R.C. Path., Albany Medical College, Albany, N. Y./USA. Formerly Professor of Pathology, Makerere University, Kampala.

Children's Tumours, p. 306

Dr. O. G. DODGE, M.D., M.R.C. Path., Consultant Pathologist, Christie Hospital, Manchester/Great Britain. Formerly Senior Lecturer in Pathology, Makerere University, Kampala, and University of Sheffield, England.

Male Genitalia, p. 132
Bones, p. 222

Professor M. S. R. HUTT, M.D., F.R.C. Path., Professor of Geographical Pathology, St. Thomas's Hospital Medical School London, S.E.1/Great Britain. Formerly Professor of Pathology, Makerere University, Kampala.

Introduction, p. 1
Liver, p. 57

Professor O. H. IVERSEN, M.D., Director of Institutt for Generell og Eksperimentell Patologi, University of Oslo, Rikshospitalet, Oslo 1/Norway. Formerly Visiting Professor, Makerere University, Kampala.

Skin, p. 180

Dr. ULLA IVERSEN, M.D., Institutt for Generell og Eksperimentell Patologi, University of Oslo. Rikshospitalet, Oslo 1/Norway.

Skin, p. 180

Dr. P. D. JAMES, M.R.C.P. (U.K.), MRC Path. Lecturer, Bland Sutton Institute of Pathology, Middlesex Hospital Medical School, London, W. 1/Great Britain. Formerly Lecturer in Pathology, Makerere University, Kampala.

Female Genitalia, p. 101

Professor M. G. LEWIS, M.D. (Lond.) M.R.C. Path. Professor and Chairman of Pathology, Memorial University of Newfoundland, St. John, Newfoundland/Canada. Formerly Lecturer in Geographical Pathology, Makerere University, Kampala.

Melanoma, p. 171

Dr. G. T. O'CONOR, M.D. National Cancer Institute, Bethesda, MD 20014/U.S.A. Formerly Senior Lecturer, Makerere University, Kampala.

Respiratory, p. 79

Professor R. OWOR, M.D. (E.A), M.R.C. Path., Professor of Pathology, Makerere University, Kampala/Uganda.

Testis, p. 132

Dr. A. SERCK-HANSSEN, M.D., Consultant Cytologist, Ulleval Hospital Oslo/Norway. Formerly Senior Lecturer in Pathology, Makerere University, Kampala.

Histiocytic Medullary Reticulosis, p. 292

Professor C. W. Taylor, M.D., F.R.C. Path., Emeritus Profes-   Ovary, p. 101
sor of Pathology. University of Birmingham Medical School,
Birmingham 15/Great Britain.

Professor A. C. Templeton, M.R.C. Path., M.R.C.P.,   Introduction, p. 1
D.R.C.O.G., Professor of Pathology, University of Minne-   Alimentary Canal, p. 23
sota, Minneapolis, MN 55455/USA Formerly Senior Lec-   Pancreas, p. 77
turer in Pathology Makerere University, Kampala.   Respiratory tract, p. 79
                                                               Breast, p. 94
                                                               Female Genitalia, p. 101
                                                               Male Genitalia, p. 132
                                                               Brain, p. 200
                                                               Eye, p. 203
                                                               Endocrine, p. 215
                                                               Soft Tissues, p. 234
                                                               Leukaemia, p. 298
                                                               Unknown Origin, p. 302

Professor D. H. Wright, M.D. (Bristol), M.R.C. Path., Pro-   Lymphoma, p. 270
fessor of Pathology, University of Southampton Medical
School, Southampton/Great Britain. Formerly Reader in
Pathology, Makerere University, Kampala.

Chapter 1

Introduction

Distribution of Tumours in Uganda

A. C. Templeton and M. S. R. Hutt

With 6 Figures

The geography of Uganda and some of the historical background of western medicine in the country are outlined. Uganda contains a wide range of climates and people and is therefore well adapted for epidemiological work. Some of the diseases prevalent in the community are pointed out.

In all, 7,347 malignant tumours were diagnosed in the period under review. This collection is surveyed briefly. Cancer of the soft tissues, penis, liver and skin were found to be the most common tumours of men, and carcinoma of the cervix, breast and skin were most frequent among women. Bias in diagnosis and registration is examined and its influence is assessed. Variations in the frequency of tumour diagnosis are examined in this light and regional variations pointed out.

Tumours are classified according to their anatomical site, cell of origin and biological behaviour. Each of the many tumours which can be derived from these axes of classification must be investigated as an entity in order to elucidate its aetiology and pathogenesis. For such research a multidisciplinary approach is essential. In the chain of investigation of environmentally determined diseases observations on individuals with the condition are usually followed by observations on groups of people living in differing circumstances. This combination of clinical and epidemiological methods may result in a hypothesis as to the cause of a given condition. This hypothesis can then be tested by experiments either in man or in animals. From time to time serendipity may reverse this process but each step provides a stimulus for and a verification of the other. Experience with cancer in immigrant groups suggests that it is mainly the differences in geographical, socio-economic and cultural background which determine the varied patterns of disease, including tumours, in different parts of the world or in different groups of people. In an individual, but only very seldom in a community, the likelihood of developing a tumour will be modified by genetic factors. In areas such as Middle Africa a wide variety of "natural experiments" occur which may be used to test the validity of observations made in Uganda or in other parts of the world. For such observations to be of value the criteria and classification of disease must be precise, for like must be compared with like. This volume attempts to follow these precepts in describing the tumour pattern of Uganda.

In most African countries demography is poor and therefore the denominator of any calculation of incidence rates is bound to be suspect. Medical facilities are largely unsophisticated and thinly scattered so that the numerator is also liable to error. Well-trained specialists are rarities and are found in only a small proportion of hospitals. In 1966 there were 642 registered doctors in Uganda (Statistical Abstract, 1969), a doctor-patient ratio of about 1 to 12,000 and Uganda is better provided for than most black African countries. It would seem therefore that any cancer study in Africa would be unlikely to produce results which could not be improved upon elsewhere. Cancer cannot be considered a major health problem for it is estimated that only about 4% of the people who die in Uganda today have a cancer present at the time and in only a proportion of these has the tumour caused death. The study of cancer cannot therefore be justified on the basis of the current medical needs of the local population.

In spite of these inherent disadvantages the contribution of doctors working in Uganda and in other similar countries in Africa have been remarkable. Some of the major observations on cancer in Uganda are outlined in Table 1. In addition a large number of important discoveries have been made in other countries by scientists working in collaboration with personnel in Uganda. These have not been mentioned in the table since we wish here to underline the importance of observational research carried out with simple techniques by small groups of individuals.

Table 1. Some landmarks in Ugandan work on cancer epidemiology

1901   "Cancer is just as frequent in Uganda" (A. Cook, 1901).

1948   Davies published a series of papers on necropsy findings in Uganda and established many of the basic facts about disease distribution (Davies, 1948).

1951   Kampala Cancer Registry set up by Professor J. N. P. Davies (Davies and Wilson, 1954).

1956   Symposium on Cancer of the Liver among African Negroes (Acta U.I.C.C., **13**, 1957).

1958   "A sarcoma involving the jaws in African children" (Burkitt, 1958).

1962   "Determining the climatic limitations of a children's cancer common in East and Central Africa" (Burkitt, 1962).

1963   The geographical distribution of carcinoma of the penis and the relation to circumcision firmly established (Dodge, Linsell, Davies, 1963).

1964   Cancer in an African community (Davies et al., 1964) showed that the proportion of cancers in Kampala had remained stable over 60 years and that cancer was therefore not a "white man's disease".

1965   Cancer in Kyadondo (Davies, Knowelden and Wilson, 1965) showed that in the middle years of life cancer was just as frequent as elsewhere and confirmed many of the impressions of previous workers.

1967   The value of a small localized cancer registry established with the demonstration of epidemic drift in Burkitt's tumour (Pike, Williams and Wright, 1967).

Development of Cancer Research in Uganda

The first observations on cancer in Uganda were made by Sir Albert Cook very shortly after his arrival in Kampala in 1897 (Foster, 1970). He realised that the apparent rarity of cancer in Africa was an artefact resulting from the extreme frequency of infectious disease and the absence of any mechanism by which cancer cases are concentrated in referrals from general practitioners and clinics (COOK, 1901). Observations from various parts of the continent showed that the proportions of different tumours occurring in Africa were different from one another and sharply distinct from the patterns seen in Europe and America (SMITH and ELMES, 1934; VINT, 1935). Analysis of autopsy data from Mulago Hospital, Kampala, showed that the pattern of cancer in Uganda was also different (DAVIES, 1948). All these observations were made on a variable sample of disease in a given area and as such were liable to error. These errors could only be minimized by the collection of comprehensive data so that the true incidence rates might be calculated. In 1951 the staff of Mulago Hospital agreed to cooperate in an effort to register all cases of cancer seen in the hospital. This was no small undertaking. Patients with no written tradition may have their names spelled in a variety of ways. Where seasonal change is not great, ages are frequently rather difficult to establish. Names change as people acquire a different status in life. No street names, house numbers, social security systems or driving licence numbers assist in tracking down patients. The elimination of errors occasioned by these background facts requires involvement and a lot of hard work. The development of this phase of the work of the cancer registry can be traced in a series of publications by DAVIES (DAVIES and WILSON, 1954; DAVIES, 1957; DAVIES, WILSON and KNOWELDEN, 1958). After a preliminary survey of hospitals in Kampala and the histological diagnoses made in the Pathology Department, Makerere University, and the Government histology laboratory, it was found that the registration rate in Kyadondo Country, which includes the city of Kampala, was higher than in the surrounding countryside. An incidence rate survey of Kyadondo was carried out over the seven-year period 1954—1960. During this time a new census was undertaken in 1959. The results of this survey (DAVIES, KNOWELDEN and WILSON, 1965) showed that the age-specific incidence rates of cancer in the middle years of life were very similar to those seen in other countries. Comparison with a survey from Johannesburg (HIGGINSON and OETTLÉ, 1960) showed in detail the points of similarity and the differences between the two African series. Tumours of the liver, cervix and penis were more common in both African series than in Europe or America, and tumours of the colon and body of the uterus were less commonly seen. Contrasts between the two series were also noted in that Kaposi's sarcoma and most types of lymphomas were much more common in Kyadondo whereas tumours of the bronchus and oesophagus were more frequently seen in Johannesburg.

The geographical variations alluded to above were seen to occur over quite short distances. CLEMMESEN et al. (1962) and THIJS (1957) showed variations in tumour patterns in Ruanda and Congo and similar changes were found to occur within Uganda. Among the first tumours found to have a marked geographical variation was the jaw tumour of childhood first noted by ALBERT COOK (COOK, 1904). In 1958 BURKITT published a paper describing the clinical feature of "a sarcoma involving the jaws in African children". This was followed by a series of papers delineating the tumours as a clinical (BURKITT and O'CONOR, 1961), radiological (DAVIES and DAVIES, 1960) and pathological entity (O'CONOR, 1961). It was shown that the marked variations in incidence appeared to be climatically determined (BURKITT, 1962). In 1963 WRIGHT further refined the diagnostic histological criteria, and in 1965 BURKITT noted the very rapid response to therapy with oral cytotoxic agents. These observations excited world-wide interest and have contributed to a reorientation of ideas in many branches of cancer research. Thus interest in the role of viruses in the aetiology of human cancer was renewed, tumour immunology was given greater impetus and hopes for successful cancer chemotherapy were rekindled. Other variations in tumour incidence were noted and some were elucidated. Carcinoma of the penis was found to correlate well with circumcision practice (DODGE, LINSELL and DAVIES, 1963). The tremendous variations in incidence of Kaposi's sarcoma were highlighted in an International Symposium held in Kampala in 1961 (ACKERMANN and MURRAY, 1963) and the different anatomical and histological distribution of salivary tumours was noted (DAVIES, DODGE and BURKITT, 1964).

Perhaps the most important discovery of this period resulted from the excellent clinical notes kept by Sir ALBERT COOK and his successors at Mengo Hospital. This hospital was the first, and, for a long period of time, the only institution caring for the local community at all levels. These records provide a unique picture of the pattern of disease present in an African community before the society had been disturbed by European influences. An analysis of the cancer patterns seen at Mengo Hospital from 1897, the time of ALBERT COOK's arrival, up to 1956 showed that the proportion of tumours occurring in the region of Kampala had remained stable over a period of 60 years (DAVIES et al., 1965). This convincingly demonstrated that cancer was a disease of the indigenous population and had not been imported by white men. It showed also that the rural African had retained most of the social and oncogenic aspects of his life essentially unaltered. The correlation between the social and oncogenic factors has been and is the major task of the Cancer Registry from that time.

In 1961 the separate Government and University histology laboratories were merged and a sustained effort to improve the diagnosis of cancer in the whole country was initiated. This was done by providing a free postal histopathology service for all hospitals in the country. This resulted in a marked increase in biopsies in each succeeding year and the number of cancers diagnosed rose rapidly (Fig. 1).

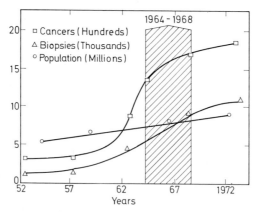

Fig. 1. Showing the cancers and biopsies registered each year and the population changes which have occurred during the lifespan of the Kampala Cancer Registry

During the period 1964 to 1968, 41,719 biopsy specimens were received in the laboratory and 6,956 cases of cancer were diagnosed. An analysis of the Kampala

Cancer Registry returns for 1964 showed that there were marked differences in cancer patterns in various parts of the country (HUTT and BURKITT, 1965). The extension and refinement of the clinico-pathological approach advocated then is the substance of this monograph. This approach demands knowledge of:

1. the country and its climate;
2. the people who live in it; their numbers, ethnic status, and social and dietary customs;
3. the medical facilities available for diagnosis and treatment;
4. the methods used in case findings and recording, together with some insight into any bias inherent in registration practice.

In order to obtain meaningful figures for uncommon neoplasms a large collection of tumours gathered under homogeneous circumstances must be available for analysis. Ideally, therefore, a study in geographical pathology should be carried out in an area small enough for all parts to be easily accessible but large enough to provide a significant collection of cases. The population should be heterogeneous but each group should be rigidly separated from the others. There should be a range of climate and other geographical features and the population should be ethnically varied. This will ensure that the sample includes similar people living under different environments and different people living under similar environments, so that control groups are available when reading the results of a natural experiment. There should be stable diagnostic criteria, best achieved if a small group of people diagnose all cases. There should be a period of political tranquillity for long enough to gather a large collection of cases. Such a country and such a period of time was Uganda in the period 1964 to 1968.

Uganda

The Period (1964—1968)

Uganda achieved independence on October 9th, 1962, after a period of 60 years as a British Protectorate. The first few years of the post-independence period were spent in manoeuvering for political position. This resolved into a conflict between two groups, on the one hand the KABAKA, head of the Baganda, who were the largest and most powerful tribe in the country, and, on the other, MILTON OBOTE, who led a loose coalition of other tribes. This rivalry finally led to a battle in May 1966, which resulted in a disintegration of the Kabakaship and to some extent reduced the domination of the Baganda in all walks of life. The period February to August, 1966 was therefore characterized by a slight lessening of surgical biopsy activity but the registration of cancers was not affected (Fig. 1). Apart from this period there was free mobility around the country and no serious disruption of daily life.

The Country

Information on the geography, geology and meteorology of Uganda is available in the Uganda Atlas (1967) and much of the information presented below is derived therefrom.

Uganda is a small country with a land area of 74,748 square miles and a further 20,000 square miles of swamp or open water. It lies astride the Equator between 4° N and 1° S and 30° and 35° E, and is very roughly 300 miles square. The altitude varies from 2,000 to nearly 17,000 feet. The southwestern plateau lies at a mean altitude of 6,000 and the country falls to 2,000 feet as one travels north and

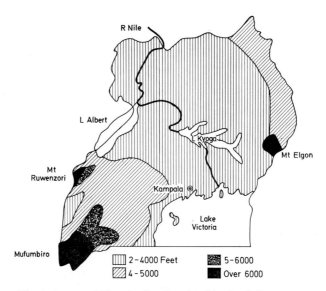

Fig. 2. A map of Uganda showing the altitude of the country

east to its lowest levels in the Northern central area (Fig. 2). The majority of people live in one of four major centres: —

1. the Kigezi plateau in the south-west of the country,
2. the crescent around the north and west of Lake Victoria,
3. the area around Mount Elgon in eastern Uganda, and
4. West Nile district.

The annual rainfall varies from 20 inches in Karamoja to over 90 inches in some of the islands in Lake Victoria. The climate ranges from desert to swamp, from tropical rain forest to alpine heath. The river Nile rises from Lake Victoria and flows northwards to Lake Kyoga, then westwards to Lake Albert where it turns sharply north once more and leaves Uganda at the Sudanese border at an altitutde of 2,000 feet. Most other river systems are essentially sluggish, swampy streams draining into the lakes of the western rift valley or Lake Kyoga. Almost 20% of the area of Uganda is occupied by lakes; these comprise Victoria, Albert, the Kyoga complex and Edward, which have a total surface area in Uganda of 20,000 square miles.

The country is divided into four administrative regions and each of these regions into districts which largely follow the traditional tribal areas. Some of the district boundaries were altered in 1968 and two new districts were formed in 1971. The boundaries used throughout this monograph are those pertaining in 1964 (Fig. 3). The administrative, commercial, communications, and medical centre of the country is Kampala. The African population of the city in 1959 was 24,000 (Uganda Census, 1959); by 1969 it had risen to 293,000 (Uganda Census, 1969). The bulk of this increase was a result of considerable broadening of the city limits. It is estimated that the city's real growth was at least 10% per year, but it has not yet acquired the extensive shanty towns which surround many other African cities.

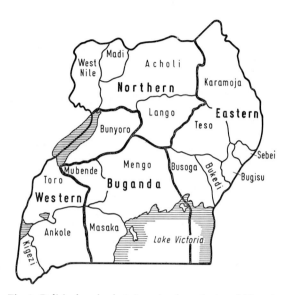

Fig. 3. Political and administrative boundaries of Uganda

The European population of the country comprises an ever-changing group of about 10,000 people, over half of whom live and work in Kampala. This expatriate group is mainly involved in teaching, administration and management. The Indian community of about 80,000 people lives predominantly in the towns and is concerned principally with commerce. Each racial group has its own distinctive pattern of cancer, as has been discussed elsewhere (TEMPLETON and VIEGAS, 1970; CHOPRA and TEMPLETON, 1971). The pattern of cancer seen in Europeans is very similar to that found in England, with a higher incidence of basal cell tumours of the face, a result of residence in the tropics. There is some evidence to suggest that the Asian community of Africa is remarkably tumour-free. It appears that they have left behind them many of the cancer hazards of India, for example, the high rate of tumours of the mouth induced by betel nut chewing. They avoid the high rates of hepatic and cutaneous carcinoma of the African and have not become heir to European cancer by virtue of skin pigmentation and lack of industrialization. This monograph is concerned with cancer in the African population.

The People and Their Social Background

The African population of the country in 1959 was 6,449,000 and in 1969 was 9,451,000 (Uganda Census, 1959, and 1969). The population of Uganda and each district at the mid-point of this study (July 1966) was calculated from these two values and is shown in Table 2. This calculation took into account the likely under-estimate of the population in the 1959 Census, and made some allowance for the immigration movements of the period (Hill, personal communication). The age and sex distribution data of 1969 is probably more reliable than those in other census

Table 2. African population by district, 1966

Buganda		2,459,700
Mengo District [a]	1,632,100	
Masaka	576,600	
Mubende [a]	251,000	
Northern		1,489,500
West Nile and Madi	617,300	
Acholi	413,300	
Lango	458,900	
Eastern		2,555,500
Karamoja and Sebei	323,500	
Teso	527,000	
Bugishu and Bukedi	866,000	
Busoga	839,000	
Western		2,097,100
Bunyoro [a]	223,400	
Toro	505,600	
Ankole	759,800	
Kigezi	608,300	
Total		8,601,800

[a] Population adapted to the old boundaries.

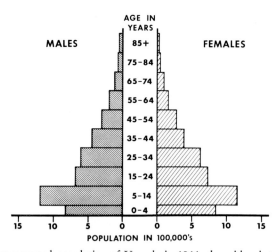

Fig. 4. The constructed population of Uganda in 1966, the mid-point of this study

returns; these ratios have therefore been applied to the 1966 calculated total and used in preference to a median figure between the 1959 and 1969 census returns. The population figures have been adapted to fit the old interdistrict boundaries, that is Buyaga and Bugangadze counties have been included in Mubende district and Singo and Busujju in West Mengo. The age distribution of the population of Uganda shows a very large number of children and a significant mortality in each succeeding decade, which produces a pyramidal histogram (Fig. 4). This curve is essentially similar in all tribes and in rural areas of the country. The male-female ratios differ slightly in different districts. However, in the towns, particularly Kampala, there are fewer children and old people, with an excess of young adult males (DAVIES, KNOWELDEN and WILSON, 1965). The population of Uganda grew at a rate of 3.2% per annum between the censuses of 1959 and 1969. Part of this increase of about three million people was probably an artefact of a more efficient census. A further portion was a result of immigration from neighbouring countries, Ruanda, Congo and Sudan, all of which have had major civil disturbances within the past decade. In addition, a number of people, particularly from Burundi and Kenya, have come to Uganda to find work. Nonetheless, the natural rate of increase is high and it is estimated that about 330,000 deliveries occur each year in Uganda (TRUSSELL, GRECH and GALEA, 1968). Infant mortality, which results from malnutrition combined with a whole range of parasitic and infectious diseases, is falling but is still high.

Uganda lies at the crossroads of many of the migrations of people into Africa, most of whom have used the Nile Valley as the route of travel. At present there are

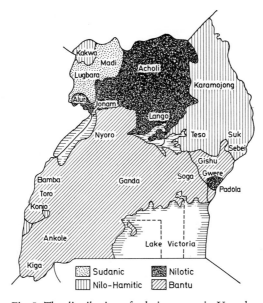

Fig. 5. The distribution of ethnic groups in Uganda

representatives of four major ethnic groups resident in Uganda, the Sudanic, Nilotic, Nilo-Hamitic (or Para-Nilotic) and Bantu. The majority of the population are Bantu mostly living in the southern half of the country (Fig. 5). The Nilotic peoples comprise two major tribes, the Acholi and Lango who live in the northern central area, and three smaller groups, the Alur and Jonam in southern West Nile District and the

Padhola (Dama) who live in the southeast corner of the country. All these tribes are closely related to the Luo of Western Kenya. The Sudanic tribes (Madi and Lugbara) are resident in West Nile District. The Para-Nilotic people, the traditional nomadic cattle herding tribes, have migrated to many parts of Uganda and live mainly in the north and east of the country. The precise ethnic status of the Teso is under dispute but many authorities regard them as of Nilo-Hamitic origin. The Bahima people of Buganda and Ankole and the Watutsi of Ruanda are probably also Nilo-Hamitic as are the Kakwa of West Nile District. The divisions used above are largely based on linguistic relations but there is some anthropomorphic and genetic distinction. The tall, slender Nilo-Hamitic with fine features is instantly distinguishable from the shorter, fatter and flatter-featured Bantu. The Nilotic and Sudanic peoples, by comparison, are tall but well-built. Each tribe has retained its identity to a great extent, and in most rural areas just by knowing someone's name it is possible to predict accurately his tribe, diet, housing style, circumcision status, climate he has lived in and roughly which infectious diseases he is likely to have suffered from. The pattern is breaking up under the onslaughts of education, better transport, radio and the drift to the towns, but if one assumes that the incubation period for many cancers is a long one then the important period of time from the point of view of aetiology is ten or more years ago when the divisions were more rigid.

Approximately 95% of the African population are rural dwellers involved in agriculture. Cash crops such as coffee, cotton and tobacco provide the bulk of income. Cigarette smoking is not yet widely practised. Males in Ankole and Kigezi and females in Buganda smoke pipes but chain smoking as seen in Europe and America is not found in Uganda outside a tiny elite class. Most foodstuffs are grown on the home plots of land. The staple diet of the Baganda and many of the Bantu people is the cooking banana (*musa* sp.). Millet (*Eleusine caracana*) is grown in the east and north of the country and widely favoured by Para-Nilotic tribes. Sorghum is grown and eaten in Karamoja and Kigezi and outside this area is most often used mixed with cassava flour. Cassava is widely eaten in the west and north of the country. Sweet potatoes are grown in most regions but the highest concentration occurs in Kigezi District. These staple foods are usually taken with a sauce made from simsim or pigeon peas (*cajanus* sp.) in the north, groundnuts in the east and south, cow peas (*vigna* sp.) in Teso and field peas (*pisum* sp.) and beans (*phosidus* sp.) in Kigezi. Alcohol consumption is high in most areas of the country, particularly among men, and is usually brewed from the staple crop of the area. More detailed information on dietary habits can be obtained in a book by McMASTER (1962).

Children are almost invariably breast-fed for the first year or eighteen months of life unless displaced by a younger sibling or separated from the mother. There are virtually no traditional weaning foods in Uganda so that the child has to make a rapid adaptation from breast milk to an adult diet. This transition period is often marked by some degree of malnutrition, particularly in banana-eating parts of the country.

Manufacturing industry is in its infancy and occurs only in Kampala, Tororo and Jinja, and there is no large scale heavy manufacturing industry. Copper mining in the Ruwenzori is an important revenue earner and some 7,000 persons are employed in mining activities in the whole country. Fishing is a developing industry, both an the lakes and in ponds and dams. Cattle rearing is a way of life to Nilo-Hamitic people and an important source of protein for other tribes. None of these industries seems to be important in the development of cancer.

Housing is usually built by the owner-occupier and is made of local materials, mainly mud and wood. Roofing is usually of thatch but corrugated iron is now being used more frequently. In the towns and close to main roads concrete construction is used extensively but the majority of the population live between earthen walls on an earthen floor. Open fires are used for heating and cooking. These are often found in the house itself so that many people, particularly women, live long periods in an atmosphere of smoke. Sanitary facilities are primitive and where they exist at all largely consists of long drop latrines. Water is usually gathered from a neigbouring stream or pool, except in the drier areas of the country where bore-holes have been sunk. Piped water supplies are largely confined to the towns.

Clothing habits vary markedly in different parts of the country. The Karamojong and Lugbara have only recently started to wear trousers or skirts. Most men in most parts of the country wear a pair of trousers and a shirt of varying age and state of repair. Women usually wear a knee length dress except in Buganda where the full length Busuti is widely used. Clothing above the waist is worn by everyone except in Karamoja. Children are often not clothed until the age of four or five and thereafter wear a dress or a shirt and shorts. Shoes are now being worn more frequently but a large proportion of the population go barefoot.

Transport by bus is cheap but not prolific and it is relatively easy to travel between towns. However, most people reside in small villages and may be many miles from the nearest bus route. Owning a bicycle used to be a luxury item for many families but is becoming within the reach of more and more people. Such bicycles are used to transport food to market, and furniture and the family either separately or even at the same time. The majority of people walk wherever they want to go and the range of activity is therefore small. This has resulted in tight-knit communities who are concerned with and limited to a tribal horizon. Therefore, intertribal marriages are rare. Social custom varies little within a tribe but is markedly different between tribal groups.

Marriage is usually arranged by the parents. Money or goods are often given to the bride's parents by the bridegroom and the amount varies with the beauty and accomplishments of the lady in question. Pre-marital sexual relations are therefore discouraged by parents but with only limited success (as in other lands). Male circumcision is practised by a minority of tribes and by Muslim Africans who between them account for about 15% of the population. Female circumcision has largely been abandoned but was common among the Karamojong earlier.

Medical Facilities

In 1966, the mid-year of this study, there were 642 registered doctors and 8,716 hospital beds in the country. 139,000 people were treated as in-patients and 2,435,000 were seen in out-patient departments (Statistical Abstract, 1969). The doctor-patient ratio was about 1 : 12,000, about 15 times as many patients per doctor as in most Western European countries. Throughout the five-year period transport facilities and basic education improved steadily. A number of new hospitals were built but most of these did not open until 1969. The total number of hospital beds in the country rose from 7,829 to 9,370 but the majority of this increase occurred in hospitals which were not open to the average African (e. g. military hospitals, private clinics, etc.). The number of doctors in the country rose from 538 in 1964 to 797 in 1968 (Statistical Abstract, 1969). This was largely due to increases in the staff of the University Hospital in Kampala and once again, most rural Africans did not immediately benefit.

New Mulago Hospital, Kampala, was completed in 1962 and has 960 beds. The hospital serves as the teaching hospital of Makerere University, the general treatment hospital of Kampala and the referral centre for problem cases from other hospitals in the country. Mulago Hospital is reasonably well staffed with doctors, a full range of specialist opinion is available and diagnostic facilities are reasonably comprehensive. A large proportion of the hospital beds, a large proportion of the doctors, almost all specialists and 50% of the medical budget for the country are deployed in Kampala. By comparison facilities outside the capital are severely strained and only a limited range of diagnostic and therapeutic methods is available. Radiotherapy is not available anywhere in Uganda.

Prevalent Diseases [1]

The relationship between cancer and other disease is largely unknown, or at most hypothetical. A number of possible associations have been mooted but in no cases has the relationship been definitely established. Nonetheless, the presence of different diseases has such a widespread effect upon the host that it is highly probable that this would influence tumour formation.

Malaria is extremely common in Uganda and is almost entirely due to *P. falciparum*. The incidence is low in Kigezi, Ankole and parts of Toro district. It is holoendemic in a small area of Acholi and hyperendemic in West Nile and the whole of the north, central and eastern areas except around the high mountains in the northeast of the country. The incidence is mesoendemic in Buganda. It has been suggested that since this distribution closely parallels the frequency of Burkitt's lymphoma, malaria may be important in the development of the tumour (BURKITT, 1969; O'CONOR, 1970). Other lymphomas, particularly histiocytic medullary reticulosis, might also result from long-standing particulate stimulation of the reticuloendothelial system such as occurs in malaria (SERCK HANSSEN and PUROHIT, 1968).

Schistosomias is found along the Nile and all the major lakes in Uganda (BRADLEY, 1968). *S. haematobium* has been implicated in the development of bladder cancer, particularly squamous type. The majority of bladder cancer in Uganda is of squamous type (Chapter 8) but there does not appear to be any correlation between the distribution of cancer and schistosomiasis. Similarly, no correlation has been found between S. mansoni infection and tumours of the bowel, liver or bile ducts. A relationship between schistosomiasis and lymphoreticular tumours has been found in Egypt (el GAZAYERLI et al., 1964) and Nigeria (EDINGTON and MACLEAN, 1964) but in Uganda the correlation is less convincing. Other parasitic infections are very common indeed. Ascaris is common but the intensity of infection is rather lower than in many

---

1 Much of the information discussed below is derived from the Uganda Atlas of Disease Distribution, an invaluable review of many aspects of the interplay of geography on medicine (HALL and LANGLANDS, 1968).

countries. For example, intestinal obstruction due to boli of worms is very rarely seen in Uganda. Hookworm (*Necator americanus* predominates) is common, particularly in children, and is a frequent cause of anaemia. Other intestinal parasites such as *Taenia saginata, Strongyloides stercoralis,* and *trichuris* are frequently seen. Systemic filarial infections are common. Onchocerciasis is now limited to the Western rift valley and the area around Mount Elgon but was previously found in the Nile valley. *D. perstans* is regularly seen in blood films and smears from pleural fluids but appears to be innocuous.

Viral infections are extremely common and a large number of new organisms have been isolated at the Virus Research Station, Entebbe. Viruses thought to be involved in human cancer in Uganda include a variety of Herpes viruses. Epstein-Barr virus is isolated regularly from Burkitt's tumour cells (EPSTEIN, 1970), Herpes simplex (genitalis) may be involved in the development of carcinoma of the penis and cervix uteri (British Medical Journal, 1970) and a new Herpes virus has been isolated from tumours of the post-nasal space (ACHONG et al., 1971).

Tropical ulcers are extremely common and usually occur on the skin. Carcinoma of the skin frequently develops in association with these ulcers. But whether this is a result of the disease, its attempted cure, or the scar following partial healing is a matter for debate (see Chapter 10).

Malnutrition in the immediate post-weaning period is widespread. In southern Uganda this usually takes the form of kwashiorkor which results from a relative protein deficiency in a diet of adequate calorie intake. In the north of the country marasmus, which results from a low intake of calories, is more common. This is largely due to cultural practices rather than a shortage of food, particularly in the Buganda region. The influence of this period on the liability to develop cancer is speculative.

Venereal disease is widespread. At present some 120,000 new patients with gonorrhoea are seen each year in the clinics of Ugandan hospitals (Medical Services Statistical Records, 1968—69). The relationship between gonorrhoea, stricture formation and bladder cancer has been suggested as one reason why squamous cancers of the bladder are common in Buganda (DODGE, 1964).

Cancer Registration Practice

Cases were classified by anatomical site using the World Health Organisation sponsored International Classification of Disease (I.C.D., 7th edition, 1955). Histological coding followed the Manual of Tumor Nomenclature and Coding (American Cancer Society, 1956). Details of the anatomical site, histology, grading and staging of each tumour was inserted on a card together with the patient's name, age, sex, tribe, address and hospital. A brief summary of the patient's clinical history was also included. Duplicate registrations were avoided by cross reference files based on name, diagnosis and hospital registration number. The histological diagnosis of every case was reviewed by the senior author of each chapter and the editor and any necessary alterations in coding made. Punch cards from the Cancer Registry data were prepared and the data encoded on computer. The computer stored information on the Cancer Registry number, year of diagnosis, site, histology, age, sex, tribe, race, hospital, address and method of diagnosis in each case.

The majority of cases recorded in the Kampala Cancer Registry are derived from the returns of the Department of Pathology. 7,347 cases are included in this survey of which only 391 were without histological confirmation. In these "clinical cases" there was adequate evidence of diagnosis. This was obtained by scrutiny of case notes, interviewing medical attendants or by means of chemical, haematological or radiographic evidence. For these reasons case registration without biopsy is effectively restricted to Buganda, and only 67 cases were registered from other regions of the country. It is in Kampala that the biopsy rate is likely to be highest. Therefore the number of cases added was small, but limitations of personnel and time precluded any other approach. Tumours diagnosed without histological confirmation were largely those which produced readily recognizable symptoms and signs (Table 3).

Table 3. Histologically unconfirmed cases of cancer compared with the number histologically identified

	No histology	Histology	% Histological confirmation
Oesophagus	26	93	77
Stomach	21	160	88
Liver	41	558	93
Breast	37	318	89
Cervix	88	663	88
Prostate	28	112	80
Penis	15	459	97
Bladder	14	170	92
Burkitt's	32	272	90
Unknown	19	363	95
Others	70	3,715	98
All cancer	391	6,956	95

It is probably the single greatest weakness of the Registry that only a very few tumours without histological verification are included. There are advantages and disadvantages of including histologically unconfirmed cases (Burkitt, Hutt and Slavin, 1968) but in many instances the inaccuracies of leaving out such cases far outweigh the possible inaccuracies of diagnosis. In most cases a much closer approximation to the true distribution of tumours in the country will be found if clinically diagnosed cases are included in registry returns. For example, the diagnosis of hepatocellular carcinoma can be made with 80% chance of being correct on clinical grounds alone (Davies and Owor, 1960), whereas it is probable that only about 50% of clinically diagnosed cases are biopsied (Cook and Burkitt, 1971). Only 7% of liver cancers included in this survey were not histologically confirmed (Table 3). The accuracy of clinical diagnosis at other sites such as cervical, penile or oesophageal cancer and Burkitt's tumour of the jaw is probably greater than 90%.

4.1% of histologically confirmed cases were of uncertain origin. The reasons why such a large proportion should occur are discussed in Chapter 18. About half these cases were diagnosed from lymph node secondary deposits where the primary site was unknown. 60% of the remainder were widespread intra-abdominal neoplasms with extensive peritoneal swellings. Some estimate of a likely primary site is possible in some cases. This suggests that tumours of the bronchus, pancreas, stomach and ovary account for a considerable proportion of cases and are likely to be under-estimated in a histological survey.

Studies on the distribution of cancer using returns from many hospitals in East Africa which include a large number of cases without biopsy, has shown how markedly the proportions of tumours vary in different areas (COOK and BURKITT, 1970). There are considerable advantages to be gained from a broad look at cancer in a continent such as is provided by these surveys (COOK and BURKITT, 1971). They provide information as to where more detailed studies on particular tumours might best be carried out. Such an overview of Uganda has already been carried out and the time has now arrived to undertake the detailed analysis suggested.

One method of achieving a more detailed knowledge is to study the tumours occurring within a small area. A good example of this method is to be found in the Cancer Registry of Dr. E. H. WILLIAMS working at Kuluva Hospital in West Nile (WILLIAMS, 1967). The diagnosis, personal details and address of each case of cancer presenting at hospital are noted. This personal registry includes a greater proportion of clinically diagnosed cases than is found in the Kampala Cancer Registry and prob-ably reflects more accurately the relative frequency of tumours occurring in the area. This approach has led to a whole stream of stimulating ideas on a wide variety of subjects such as the epidemic drift of Burkitt's tumour (WILLIAMS, SPIT and PIKE, 1969) and the association of Kaposi's sarcoma and onchocerciasis (WILLIAMS and WILLIAMS, 1966). A similar registry has been set up at Ishaka Hospital in Ankole District (BUCKLEY, 1967). Another area which has been subjected to a similar detailed scrutiny has been Kyadondo County. Incidence survey have been carried out twice in the past 20 years (DAVIES et al., 1965; TEMPLETON, BUXTON and BIANCHI, 1972). Such intensive surveys, however, are quite impracticable in more than a few small areas under present conditions in Africa. In the future it is probable that the best in-formation on tumour incidence will come from small registries in sharply delineated areas and semi-rural conditions. All medical schools in Africa are set in the highly artificial background of a rapidly growing shifting urban population. In such circum-stances the bias in registration is very large and is likely to get larger as the cities grow. Accurate population data will become increasingly difficult to obtain and the environment will become progressively more heterogeneous. Conversely, the facilities for diagnosis in smaller towns are poorer and staffing is less adequate. Nonetheless the application of a limited amount of funds and personnel to such a rural area would result in extremely valuable data unavailable in larger towns.

Another approach is to take an admittedly incomplete series and accurately define each entry by a number of parameters. For example, the site of origin and histo-logical appearance of the tumour, and the geographical origins and the sex and age of the patient. This method will determine whether any parameter varies independently of any other. If a disease is an entity then it should have aetiological factors which are distinctive. The age, sex, anatomical, histological and geographical distribution should be unique to that disease. In other words a disease entity can only be defined as such when it is homogeneous when inspected from a number of different view-points. If a disease can be split into a number of subdivisions by the use of a single parameter it may be that the pre-existing definition in fact covers a number of

entities. The method of testing the validity of a division of an apparent entity is to
see whether there is a correlation with other parameters. Thus, to take an obvious
example, in most cancer registries tumours of the eye are all classified together under
I.C.D. rubric 192. Histologically such tumours show a wide range of appearances.
Retinoblastomas are easily distinguishable from squamous carcinomas of the conjunctiva. Inspection using other parameters shows them to have a different site of origin,
age of onset, behaviour, prognosis and geographical distribution. We therefore call
them different diseases and expect that the aetiology will be different. If an epidemio-
logist is to present an experimentalist with a testable hypothesis then he must be sure
he is dealing with a homogeneous disease entity, because it is unlikely that an aetiological factor will be incriminated if retinoblastoma is confused with squamous
carcinoma of the conjunctiva. Similarly, very little of the exciting work on the aetiology of Burkitt's lymphoma would have been possible if there had not been methods
of separating this tumour from other lymphomata. If such obvious differences are
seen within groups of tumour previously classified together, it seems probable that
other less obvious differences will be found if actively sought. For example, do
tumours in different parts of the colon show a different age, histological or geographical distribution? If it appears that all these parameters vary together then one
is dealing with a single disease entity. But if, for example, tumours of the caecum
occur at a different age, and are histologically distinct from tumours of the sigmoid,
and if the relative frequency at these sites varies in different countries, then these are
grounds for supposing that they are not the same disease. If the disease is different
then it is possible that the aetiology will be different. If one accepts that the aim of
geographical studies is to provide hypotheses capable of experimental clarification
then these hypotheses must be based on solid data. If the data provided relate to a
number of entities, in other words if they are contaminated by irrelevant material,
then such hypotheses are unlikely to be provable, or for that matter disprovable.

Data as published from most cancer registries are entirely inadequate for such
studies. Many rubrics are an amalgam of disparate entities having nothing more in
common than chance anatomical juxtaposition. Attempts have been made to remedy
this situation in regard to tumours of the ovary, testis, bladder and thyroid and to
leukaemia by comparing the proportions of each histological type of tumour in different registries (Tulinius, 1970). In this monograph we have applied this degree of
precision to all rubrics and have also used other parameters such as anatomical site
and geographical distribution. Many unexpected anomalies of distribution have been
discovered by this process. It is only after demarcating true disease entities which are
distinct from one another that one can start to use the potential of the geographical
approach. We believe that such a technique is capable of asking stimulating questions
susceptible to experimental testing and that the answers are of supreme importance.

Tumour Patterns in Uganda

The total number of cases diagnosed in this five-year period is shown in Table 4.
The registration of malignant tumours is incomplete, particularly in the more sparsely
populated areas of the country remote from larger hospitals. Benign tumours are
grossly underestimated since the majority of patients with such lesions are likely to be
dealt with at home or at dispensaries. It is also probable that some of the tumours

which are excised in hospital are not submitted for histological examination. With malignant tumours the proportion of specimens submitted is higher and we believe that virtually all excised material is referred to the laboratory. Only about 1,200 post-mortem examinations are performed in the country annually (virtually all in Kampala) and therefore registration of internal benign tumours will occur only when symptoms are produced.

Table 4. Total number of tumours registered in 1964—1968

W.H.O rubric		Site	Malignant	Benign	Total
140—148 (except 146)	210	Mouth and Pharynx	185	216	401
146+160—162	212	Respiratory tract	243	52	295
150—154	211	Gastro-int. tract	476	51	527
155—157		Liver, Pancreas	629	2	631
170	213	Breast	355	104	459
171—176	214—217	Female genitalia	1,180	1,387	2,567
177—179	218	Male genitalia	635	75	710
180+181	219	Urinary tract	268	12	280
190+191	220—222	Skin and melanoma	893	86	979
192+193	223	Brain and sense organs	143	82	225
194+195	224+250	Endocrines	114	58	172
196	225	Bone	129	134	263
197	226+7+8	Soft tissue	670	1,339 [a]	2,009
198, 9, 159, 163, 164		Unknown primary	363	—	363
200—203		Lymphoma	860	—	860
204+205		Leukaemia	204	—	204
All neoplasms			7,347	3,598	10,945

[a] Excludes tumours in genital and alimentary tracts.

The registration rate of cancer in the region immediately around Kampala (Kyadondo County) is higher than elsewhere in Buganda (DAVIES et al., 1965; TEMPLETON et al., 1972). The registration rate in Buganda in turn is higher than in other regions (TEMPLETON and BIANCHI, 1972 a). Even in Kyadondo County diagnosis and regisration is probably deficient, particularly among old people, but if the rates found in Kyadondo are applied to the country as a whole then some indication of the extent of underregistration in rural areas is obtained (Table 5). In each region females are registered much less efficiently than males. It seems that this is largely a result of unwillingness or inability to come to hospital. This follows from the traditional inferior position of women in Ugandan society and lack of awareness of the benefits of western medicine (TEMPLETON and BIANCHI, 1972 a). Where facilities are thinly scattered only fairly fit sick people will be able to make the journey to hospital and in some areas there are very few medical personnel so that many patients will be unable to see a doctor. There is a tendency, therefore, for the proportion of slowly growing superficial non-disabling tumours to be higher in poorly staffed areas than where good transport and medical facilities are available. Thus, for example, the majority of patients with adamantinoma are likely to reach hospital and to be operated on, whereas only a small proportion of patients with hepatocellular carcinoma will actually have a biopsy taken. In those areas where specialists are not found certain tumours seem to be rare. Thus cerebral tumours are rare in the absence of a neurologist or neurosurgeon; tumours of the post-nasal space are rare where no speculum is available. Hepatocellular carcinoma closely follows the availability of biopsy needles (Alpert, Hutt and Davidson, 1968) and bladder tumours are found where there are cytoscopes. In this respect it is interesting to compare diagnoses made at Mulago Hospital with those made at other hospitals. In Mulago a full range of

Table 5. Cases registered compared with cases expected in each region in 1969. Expected cases were calculated with reference to age-specific incidence rates in Kyadondo County

	Cases registered	Cases expected	Proportion registered
Males			
Buganda	444	705	66
Northern	196	495	40
East	218	667	33
West	149	603	25
Total	1,007	2,470	41
Females			
Buganda	413	797	53
Northern	160	556	29
East	195	754	26
West	138	684	20
Total	906	2,791	33

diagnostic methods of investigation is available whereas other hospitals are often short of personnel and equipment. The proportion of registered cases of a given tumour diagnosed at Mulago Hospital will vary in proportion to the sophisticated equipment necessary for the diagnosis (Table 6). Thus 25 out of 32 brain tumours were diagnosed at Mulago compared with 6 out of 34 tumours of the lip.

The apparent incidence of tumours in different tribes is similarly biased. The Baganda reside in that part of the country in which medical facilities are most prolific and transport is easiest. Thus the Baganda account for a much greater proportion of tumours overall (29.5%) than their contribution to the population (16.3% in 1959). The ratio between these two figures is a rough indication of the efficiency of diagnosis in different tribes (Table 7). (These calculations assume that the proportion of the population derived from each tribe was similar in 1966 to that found in 1959). The lower the diagnostic efficiency the greater the possible registration bias. For this reason figures for immigrants from Ruanda and Burundi or in the Karamojong should be interpreted with caution.

Examination of the bias in diagnosis and registration in Uganda has shown that tumours in women and tumours in inaccessible sites are selectively under-diagnosed. The extent of this under-diagnosis was calculated by reference to the registration pattern found in Kyadondo County in 1969 (Templeton and Bianchi, 1972a). It was suggested that correction of data from rural areas using Kyadondo as a standard would give more reliable information as to the true distribution of disease than either proportional rate studies or incidence data. As a rule of thumb the number of tumours in women at the time of this survey should be doubled in order to be comparable with male rates. Similarly tumours in inaccessible sites should be doubled when comparing them with tumours of superficial locations.

Age-specific incidence rates for tumours overall are shown in Fig. 6. In both males and females the incidence in Kyadondo County is considerably higher than in the

Table 6. The proportion of cases first diagnosed at Mulago hospital at different sites

Males	%	Females	%
Oesophagus	78	Oesophagus	80
Brain	73	Brain	77
Pancreas	65	Pancreas	70
Leukaemia	60	Leukaemia	52
Prostate	58	Stomach	45
Bladder	55	Bladder	40
Stomach	51	Breast	38
Liver	36	Cervix	37
Colon and Rectum	35	Colon and Rectum	36
Mouth	35	Liver	36
Lymphoma	32	Mouth	31
Breast	30	Lymphoma	31
Penis	25	Ovary	29
Kaposi	23	Kaposi	17
Skin	20	Burkitt's	16
Burkitt's	17	Skin	11
All cancer	33%	All cancer	33%

Table 7. Diagnostic efficiency index in the major tribes of Uganda. The index is calculated by dividing the percentage contribution of each tribe to the population by the contribution to the cases at each site

	Total cases	% of total cancer	% of total population	Index
Ganda	2,172	29.5	16.3	1.8
Acholi	373	5.1	4.4	1.2
Toro	256	3.5	3.2	1.1
Lango	402	5.5	5.6	1.0
Banyoro	218	3.0	2.9	1.0
Lugbara	234	3.2	3.7	0.9
Soga	471	6.4	7.8	0.8
Ruanda/Rundi	474	6.5	8.1	0.8 [a]
Ankole	465	6.3	8.1	0.8
Teso	460	6.3	8.1	0.8
Riga	360	4.9	7.1	0.7
Gishu	202	2.7	5.1	0.5
Karamojong	54	0.7	2.0	0.3
Others and unknown	1,212	16.4	17.6	0.9

[a] This figure is the least reliable since the population of immigrants is very difficult to estimate.

country as a whole. The distribution of the curves for Kyadondo show a rise in middle age with a peak at the age of about 60 and a fall thereafter. Caucasian series all show a steadily rising curve (Doll, Muir and Waterhouse, 1970), so do the Indian and Caucasian population of Uganda (Templeton and Viegas, 1970). Part of this difference is because tumours which are common in Uganda are not those which show an exponential rise with age. For example, carcinoma of the cervix rises to a

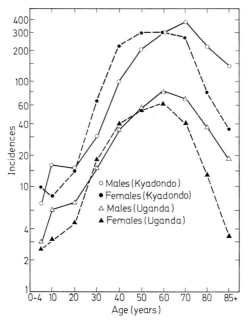

Fig. 6. Age specific incidence rates in Kyadondo County and Uganda (mean annual incidence of cases per 100,000 persons)

plateau by the age of 40 years and does not rise significantly thereafter. But the major difference is probably a result of inability or unwillingness to come to hospital on the part of older people. In the country as a whole the incidence of tumours is lower in all age groups but is closer to the Kyadondo figure among young people, registration rates fall progressively behind in older age groups. It follows, therefore, that if crude figures are inspected there will appear to be an exaggeration of tumours of young people. Even if a correction for the population structure is applied there will still be a tendency for tumours prevalent in older people to be under-represented. Proportional rates of some of the more common tumours are shown in Table 8. This illustrates the very marked difference in the distribution of Burkitt's lymphoma in different tribes, which is undoubtedly not a result of diagnostic artefact. Other apparent differences might be ascribable to such an artefact. For example, the excess of oesophageal tumours in the Baganda might be a result of proximity to Mulago Hospital. Conversely, the increased rate of superficial tumours in the Bakiga might be in part explained by a reduced diagnosis of deeply placed neoplasms. By contrast comparisons between Kiga and Toro or between Lugbara and Acholi are justified, since both have a similar diagnostic bias. For all these reasons comparison of tumour incidence in different parts of the country is a hazardous procedure. Nonetheless, provided that the limitations are understood, comparisons are both valuable and valid.

Table 8. Proportional rates of selected tumours in some major tribes of Uganda. Figures which are markedly different from other tribes are in heavy type

	All tribes	Ganda	Kiga	Toro	Lug-bara	Acholi	Teso	Ruanda/Rundi
Males								
Oesophagus	1.7	**3.4**	2.4	0.7	0.7	1.6	2.1	**0.3**
Stomach	3.0	4.0	2.4	3.5	1.5	1.0	1.3	**8.1**
Liver	11.0	**6.2**	7.7	7.8	14.8	10.5	8.1	**16.3**
Penis	12.0	12.0	4.2	**31.2**	**3.0**	10.5	25.1	10.7
Bladder	4.0	**10.3**	—	2.8	—	1.0	0.9	1.2
Skin	9.9	**4.4**	21.4	10.6	12.6	6.3	11.1	13.8
Kaposi	8.0	6.9	12.5	12.8	**14.8**	5.2	**3.8**	5.9
Burkitt	5.0	1.4	—	0.7	**14.8**	12.6	8.9	2.8
Females								
Oesophagus	1.5	**4.0**	1.6	—	—	0.6	0.4	—
Stomach	1.8	1.6	2.1	**5.2**	—	1.1	—	**5.8**
Breast	9.3	10.8	7.9	12.2	9.1	**5.0**	9.3	9.7
Cervix	22.3	27.3	14.8	24.3	**10.1**	30.9	20.9	17.5
Ovary	6.5	7.7	0.5	4.3	1.5	2.8	0.4	0.6
Melanoma	2.9	**1.5**	4.8	6.1	*7.1*	2.8	1.8	3.2
Skin	9.0	**2.2**	31.7	4.3	18.2	6.1	6.2	15.6
Burkitt	3.2	1.1	0.5	0.9	**13.1**	6.1	4.4	2.5

Table 9. The 15 most frequently diagnosed tumours in Uganda. The figures represent the proportion of total cancer in each sex

	Males (%)	Females (%)	Both sexes (%)
1.	Soft tissue 12.2%	Cervix 22.3%	Cervix 10.2%
2.	Penis 12%	Breast 9.3%	Skin 9.5%
3.	Liver 11%	Skin 9.0%	Soft tissues 9.1%
4.	Skin 9.9%	Ovary 6.5%	Liver 7.9%
5.	Lympho/Reticulo 6.6%	Soft tissues 5.6%	Penis 6.4%
6.	Burkitt's 4.5%	Liver 4.3%	Lympho/Reticulo 5.0%
7.	Bladder 4.0%	Lympho/Reticulo 3.2%	Breast 4.8%
8.	Prostate 3.5%	Melanoma 2.9%	Burkitt's 3.8%
9.	Stomach 3%	Burkitt's 2.9%	Ovary 3.0%
10.	Leukaemia 2.9%	Leukaemia 2.5%	Leukaemia 2.7%
11.	Hodgkin's 2.5%	Vulva/Vag 2.3%	Melanoma 2.7%
12.	Melanoma 2.4%	Chorio Ca 2.0%	Bladder 2.5%
13.	Eye 1.8%	Stomach 1.8%	Stomach 2.5%
14.	Oesophagus 1.7%	Thyroid 1.6%	Prostate 1.9%
15.	Bone 1.6%	Oesophagus 1.5%	Hodgkin's 1.8%
Total cases	3962	3361	7347 [a]

[a] Includes 24 patients of unknown sex.

Raw data from Uganda requires to be interpreted with all the above factors in mind. Nonetheless it is interesting to have some overview of the frequency with which various tumours are seen. Table 9 shows the 15 most frequently diagnosed tumours. This is not to say that these are the 15 most frequently occurring tumours. As pointed out above, deeply placed neoplasms are less readily diagnosed than superficially placed tumours. Thus gastric bronchial and pancreatic neoplasms are un-doubtedly markedly underestimated. An attempt has been made to calculate the true incidence of cancer in Uganda taking the known bias in registration into account (TEMPLETON and BIANCHI, 1972 b). In this study it was concluded that hepatocellular carcinoma was probably the most frequently occurring cancer in Uganda, followed by tumours of the cervix. Tumours of the skin and penis and Kaposis sarcoma are probably somewhat over-represented since they are superficial and have a long history which would almost inevitably bring the patient to hospital.

This chapter has dwelt at length on the disadvantages of cancer registration in Uganda. This has been done so that interpretation of data should be as accurate as possible. The advantages of the Kampala Cancer Registry have not been emphasized but are numerous. Cases are collected, diagnosed, classified, encoded, reviewed and written about entirely homogeneously. No other registry in the world handling as many cases has these advantages in quite such full measure.

Chapter 2

Tumours of the Alimentary Canal

A. C. TEMPLETON

With 7 Figures

Tumours of the alimentary canal account for a rather smaller proportion of cancer overall than in many countries. Carcinoma of the mouth and oropharynx is unusual. Salivary tumours overall are about as common as in other countries but are found relatively more frequently outside the parotid gland than in Caucasian peoples. The palate and submandibular gland are frequently the site of tumours. Tumours of the oesophagus are found in Buganda and Eastern region and the incidence appears to be rising rapidly. Tumours of the pylorus are found in people from the west of the country. Carcinoma of the colon is unusual in Uganda and cancer of the rectum and anus is relatively much more frequent. The low frequency of colonic cancer correlates with the rarity of diverticular disease and polypi and all these conditions may be modified by dietary factors.

Tumours involving the alimentary canal are shown in Table 1. Lymphomas and soft-tissue tumours are discussed in Chapters 16 and 15 respectively. Benign tumours at all sites are markedly under-represented for a variety of reasons. This chapter is therefore mainly concerned with malignant epithelial tumours.

Cancer of the alimentary canal accounted for 9.1% of malignant tumours in this survey. This is a much smaller proportion than is found in most other countries (Tables 2 and 3). This low figure is partly a result of deficient registration of deeply placed neoplasms, particularly in rural areas. The proportional rate of alimentary tumours in Kyadondo County was 15%, which indicates that under-registration is occurring in other parts of the country.

The relative frequency of tumours occurring in different parts of the alimentary canal vary in different countries (Tables 2 and 3). Tumours of the mouth and tongue are unusual in Africa. Most such patients would be expected to come to hospital eventually and significant under-diagnosis is less likely to occur than at other sites. The incidence of salivary gland tumours is difficult to compare since there are varying practices in their classification. Carcinoma of the oesophagus probably has a greater variation in different countries than any other tumour. This variation may occur over quite short distances and over very short time periods (OETTLÉ, 1963 a). Ten years ago oesophageal cancer was not commonly seen in any area in Uganda and was decidedly rare in western and northern parts of the country. Cases were seen from time to time in eastern parts of the country. More recently there has been a marked rise in incidence in the region around Kampala, particularly among women (Templeton, Buxton and Bianchi, 1972).

Table 1. Tumours of the alimentary canal

Lip, Mouth and Oropharynx (140—145)		248
Malignant epithelial tumours	137	
Other malignant tumours	19	
Benign epithelial tumours	22	
Other benign tumours	70	
Major Salivary Glands (142)		139
Malignant	43	
Benign	96	
Hypopharynx and Oesophagus (148 and 150)		127
Malignant epithelial	121	
Leiomyoma	6	
Stomach		199
Carcinoma	179	
Other malignant tumours	12	
Benign connective tissue	8	
Small intestine		57
Carcinoma	10	
Sarcoma	25	
Lymphoma	7	
Benign connective tissue	15	
Colon and Rectum		206
Carcinoma	148	
Sarcoma	17	
Lymphoma	12	
Benign epithelial tumours	23	
Benign connective tissue	6	
Anus		23
Carcinoma	18	
Other malignant tumours	5	
		999

Table 2. Percentage of tumours overall occurring in the alimentary canal in different countries (males). (All figures outside Uganda are taken from Doll, Muir and Waterhouse, 1970)

Site	England	Colombia	Japan	India	Nigeria	Uganda (all areas)	Uganda (Kyadondo)
140—148 [a]	3.3	4.2	1.4	27.7	4.6	2.4	2.7
150	1.9	1.8	7.1	8.5	0.5	1.7	5.7
151	10.1	21.7	50.0	6.4	7.8	3.0	2.7
152	0.2	0.3	0.1	0.1	—	0.2	0.3
153 and 154	11.8	3.2	4.6	5.5	2.4	2.5	2.4
140—154 [a]	27.7	32.2	62.5	50.0	15.6	10.0	14.0
No. of cases	20,849	1,698	4,082	5,852	707	3,964	290

[a] Excludes 146 (Nasopharynx).

Gastric cancer is considerably under-diagnosed in Uganda. Symptoms may only occur late in the course of the disease and many patients will probably die before a diagnosis has been established. In patients with advanced intra-abdominal neoplasia it may be difficult to distinguish the precise site of origin.

Table 3. Percentage of tumours overall occurring in the alimentary canal in different countries (females). (All figures outside Uganda are taken from DOLL, MUIR and WATERHOUSE, 1970)

Site	England	Colombia	Japan	India	Nigeria	Uganda (all areas)	Uganda (Kya-dondo)
140—148 [a]	1.6	2.4	1.1	11.1	2.6	2.7	1.0
150	1.9	0.4	3.3	7.5	0.2	1.5	6.7
151	13.5	8.6	31.2	3.9	3.7	1.8	3.7
152	0.1	0.2	0.3	0.2	0.1	0.1	0.3
153, 154	13.9	2.4	6.2	4.3	2.2	2.0	4.3
140—154	25.6	14.2	43.4	27.7	9.2	8.1	16.0
No. of cases	21,064	2,441	3,623	3,851	718	3,364	306

[a] Excludes 146 (Nasopharynx.)

Tumours of the small intestine are unusual in all countries and Uganda is no exception. Tumours of the lower bowel are also uncommon in all African countries. Rectal neoplasms are more common than colonic tumours in Africa whereas in Europe the reverse applies.

These general findings are very similar to those reported by HUTT, BURKITT and SHEPHERD (1967) in a survey of Uganda carried out in the years 1961—1964. There is also a close resemblance to the distribution of tumours of the alimentary tract found in other African countries which were presented at the same symposium, held in 1965 (MURRAY, 1967).

Tumours of the Lips

37 cases of malignant tumours of the lips were seen; this is only 0.5% of malignant tumours, an incidence of 0.08 cases per year per 100,000 of the population. 31 of these tumours were squamous cell carcinomas; 2 cases were not biopsied but are presumed to have been epithelial tumours. There was one case each of basal cell carcinoma, histiocytic lymphoma, Kaposi's sarcoma and melanoma. The latter three cases will be dealt with under their respective headings and the remainder of this section refers to the 34 epithelial tumours only. Benign tumours were very seldom seen and included 3 pleomorphic adenomata, two on the upper lip and one on the lower.

The incidence of carcinoma of the lip is considerably lower than in Western European countries but is similar to that found among South African Bantu, in Nigeria and in Japan (DOLL et al., 1966 and 1970). The age ranged from 30—78 years with a mean of 44.5 years. Tumours were most frequently seen in the 4th and 5th decades of life but the incidence was greatest in the 6th. 14 patients were females and 18 males. In most parts of the world there is considerable male excess in such tumours. In view of the deficient registration of many tumours in females in Uganda, these figures might suggest that the disease is in fact more common in females than in males.

Tumours seem to be more common in northern districts particularly in the Lango tribe. No cases were seen from the south west of the country among Batoro, Ankole or Bakiga people. This variation in incidence follows the amount of tobacco grown in the different areas. However, no details of smoking or chewing habits in these patients are available.

Five tumours were located on the upper lip, 14 on the lower lip and 11 at the commissure. In 4 cases the site was not stated. There were no differences in age, sex or histological appearance between the tumours at the different sites, except that the verrucoid pattern was seen most frequently at the commissure. The excess of tumours on the lower lip is usually explained as a function of the greater amount of ultra-violet light incident on that surface. In these cases no elastotic degeneration of the collagen was seen underlying the tumour as is usually found in solar-induced tumours. Actinic causation in these cases is therefore doubtful.

Nineteen of the tumours were ulcerative and 7 appeared proliferative; four showed a verrucoid appearance (ACKERMAN, 1948 a). Verrucoid carcinoma did not appear to be associated with tobacco chewing or with increased age in our cases. Three were located at the commissure, which was the site of most of the tumours reported by COOKE (1969) from New Guinea. In New Guinea the development appeared to be associated with application of lime to the lips. There is no such habit in Uganda.

Table 4. Showing the relationship between the grading and behaviour of carcinomas of the lip

Histological differentiation	Number of cases	Lymphatic metastases	History (mean duration)
Good	9	1 (11%)	15 months
Average	14	7 (50%)	12 months
Poor	8	3 (37%)	2 months

There were 31 squamous carcinomas, which were histologically graded as shown in Table 4. Average-grade tumours had a significantly higher incidence of metastasis to the lymph nodes than well differentiated tumours. None of the four verrucoid carcinomas had given rise to metastasis. The stroma underlying poorly differentiated tumours showed a much more marked inflammatory response than was found in well differentiated tumours. The length of history in patients with poorly differentiated tumours was much shorter than in those with better differentiated varieties (Table 4).

Basal cell carcinoma (THACKRAY, 1951) and melanoma of the lip (BAXTER, 1941) have been previously reported but are both extremely rare. Kaposi's sarcoma of the lip does not appear to have been previously reported, and lymphoma involving the lip is also very rare.

Tongue

Twenty cases were seen, that is 0.3% of all malignant tumours, an incidence of 0.046 cases per 100,000 persons per year. These figures are considerably lower than those reported in Caucasians (HARNETT, 1952).

In one case the tumour arose in a 6½-year-old boy suffering from xeroderma pigmentosa. He later developed squamous cell carcinomas of his face and lips. Apart from this case the age ranged from 30—70 with a mean of 50.3 years. There were 13 males and 6 females. Most tumours arose on the tip of the tongue or on the lateral margins.

The numbers are too small to make valid conclusions as to variations in different parts of the country, but 8 of the 19 patients came from Nilo-Hamitic tribes which is a two-fold greater proportion than their contribution to the total population.

No biopsy was taken in one case but all the remainder were squamous cell carcinomas. Eight were assessed as low-grade, 8 as average-grade and 3 as high-grade malignancy, and 2 of the 3 high-grade tumours occurred in the posterior part of the tongue. At the time of presentation 3 cases showed involvement of cervical lymph nodes proved histologically, and in a further 3, large lymph nodes were palpable clinically and were assessed as inoperable.

Conditions known to be associated with the development of carcinoma of the tongue include poor oral hygiene, syphilis, and use of tobacco. Tobacco is not widely used and has only recently been introduced in many parts of the country. Oral hygiene is better than in most countries, and the incidence of dental caries is lower. It seems likely that the incidence will rise as both tobacco and caries increase in frequency. Although syphilis is extremely common in Uganda the changes of chronic glossitis have not been noted in clinics and were not present in patients with cancer.

Tumours of the Oral Cavity

Tumours involving this region (I.C.D. 143 and 144) are shown in Table 5. The discussion is concerned with epithelial tumours; others are shown in the table but are considered in detail elsewhere.

Table 5. Showing the frequency of tumours and tumour-like conditions of the oral cavity

Malignant tumours	
Epithelial tumours (all types)	65
Melanoma	7
Adamantinoma	32
Burkitt's tumour	143
Other non-epithelial tumours	9
Benign lesions	
Giant cell lesions and ossifying fibroma	61
Pleomorphic adenoma	22
Congenital myoblastoma	6
Granuloma pyogenicum	17
Epulides	64

Seventy malignant epithelial tumours were seen, 1% of all malignant tumours; these encluded 49 squamous cell carcinomas and 16 derived from minor salivary glands. In five patients with obviously malignant tumour no biopsy was taken.

Benign tumours included two papillomas and 22 pleomorphic adenomata, 18 of which arose on the palate.

In 25 of the 49 cases of squamous carcinoma the tumours were well differentiated; differentiation was average in 11 and poor in 8. No typical example of verrucoid carcinoma was seen but in many cases the biopsy taken was too small to exclude such a tumour. All cases were advanced at the time of presentation and most showed invasion of bone. In one case the tumour was located centrally in the ramus of the mandible; such tumours are extremely rare but well recognized (STOLL et al., 1957). Lymph node metastasis was clinically apparent in 30% of cases when they were first seen.

A wide variety of tumours of minor salivary glands was seen. Adenocarcinomas were virtually all poorly differentiated. In a number of cases crystalline marked inclusions were seen in the cytoplasm of tumour cells. Such inclusions were seen quite commonly in salivary neoplasms in Uganda but their nature is unknown. Adenoid cystic carcinoma was diagnosed in 8 cases and in 2 the tumour appeared to have arisen in a preexisting pleomorphic adenoma. Three well differentiated mucoepidermoid tumours were seen, all on the hard palate.

Eighteen of the 22 intra-oral pleomorphic adenomata occurred on the palate. These showed the usual variety of structure seen in these tumours though no case was seen in which pseudocartilage occurred. Encapsulation was always defective and recurrence after enucleation was common, asthese tumours often had a close relation to bone.

Many tumours were well advanced at the time of presentation so that it was difficult to be certain of the precise site of origin. Twenty-three cases of squamous carcinoma arose on the floor of the mouth or lower gingival margins, 23 on the palate and 3 on the inner aspect of the cheek.

Twenty-nine of the 35 tumours of salivary origin arose on the palate, most of them at the posterior part of the hard palate where mucous glands are most frequent.

The age range of patients with squamous carcinoma was 27 to 90 with a mean of 50.7 years. Salivary tumours occurred at a distinctly younger mean age of 35 years with a range of 8 to 52 years.

The sex distribution was markedly different from that seen in other countries. Squamous cell carcinoma was seen in 32 females and 17 males. SHEDD, VON ESSEN, CONNELLY and EISENBERG (1968) quote a number of series in all of which males outnumber females by at least 1.5 to 1 and the excess is more usually in the region of 4 or 5 to 1. Salivary tumours in the oral cavity also showed a female excess, 11 males and 24 females, a ratio of 2.2 to 1. And in some types of tumour the female excess was even more pronounced, for example, 7 of the 8 patients with adenoid cystic tumours were female.

Some series in Uganda have shown a slight excess in northern tribes (TEMPLETON et al., 1972) but no marked variations in the incidence in different regions were found in the present study.

Factors which appear to be important in the development of tumours of the mouth include tobacco, alcohol, syphilis, heat, nutritional deficiencies and advanced age (WYNDER, BROSS and FELDMAN, 1957). The decreased incidence in Uganda may be a result of rather less frequent use tobacco and the age structure of the population. Alcohol is widely taken in large quantities and syphilis is an extremely common disease but seldom seems to be associated with the development of oral manifestations. Arsenicals have never been widely used in treatment. None of the above factors adequately explains the excess in females. Women smoke tobacco as frequently but probably no more than males. None of the other factors mentioned above affects women more than men. There is a strong association between iron deficiency anaemia, Paterson Kelly syndrome and oropharyngeal cancer. Iron deficiency, however, results in changes in the oral mucosa (BAIRD, DODGE and PALMER, 1961) rather than in the postcricoid and oesophageal regions. Unfortunately no haematological data are available on these patients but iron deficiency anaemia is extremely common among the Ugandan population and this association would be worthy of investigation. It should be noted, however, that sideropenic dysphagia has not been noted in Uganda and that post-cricoid carcinoma is rare and is a disease of men. This is in marked contrast with the findings in Sweden (WYNDER, HULTBERG, JACOBSSON and BROSS, 1957) and suggests that some factor in addition to iron deficiency might be responsible for the changes found in Sweden.

Tumours of intraoral salivary tissue are frequently seen in Uganda, particularly in the palate (DAVIES, DODGE and BURKITT, 1964). No reason for this or for the marked female preponderance has been suggested. It is interesting to note that adenoid cystic carcinoma occurring on the palate was mainly a disease of females but in the nose this tumour occurred as commonly in males. Tumours of the major salivary glands, on the other hand, show an equal sex incidence. Childhood malnutrition, which occurs very commonly, influences salivary function markedly and it may be that these differences in tumour incidence are similarly modified. Two of the tumours occurred in children, one adenoid cystic carcinoma in an 8-year-old girl and a mucoepidermoid tumour in a 12-year-old boy.

In advanced cases of cancer it is sometimes difficult to tell whether a given tumour arose from palate or antrum but the histories of all these patients suggest that an ulcer or mass on the palate occurred well before any symptoms referable to the nose were noted. Squamous carcinomas of the palate account for a far greater proportion of oral cancer than in Connecticut. Out of 2,268 patients with oral cancer in Connecticut, 8% had lesions on the palate (SHEDD et al., 1968), compared with 32% of oral squamous carcinoma in Uganda. If salivary tumours are included the preponderance of palatal tumours was even more marked. Other tumours arising in the palate included 2 cases of lymphosarcoma and a case of fibrosarcoma. There is no such habit as "wrong-way-round" cigarette smoking to explain the relative frequency of tumours at this site. By contrast, tumours of the buccal lining of the cheek appear to be particularly unusual, as is leukoplakia of this region, possibly a result of the rather better dental hygiene prevalent until recently in Ugandans.

Tumours of Salivary Tissue

Salivary tissue may produce a bewildering range of tumour types. There is no internationally agreed nomenclature available as yet and little agreement on defining the limits between histological entities. Even if histological diagnosis is uniform classification practice varies widely. Some registries include pleomorphic adenomata under rubric 142 whereas others exclude these cases which are then found under 210. Some registries classify neoplasms derived from the mucous glands of the palate under 142, others under 144 along with other tumours of the mouth. We shall discuss all tumours of mucous and serous glands in the head and neck in this section. Pleomorphic and monomorphic adenomas were not classified as cancers. Rubric 142 was reserved for malignant neoplasms of the submandibular and parotid glands, tumours of glands in the palate, nose or lacrymal apparatus were classified with other malignant tumours of the mouth, nose and eye respectively.

Table 6. Site of origin of 211 salivary and mucous gland tumours

	Males	Females	Both sexes	% of all sites
Parotid	42	53	95	45
Submandibular	23	20	43	20
Palate	12	21	33	15
Lacrymal	6	8	14	7
Nose	10	6	16	8
Other and unknown	2	8	10	5
Total	95	116	211	100%

Tumours of salivary tissue were diagnosed in 211 cases. The sites of origin are shown in Table 6. Tumours of the parotid accounted for only 45% of the total. This is a considerably smaller proportion than that found in Caucasian series where a rule of thumb has long been applied that 75% of tumours occur in the parotid and 75% are benign. This distribution is almost exactly the same as that found by DAVIES, DODGE and BURKITT (1964), in Uganda and HIGGINSON and OETTLÉ (1960) in South Africa. It is difficult to be certain whether this variation in proportion is a result of decrease in the incidence of parotid tumours or increase in the tumours of other sites because of the variations in registration alluded to above. American negroes at Memorial Hospital show a tendency to more frequent involvement of the submandibular gland than whites (BERG, 1971, personal communication). No explanation of this anomalous distribution is forthcoming.

Tumours of all sites except the nose and submandibular were marginally more common in females (Table 6). The age distribution is shown in Table 7. The largest number of cases was seen in patients in the third decade of life but when correction for the population at risk is applied the highest incidence is seen to occur in the very old. Eleven malignant tumours occurred in children under the age of 19 years, 9 of which were mucoepidermoid tumours. Ten benign lesions were diagnosed in this age group, most of which were found in the submandibular gland and the mean age of patients with pleomorphic adenomata at this site was much younger than patients with adenomata of the parotid. This factor might partially explain the relative preponderance of submandibular tumours occurring in the youthful population of Uganda.

Examples of all the recognized varieties of salivary neoplasms were seen, with the striking exception of adenolymphoma (Table 8). Only one case of this tumour has been seen in Uganda in a 15-year period out of a collection of some 400 salivary tumours, and that occurred in an expatriate Englishman. No reason for the absence of this tumour in Africans is apparent. The oncocytic appearance of cells which is

Table 7. Age distribution of mucous gland tumours at all sites

Years	Benign	Malignant	Total
0— 9	3	1	4
10—19	7	10	17
20—29	24	14	38
30—39	31	5	36
40—49	22	12	34
50—59	8	14	22
60—69	12	9	21
70+	2	7	9
Adults	25	5	30
Total	134	77	211

Table 8. Histological types of mucous gland tumour diagnosed at different sites

	Parotid	Subman-dibular	Palate	Lacrymal	Nose	Others	Total
Adenomas	57	39	18	10	4	4	134
Carcinomas	38	4	14	4	12	5	77
Adenoid cystic	5	3	6	1	9	1	25
Mucoepidermoid	10	1	5	1	2		19
Acinic cell	5						5
Squamous	5						5
Adenocarcinoma	1				1	2	4
Ca. in P.A.	12		3	2		2	19

seen so frequently in salivary tissue in older European subjects is conspicuously absent in Africans. Salivary oncocytomas are not seen and oncocytic change in the thyroid has not yet been recorded.

Adenomas account for 64% of tumours seen. Histologically they display the same range of epithelial components as seen in other countries. Squamous differentiation occurred frequently and was particularly common in tumours from the submandibular region. The stroma was usually myxoid, hyalisation of collagen was noted frequently but apparent cartilagenous differentiation was seen only rarely and was found almost exclusively in tumours from the submandibular region and in two cases boney metaplasia had occurred. One hundred and eighteen tumours conformed to the general pattern of pleomorphic adenoma. In 16 cases, however, there was no stromal induction and the epithelial component comprised the overwhelming bulk of the tumour. These cases were diagnosed as monomorphic adenomas. In the majority of cases these had a marked tubular pattern, usually with a distinct myoepithelial component (Fig. 1). These tumours occurred more frequently in women than in men (11 females, 5 males) and 14 of 16 cases occurred in the parotid. The patient was usually 40 or 50 years old and gave a history of a slow-growing painless mass which had been present for a long period of time. The tumour was always sharply demar-

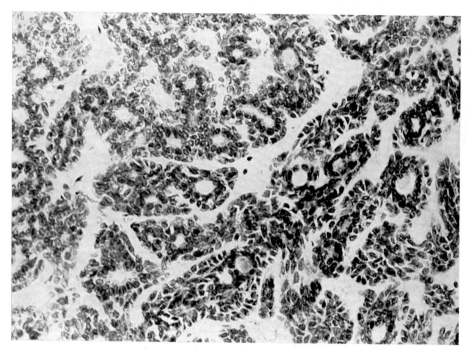

Fig. 1. Monomorphic tubular adenoma. Each tubule is regular and has a double lining of cells. There is minimal stromal tissue in between tubules

cated from the surrounding tissue and was often cystic (Fig. 2). Histologically the differentiation from adenoid cystic carcinoma (Fig. 3) may be problematic. The general uniformity of the cells and the tubular arrangement closely resemble that tumour. The macroscopic arrangement, the prominent single cell myoepithelial layer and lack of signs of invasion or necrosis all help to differentiate this entity. Recurrence of pleiomorphic adenoma was seen quite frequently; this was a result of inadequate primary excision leaving small nodules around the periphery of the original tumour which then regrew (Fig. 4).

Mucoepidermoid tumours occurred at an exceptionally youthful age. Twenty cases were seen, 12 of which occurred under the age of 25 years. Four were noted under the age of 15 years. Tumours were well differentiated and prone to local recurrence, for example, five attempted excisions were carried out on one child before there was evidence of lymphatic metastasis.

Carcinoma arising in pre-existing pleomorphic adenoma was seen relatively frequently. This is possibly a result of the long delay in seeking treatment which is

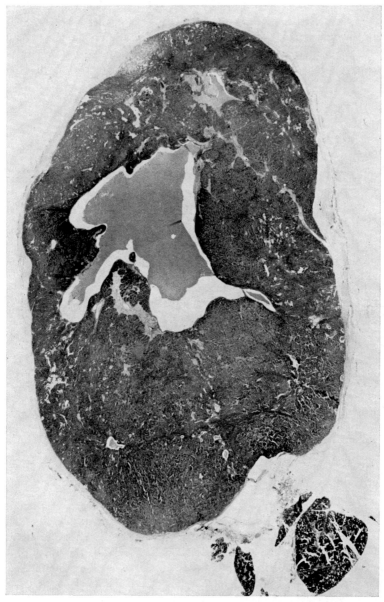

Fig. 2. Monomorphic tubular adenoma showing the sharp demarcation from surrounding tissue and central cystic degeneration

characteristic of medical practice in Africa. Other tumours showed no marked histological differences from the patterns seen in other parts of the world.

The proportion of tumours occurring at different sites showed quite marked differences (Table 8). Tumours of the submandibular gland were common and accounted for 20% of the total series. The proportion of benign tumours at this site

34 A. C. TEMPLETON

was higher than in other glands. This finding is in direct contradistinction to that occurring in Caucasian subjects, where the incidence is smaller but the proportion of malignant tumours is much higher (SIMONS, BEAHRS and WOOLNER, 1964). By contrast, in Ugandan patients the parotid occupies a much lower proportion of cases but the percentage of malignant tumours (40%) is much higher than in Caucasians.

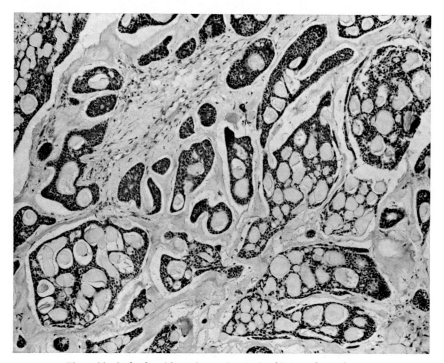

Fig. 3. Typical adenoid cystic carcinoma in this case from the nose

Tumours of the palate occurred frequently and were usually located on the posterior part of the hard palate. Rather less than half the tumours were histologically malignant. However, pleomorphic adenomas at this site were very prone to recur, probably because of the close proximity to bone. The relative frequency of adenoid cystic tumours at this site, all of which occurred in females, is unexplained. Adenoid cystic tumours were also frequently seen in the nose and sinuses but at this site the sex incidence was equal. Lacrymal gland tumours occurred relatively frequently and the proportion of different histological types was similar to that reported in other countries (BÖCK and FEYRTER, 1966).

The incidence of this group of tumours is difficult to compare with other countries but there is little evidence to suggest they are more frequent than in Caucasian subjects. Salivary tumours in African have a reputation of being both common and highly malignant. This impression is erroneous and probably resulted from memories of the extreme size and longevity of the tumours which would be exaggerated by the process of "cropping" of long-standing cases when new hospitals were opened in

Africa. Explanations of the very different distribution of tumours in Africans have usually invoked the effect of malnutrition but all are unsatisfactory (summarized by DAVIES et al., 1964). The varied distribution, both anatomically and geographically, requires explanation but there is no reasonable hypothesis currently available to explain aetiology or distribution of any of these tumours.

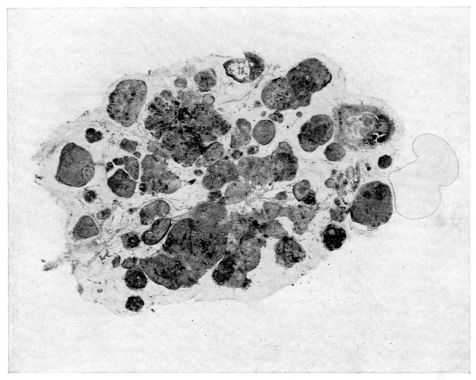

Fig. 4. Re-growth of small satellite nodules of pleiomorphic adenoma giving rise to recurrence

Tumours of the Tonsil and Oropharynx

13 cases of squamous carcinoma of the tonsil and fauces were seen, comprising 0.2% of tumours overall. In addition there were 19 cases of lymphoma arising in this region. Although Burkitt's tumour often occurs in the maxilla and mandible, involvement of the tonsils was not seen. Why this should be is not known but it seems possible since the thymus, tonsil and appendix are all very seldom affected by Burkitt's lymphoma that some form of immune resistance is active in these areas. Kaposi's sarcoma was seen to involve the tonsil in at least 5 cases but was never biopsied from that site. Patients with squamous carcinomas ranged from 30 to 70 years (mean 39 years) and the age range of patients with lymphoma was 12 to 90 years (mean 44 years). This age distribution is rather younger than that found in other countries.

Sex distribution showed a male preponderance that was slightly more marked in the case of lymphomas than with carcinomas. There were 10 males and 3 females with squamous carcinoma and 16 males and 3 females among 19 cases of lymphoma. The only E.N.T. specialists in the country work at Mulago Hospital, where ten of the 13 squamous carcinomas were diagnosed. This factor probably largely accounts for the fact that 7 out of 13 patients with squamous carcinomas in this group of tumours and 6 out of 19 patients with lymphomas were Baganda. In general, lymphomas are relatively more frequent in northern tribes but in the particular case of lymphoma of the tonsil this regional distribution of cases appeared to be equal. However, the distortion induced by diagnostic practice and the small number of cases make it difficult to be dogmatic.

Biopsy material from 10 of the squamous carcinomas was gradable, 3 were well differentiated keratinizing tumours, 4 were average-grade and 3 poorly differentiated. No case of transitional cell or lymphoepitheliomatous tumour was seen in the tonsil, a marked contrast to the situation with tumours of the nasopharynx, which were virtually all of this type. Six of the 11 cases had clinically obvious lymph-node metastases but since none of the tumours was considered operable no biopsies were taken from the nodes. Well differentiated tumours involved nodes as frequently as anaplastic tumours. Tumours were usually very extensive at the time of presentation and it is very seldom that surgery is feasible in such patients. Radiotherapy is not available in Uganda, and nitrogen mustard infusion into the carotid artery offers the best hope of regression. Gratifying short-term results have been obtained with this method but recurrence is inevitable. A good response to chemotherapy was more frequently seen with lymphomas.

Carcinoma of the Hypopharynx and Oesophagus

Tumours of the lower part of the oesophagus are much more frequent than those in the upper part and in many respects were very different from those of the upper third. In terms of clinical, histological and epidemiological parameters, tumours of the upper oesophagus were more closely related to hypopharyngeal tumours than to those of the lower oesophagus. The region has therefore been divided in a rather unconventional fashion, although in the tables in the introduction the classification has followed the recommendations of the I.C.D. 7th edition.

1. Tumours above the Level of T2

The hypopharynx and upper part of the oesophagus were only rarely the seat of neoplastic growths. Six squamous carcinomas were found in the hypopharynx and 9 in the upper oesophagus, compared with 110 in the lower oesophagus und 13 involving the oropharynx. Three lymphomas occurred in the hypopharynx, one case of Hodgkin's disease and 2 reticulum cell sarcomas. One additional patient was noted to have a tumour of the "pharynx" but the site was not specified more closely. Only the 15 epithelial tumours are considered further here.

The mean age of patients was 54 years (range 37 to 78). The three patients with lymphoma were aged 16, 28 and 38 years. There were 9 males and 6 females, and there was no significant age difference between male and female patients.

Since 11 out of 15 cases were diagnosed at Mulago Hospital information as to tribal and geographical variation requires cautious interpretation. Four patients were of the Baganda tribe and the other eleven came from widely different parts of the country. Four were from Eastern region, five from Western region and four from the North. There was no excess among tribes of Eastern Uganda as was seen with tumours of the lower oesophagus.

All four squamous carcinomas of the hypopharynx which were biopsied were poorly differentiated tumours. Only one showed keratin formation, one showed a basaloid appearance and the third was composed of large vesicular cells arranged in clumps very similar to nasopharyngeal tumours in appearance (Chapter 4).

Eight of the 9 epithelial tumours in the upper oesophagus were squamous carcinomas. Two were well differentiated, 3 of average grade and 3 poorly differentiated. The stroma in one case showed a pseudosarcomatous proliferation. The ninth case showed a rather strange picture with islands of small dark cells surrounded by a layer of more elongated cells, rather in the fashion of a basal cell carcinoma. PAS-positive diastase-resistant material was present in the columnar cells and there was no evidence of keratinization. This tumour probably developed from the duct of a mucus gland of the pharynx.

The prognosis in these patients was poor. Four died in hospital within a few weeks of diagnosis. Others were discharged but survival was never prolonged.

2. Tumours of the Middle and Lower Oesophagus

For descriptive purpose it is customary to divide the oesophagus into upper, middle and lower thirds. Tumours of the lower oesophagus were frequently so large that it was difficult to be certain in which area a given tumour arose. After some rather arbitrary assessment of cases had been made, 43 tumours appeared to have arisen in the lower third and 39 cases in the middle third of the oesophagus. Since these two groups did not differ in age, sex, geographical, tribal or histological distribution they are considered together for the purposes of this review. Adenocarcinomas of the cardia, however, appeared histologically and geographically distinct and so are treated separately under the general heading of tumours of the stomach.

Squamous carcinoma was histologically confirmed in 84 cases and a further 26 cases were diagnosed by other means without biopsy. This represents 1.5% of malignant tumours overall. This proportion is considerably smaller than in most countries of the world. COOK and BURKITT (1970) have shown that the biopsy rate in patients with oesophageal cancer in East Africa is low, so that this figure is almost certainly an underestimate of the true incidence. There is evidence that the incidence of oesophageal cancer in Kyadondo County has recently increased rapidly (TEMPLETON et al., 1972). The situation in the country is now somewhat analogous to that pertaining in South Africa in 1950 (OETTLÉ, 1963 a), when that country experienced the start of what proved to be an epidemic of oesophageal cancer. The rise in incidence in Uganda appears to have been a result of tumours developing in the lower parts of the oesophagus only and has mainly affected women.

The mean age at presentation was 52 years, with a range of 32 to 90 years. There were 65 male patients and 47 female. This apparent male excess is in part a result of registration bias. For example, among residents of Mengo district, Baganda patients showed a slight female excess of 27 males to 30 females, whereas all 12 patients of other tribal origins were male. Whether this equal sex ratio in one tribe is representative of the country as a whole or not is difficult to say but it seems most unlikely that the true sex distribution in other tribes is in fact 12:1. Non-Baganda males resident in Mengo district heavily outnumber females because men coming to find work in Kampala tend to leave families behind. Among patients referred from up-country there was a male excess of 11 males to 2 females. This is probably a result of the greater willingness of male patients to travel to hospital and undergo diagnostic procedures (Templeton and Bianchi, 1972 a). In spite of these figures there are good reasons to suppose that the sex distribution in Uganda is unlikely to show the great male preponderance recorded in other parts of Africa.

Baganda patients accounted for 77 out of 110 cases. This gross excess is to some extent a result of bias in diagnosis but there appears to have been a rapid rise in incidence in recent years among Baganda patients which has not affected other tribes resident in the same area (Templeton et al., 1972). When patients from other parts of the country were considered there was a pronounced tendency for patients to come from eastern rather than western tribes, northern tribes occupying a median position (Table 15). This distribution contrasted with the findings in cases with tumours of the upper oesophagus or cardia and is therefore very unlikely to be a result of diagnostic bias.

All but two biopsied cases were squamous cell carcinomas and most showed marked keratinization. Thirteen were well differentiated, 42 average and 17 poorly differentiated tumours. One squamous carcinoma showed a spindle pattern reminiscent of fibrosarcoma. In only two cases was there evidence of extensive in-situ change in the mucosa above the tumour. There was a slight tendency for females to have rather better differentiated tumours than males. Six squamous carcinomas were found to involve the cardia and had spread down to invade gastric mucosa, compared with 23 adenocarcinomas which had arisen in this region. Adenocarcinomas of the cardia have all been classified as gastric neoplasms even though some of these tumours arose in oesophageal glands.

Two tumours were noted which were not squamous carcinomas. One in the middle third of the oesophagus had the structure of an oat-cell carcinoma. Post-mortem examination showed no evidence of tumour in the lungs or bronchi and it probably arose from mucous glands in the wall of the oesophagus. The second case was probably also a mucous gland tumour and showed both glandular and squamous neoplastic elements. This tumour type has been labelled mucoepidermoid, but although this is a reasonable description of the findings in such cases, the tumour of major salivary glands which is also called mucoepidermoid has an entirely different appearance. For this reason some other term, such as adenosquamous carcinoma, is advocated.

Patients with carcinoma of the oesophagus present late in Uganda, and death is rapid and almost inevitable. Thirty-six patients died in hospital within a few days of diagnosis. A further 27 patients died at home within a few months of discharge, and only two patients are known to have survived one year. The remaining 17 patients were lost to follow-up.

Post-mortem examination was performed in 32 cases. The cause of death was most often found to be aspiration pneumonia; three patients died in the immediate post-operative period, 2 died as a result of massive bleeding following erosion of the aorta, two developed mediastinitis following perforation and one had a massive pulmonary embolus. In 13 cases (40%) there was no evidence of metastasis; in all the others involvement of local lymph nodes was found and in 10 cases lymph nodes below the diaphragm contained deposits. Metastasis to the liver was found in four cases, in two of which the tumour was located in the middle third of the oesophagus. The lung was involved either by direct spread or metastasis in the majority of cases. Other organs more rarely involved included bone, kidney and adrenals. In two cases multiple strictures were found but since each area showed a similar histological appearance and there was no surrounding epithelial dysplasia it was assumed that this represented metastatic involvement probably via intra-mural lymphatics rather than multiple sites of origin. The tumour itself was always large and extended over at least 5 cm in length, in most cases involving the full circumference of the wall. Spread downwards to involve the stomach was seen in 6 cases of squamous carcinoma but more often the growth ceased at the level of the cardia. Hepatic cirrhosis was found in only one case (3%), whereas the overall incidence of cirrhosis at post-mortem in Kampala in 1968 was 4%. This contrasts with the findings of STEINER (1954) who found a positive correlation between cirrhosis and oesophageal carcinoma. It is probable that alcoholism is a rare cause of cirrhosis in Uganda.

Discussion

The incidence of carcinoma of the oesophagus varies widely in different parts of East Africa (COOK and BURKITT, 1970). The incidence may change very rapidly in very short distances, for example, a very high rate has been found at Kisumu whereas close by, the incidence is much lower (AHMED and COOK, 1969). In Uganda overall the incidence seems to be relatively low (2.8 cases per million per year) but the biopsy rate in such tumours is low and probably many cases are missed. Cases referred to Kampala from outside Mengo district came predominantly from the Eastern region towards that part of Kenya where the incidence is known to be high. Referrals of cases from the Western region, where the population is at least as large, were much less frequent. Ruanda, which borders on this region, also reports a low frequency (BURKITT, 1966). Five out of 6 tumours which occurred in patients from Western tribes were located in the upper third of the oesophagus although the distribution of cases overall showed a preponderance of cases in the lower two thirds in a ratio 12:1. Thus it would appear that in those parts of the country with a higher incidence whatever factors are causing the tumour act almost exclusively on the lower part of the oesophagus. Tumours of the upper part and hypopharynx are not affected by these factors and tend to predominate in their absence.

In all areas of Africa where it has been investigated, patients with cancer of the oesophagus seem to be more likely to drink alcohol and to take larger quantities than controls. It has been presumed, therefore, that some contaminant of alcohol is the cause of the disease. Suspicion has fallen on nitrosamines which are present and are known to be carcinogenic in animals (McGLASHAN, WALTERS and McLEAN, 1968). The recent rising incidence found in Baganda females affords an excellent opportunity to identify the nature of the substance. The situation affords control populations within a distance of some 200 miles of Kampala, one with a low incidence, the other a well known high incidence for comparison with a rising intermediate zone.

All tumours of the upper alimentary canal show a sex distribution that contrasts with that found in other countries. Particularly among the Baganda there is a female excess in tumours of all sites except the hypopharynx. This is the exact reverse of experience in more temperate climates and demands explanation. Iron deficiency anaemia is extraordinarily common, particularly among women, but sideropenic dysphagia is very rarely encountered. The apparently associated tumours of the hypopharynx are also rare and occur in men. Consideration of tumours of the lower oesophagus shows a slight male excess in Uganda as a whole which may be spurious. This is very different from the sex ratio seen in Kisumu, Kenya, where males outnumber females 14:1 (AHMED, 1966). This argues that the aetiology in these two areas could be different or that it is modified by social custom. Studies comparing possible differences in likely causative factors between the two regions would be worthwhile. Comparison of drinking habits between women in the two areas might be of particular interest.

Tumours of the Stomach

Malignant tumours arising in the stomach were seen in 190 cases. These included 4 lymphomas, 6 connective tissue tumours and 2 carcinoid tumours which are considered in more detail elsewhere. In 158 cases adenocarcinoma of the stomach was confirmed histologically. In a further 21 cases a diagnosis of gastric neoplasia had been made by other means. These were presumed to be adenocarcinomas although histological proof was lacking.

Carcinoma of the stomach accounted for 2.6% of tumours overall (3% of tumours in males and 1.5% of tumours in females). The crude incidence rate was 2.9 cases per million per year in women and 5.5 cases in men. These figures are a gross understatement of the true frequency of the disease in Uganda. It is estimated that in the country as a whole only about one third of deep-seated neoplasms in males and one fifth in females are actually diagnosed and registered (TEMPLETON and BIANCHI, 1972 a). In the case of gastric neoplasms the proportion is likely to be even lower. There are indications that tumours of the stomach are more common in the tribes living in the west of the country and in immigrants from Ruanda. In such people deep-seated neoplasms are diagnosed even less readily than in Buganda or in the north of the country. Also in advanced cases of intra-abdominal malignant tumours it is often difficult to be certain of the exact site of origin. Thirty-one such cases were seen during this period; it is highly likely that at least 10 arose in the stomach, but for lack of evidence they have been classified under the heading of tumours of unknown site. In Kyadondo County the incidence of gastric cancer was 27 cases per million among females and 36 cases in males (corrected for an African standard population). These figures are probably reasonably representative for the country as a whole since there are members of all tribes of Uganda resident in Kyadondo. The figure for males is very much smaller than all 60 registries from different parts of the world quoted by DOLL et al. (1970). The rate for females is very similar to that found in Nigeria, Rhodesia, and among Africans in Natal. Thus, even when under-registration is taken into account the incidence of gastric cancer in most parts of Uganda is low.

The proportional rate of gastric cancer varies widely in different parts of the country (Table 9). These variations seemed to be largely determined by tribal affiliation rather than by address. For example, Ruandans have a high proportional rate whether resident in Ruanda, Kigezi or Buganda. In these areas the rate in indigenous people varies widely. This is not to imply that environment plays no part in determining the frequency of gastric neoplasms in different areas but many immigrant studies have shown that it may require several generations before acquiring the level found in the host area.

Table 9. Showing the percentage of cancer overall made up by gastric cancer in different tribes

Tribe	Rate	Group
Ruanda/Burundi	7.8%	High rate
Ankole	4.7%	
Gishu	4.5%	
Toro	4.3%	
Konjo	3.8%	
Ganda	2.8%	Intermediate rate
Kiga	2.2%	
Acholi	1.1%	Low rate
Lugbara	0.9%	
Teso	0.7%	
Soga	0.6%	
Lango	0.2%	

It will be interesting to see whether the present high frequency in Ruandans resident in Buganda and Kigezi falls towards the level found in the indigenous tribes of these areas. The majority of Ugandan tribes in the high rate group are from the west of the country. It is known that there are very high rates recorded from Ruanda and Eastern Congo (CLEMMESON, MAISIN and GIGASE, 1962) and Northern Tanzania (BURKITT, BUNDSCHUH and DAHLIN, 1969) which border on this region. The relatively low proportion of cases among the Bakiga is therefore somewhat surprising. It is not certain whether this is a true reduction or an artefact of under-reporting. The only tribe in the high rate group that does not reside in the west of the country, the Gishu, also live high on the side of a volcanic mountain (Mount Elgon). Many of the countries with a high incidence of gastric carcinoma such as Japan, Chile, New Zealand (Maoris) and Hawaii (DOLL et al., 1970) all live in geologically young volcanic areas. Mount Kenya and Mount Kilimanjaro (both volcanoes) are also associated with higher proportional rates than the surrounding lower lying areas (COOK et al., 1970).

The site of origin of tumours was accurately known in 124 cases. In the remainder the tumour was either very extensive so that it was impossible to be certain where it arose, or the site was not accurately stated. The most common site of origin was the pylorus, but the proportion of cases occurring at different sites varied (Table 10). Tribes were divided into three groups as in Table 9. Tribes with a high proportional

Table 10. Showing the anatomical localisation of gastric tumours in the different tribal groups

	High	Inter-mediate	Low	Total
Cardia	5	13	5	23
Lesser curve	10	5	2	17
Greater curve	2	2	0	4
Diffuse	5	2	2	9
Antral	53	32	4	89
Massive or unstated	13	24	—	37
Total	88	78	13	179

rate had a greater percentage of cases occurring in the pylorus. Intermediate and low rate tribes had a larger number of tumours of the cardia. Thus changes in the proportion of stomach cancer in different tribes seems to be largely a function of alterations in the frequency of pyloric tumours. The incidence of tumours of the cardia, in contrast, remains relatively stable in different areas.

Table 11. Sex distribution of gastric cancer in different tribal groups
(1 person unknown sex)

	High	Inter-mediate	Low	All tribes
Males	56	51	10	117
Females	32	26	3	61
Total	88	77	13	179

The sex ratio overall was almost exactly 2 males to 1 females (Table 11). This ratio was not significantly different in tribes with high or low proportional rate, the sex ratio at each site was essentially similar.

The age distribution in each sex is shown in Table 12. The greatest number of patients were aged 45—54 but calculation of incidence shows a steadily rising curve except in old age where figures are unreliable. The mean age of patients was 52.7 years. There was no significant difference in age distribution in different tribes or at different sites.

Table 12. Age distribution of cases of carcinoma of the stomach

	15—24	25—34	35—44	45—54	55—64	65—74	75+	Unknown
Male	1	9	22	39	25	15	4	2
Female	—	9	14	18	13	6	1	—
Total	1	18	36	57	38	21	5	2

Adenocarcinomas of the stomach frequently show a wide range of appearances in different parts of the same tumour. Categorization is therefore often difficult. Tumours of the cardia may arise from mucous glands, stomach glands or surface epithelium either squamous or columnar. The histological appearance of tumours arising from each cell type is distinctive. Elsewhere in the stomach many attempts have been made to correlate cell of origin with histological pattern, usually without success. The classification of adenocarcinomas into two types "intestinal" and "diffuse" (LAUREN, 1965) has been widely used in epidemiological studies (MUNOZ,

Table 13. Histological types of gastric adenocarcinoma seen in different tribes

	High rate	Intermediate rate	Low rate	All tribes
Intestinal	49	26	12	87
Diffuse	28	31	12	71
Total	77	57	24	158

CORREA, CUELLO and DUQUE, 1968; CORREA, CUELLO and DUQUE, 1970; MUNOZ and ASVALL, 1971; MUNOZ and CONNELLY, 1971). These terms are unsatisfactory in many ways, but the classification has the virtues of simplicity and reproducibility and is used here. There were 160 classifiable tumours, 88 intestinal types and 72 diffuse tumours. The proportion of these two types varied in different tribes (Table 13). Thus those tribes with a high proportional rate had a high proportion of intestinal types of tumour. These differences were almost entirely a result of differences occurring at the antrum (Table 14), where intestinal patterns were more than twice as

Table 14. Histological types of carcinoma of the pyloric antrum occurring in different tribes

	High rate	Intermediate rate	Low rate	All tribes
Intestinal	31	13	1	45
Diffuse	14	10	3	27
Total	45	23	4	72

common as diffuse ones in tribes with a high proportional rate. Tumours occurring at other sites were much more evenly distributed in the different tribes. In most groups of tumours there was a male excess of 2 : 1 but among intestinal tumours of the pylorus the ratio was 23 males to 8 females. Those parts of the country where a high proportional rate of carcinoma of the stomach occurs are those in which there is an excess of male patients developing intestinal types of tumour which occur in the pyloric antrum. These conclusions are essentially similar to those found in other countries (MUNOZ et al., 1968; MUNOZ and ASVALL, 1971).

When statistics of cancer incidence from different cancer registries are published tumours of different parts of the oesophagus and stomach are not separated from one another. In many registries patients are not separated ethnically or geographically. Table 15 illustrates the valuable data which may be lost if this practice is continued. It will be seen that tumours of the upper end of the oesophagus and upper end of the stomach do not show a very significant geographical or tribal variation. Tumours of

Table 15. Non-Baganda patients with carcinoma of the upper alimentary canal (Patients from Ruanda and Burundi are classified with Western Tribes) (All figures are expressed as percentages of cases at each site)

	Total cases	Eastern %	Western %	Northern %
Upper oesophagus	13	31	38	31
Lower oesophagus	19	74	5	21
Cardia (adeno)	10	30	40	30
Pylorus	55	13	87	—

the lower end of the stomach are found in Western region and tumours of the lower oesophagus occur in the east. These tendencies would not be apparent if the bulk of cases which occur in Baganda were to be included or if the sites were not delineated.

In our material it was only rarely possible to examine tissue from the stomach to detect the presence of intestinal metaplasia, chronic gastritis or previous gastric ulcer. No conclusions can be drawn as to the relative frequency of these diseases in patients with pyloric cancer in different tribal groups. A number of facts suggest that there is a correlation. For example, patients with carcinoma of the pylorus from Northern Tanzania quite frequently presented with gastric perforation, a most unusual presentation in areas where the disease is less common. Gastric ulcer appears to be more common in Ruanda and Northern Tanzania than in Kampala, where duodenal ulcer is much more frequent. A survey of the incidence of ulceration, gastritis and intestinal metaplasia in high and low incidence areas is urgently required.

The value of investigation of predisposing lesions of carcinoma of the antral region would be enhanced by a parallel investigation of the lower oesophagus. Populations in Tanzania where the incidence of antral tumours is high and oesophagus low (BURKITT et al., 1969) and Kisumu where oesophageal carcinoma is common (AHMED and COOK, 1969) afford natural controls for one another. If the study included Kampala, where there is a changing incidence of oesophageal tumours in Baganda and the change that is likely to take place in the incidence of gastric tumours in Ruandans, the possibilities of fruitful results are increased considerably.

Tumours of the Small Intestine

Tumours affecting the small intestine were as unusual as in other parts of the world. The tumours seen during the five-year period are recorded in Table 16.

The commonest tumour occurring in the small intestine is probably Kaposi's sarcoma. Involvement of the bowel by this tumour occurs in many patients with a variety of clinical appearances and often does not produce symptoms. Most of these cases were discovered only at postmortem and a considerable number of cases with intestinal lesions remain undiagnosed. Whether the tumours in the bowel contribute to the fatal outcome or not is unclear.

Table 16. Showing the number of tumours involving the small intestine

	Male	Female	Total
Adenocarcinoma	3	2	5
Carcinoid tumour	5	—	5
Malignant lymphoma	6	1	7
Kaposi's sarcoma	18	—	18
Benign connective tissue tumours	9	6	15
Leiomyosarcoma	3	4	7
Other benign conditions	3	1	4
Total	47	14	61

Three of the carcinoid tumours occurred in the terminal ileum and the other two in the duodenum. These tumours showed all the typical features of argentaffin carcinomas. Three were found to have metastasized to lymph nodes and liver and the other two showed no evidence of metastasis at laparotomy. No case of full-blown carcinoid syndrome has been reported from East Africa and at postmortem none of the three cases showed any lesions of the right ventricle. No case of carcinoid tumour in alimentary or respiratory tracts coincident with endomyocardial fibrosis was seen.

Five cases of adenocarcinoma were diagnosed. All occurred in the terminal ileum and histologically were well differentiated or average-grade adenocarcinomas. Two showed very marked production of extra-cellular mucin (colloid carcinoma). Three patients were male and two female, and all were aged between 40 and 50 years. Three patients came from the north of the country and one from the east. The numbers are too small to make any certain deductions but it appears that carcinoma of the small intestine has an incidence at least as low as in other countries.

Diseases of the lymphoreticular system involve the small intestine quite frequently. For example, in patients with leukaemia, infiltration of the ileum may be found at postmortem in a large proportion of cases. Burkitt's tumour occurring in mesenteric nodes may give rise to involvement of the neighbouring bowel. Such cases are not recorded in this chapter, which is restricted to those lesions which appear to have arisen in the bowel rather than involving the bowel secondarily. Three cases of histiocytic lymphoma were diagnosed, two cases of Hodgkin's disease and two of lymphocytic lymphoma. Patients were aged between 14 and 50 years (mean 34 years). The sex of one patient is unknown but five of the remaining six were male. No investigation was made of the antibody-secreting function of these tumours but none were found to contain amyloid material. Thus lymphomas of the small intestine appear somewhat more common than carcinomas and occur at a younger age. Six of the 7 patients came from the north of the country where many forms of lymphomata appear to be relatively more frequent. It has been suggested that lymphomata are more common in areas where schistosomiasis is prevalent, but none of these patients had ova in the biopsy specimen examined.

Connective tissue tumours occurred relatively frequently. Benign tumours presented either as incidental findings at laparotomy or because they had produced intussusception. Malignant tumours, by contrast, had usually been palpable for some time and laparotomy was performed to assess the nature of the swelling. The age range of patients with leiomyosarcoma was 33 to 65 years, four patients were male and three female. There appeared to be no predilection as to site of origin, tumours occurring anywhere from the duodenum to the terminal ileum. The majority of patients were Baganda. Precise differential diagnosis of the benign connective tissue tumours was often difficult since many had been partially infarcted during intussusception. Most, however, appeared to be leiomyomata. Two submucus lipomas were found and three cases of neurofibroma were seen. The majority of patients were female (4 male : 11 female) and the age range was from 26 to 70 years. The geographical and sex distribution in these cases is in sharp contrast to the pattern seen with lymphomata.

Other tumour-like conditions seen included two cases where the "lead nodule" of an intussusception appeared to be an adenomatous polypoid mass. Intussusception may produce a marked heaping-up of mucosa and when the mass becomes infarcted it is difficult to be certain whether there was a preexisting lesion and, if so, what was its nature. One case of a nodule of ectopic pancreatic tissue in the jejunum was found incidentally at laparotomy.

Argentaffin (Carcinoid) Tumours

12 carcinoid tumours were diagnosed. Some of these were not argentaffin-positive but were diagnosed on the basis of the characteristic morphology of the tumour on H and E staining.

Table 17. Showing the anatomical distribution of 12 carcinoid tumours

Stomach	2
Duodenum	2
Small intestine	2
Ileocaecal region	2
Appendix	—
Colon	—
Rectum	4

The distribution of cases was somewhat different from that seen in other countries (Table 17). In particular no appendicular carcinoid tumours were found during this period. More recently, a small number of such cases have been seen in Ugandan Africans but there seems to be a real deficiency in incidence. Appendicitis is uncommon so that relatively few appendices are examined surgically and it is probable that many cases could be missed at necropsy. The greatest number of cases were found in the rectum. These were all argentaffin-negative and showed the adenoid appearance typical of hind-gut carcinoid tumours. Two tumours were located in the duodenum and only two in the ileum. Two of these patients had developed hepatic metastasis but no case of full-blown carcinoid syndrome was described. Two patients had masses in the ileocaecal region. One was a 40-year-old male who gave a history of colic and diarrhoea for two years. At operation he was found to have a carcinoid tumour surrounded by a mass of dilated lymphatics exactly similar to a benign lymphangioma. The other patient was a 67-year-old male whose tumour was the only one in this series to show extensive elastosis of the surrounding vessels (ANTHONY and DRURY, 1970). It may be significant that this man came of a rich family and had adopted a western style of life and also had an adenoma of the caecum.

Tumours of the Colon and Rectum

One of the great problems in comparative studies of tumour incidence in different countries has been the lack of agreed distinction between the rectum and colon. In parts of the world where the colo-rectal area is a common site for tumours, slight changes in definition will result in considerable changes in the relative proportion of these two sites. In 1965 a Symposium on tumours of the Alimentary Tract in Africans (MURRAY, 1967) endorsed the recommendations of the OMGE Research Committee (1964) that the classification used should be into tumours of the right and left colon, using the splenic flexure as the dividing point, rather than into rectum and colon as was more usual. Although there is much to commend this system it is not widely used. In this section all tumours of the lower bowel are considered together (WHO rubrics 153 and 154) and the material presented is divided into three groups:
  (i) right colon from caecum to splenic flexure
  (ii) left colon from splenic flexure to the pelvic brim
  (iii) rectum below this point.
These groups can be combined to conform with either system. Tumours around the anus which are adenocarcinomas are classified with rectal neoplasms since this is done in other series. Reasons will be given to suggest that this practice is not necessarily correct in all cases.

Table 18. To show the site and sex distribution of tumours of the lower bowel
(Histologically unconfirmed cases are in brackets)

	Male		Female		Total	
Right colon	19	(2)	14	(2)	33	(4)
Left colon	18	—	5	(1)	24[a]	(1)
Rectum	51	(3)	30	(2)	81	(5)
Anal canal	4		6		10	
Perianal	2		6		8	
Total	94	(5)	61	(5)	156	(10)

[a] The sex of 1 patient was not stated.

One hundred forty-eight epithelial tumours were seen arising in the colon and rectum, that is 0.4 cases per 100,000 per year, or 2.0% of malignant tumours overall. The incidence in Kyadondo County over this period was 2 cases per 100,000 per annum, which indicates the extent of loss of cases from up-country areas. In addition to registered cases a number of very advanced cases of abdominal malignancy was reported, some of which undoubtedly arose in the colon but the evidence available was insufficient to distinguish between neoplasms of stomach, colon or ovary in these cases.

Adenocarcinoma was confirmed by histological examination in 133 cases; in addition 12 lymphomata, 5 carcinoid tumours and 5 leiomyosarcomas were seen. Four of the five carcinoid tumours occurred in the rectum and only one in the caecum. By contrast, ten of the twelve lymphomas involved the region of the caecum. Epithelial tumours were considerably more frequent in the right colon than in the left. Twenty-three tumours were found involving the caecum, 9 in the ascending colon, 1 at the splenic flexure and 3 in the transverse colon. There were 21 tumours in the region of the sigmoid and only 4 were found in the descending colon. Tumours of the rectum were more frequent than those of the colon (82:62). This ratio is similar to that found in other series from Africa but is approximately the reverse of the situation in Caucasians (DOLL et al., 1966).

Tumours of the left colon and rectum both showed a marked excess of males whereas tumours of the right colon showed an equal sex distribution (Table 18). Tumours of the right colon occur in younger patients than those of the left colon (Table 19). Tumours of the rectum and left colon show a similar age distribution with

Table 19. Showing the age distribution of adenocarcinomas in different parts of the lower bowel

	Right colon	Left colon	Rectum	Total
15—24	3	1	—	4
25—34	1	2	6	9
35—44	10	5	15	30
45—54	12	6	18	36
55—64	6	7	26	39
65—74	2	4	13	19
75+	1	—	3	4
"Adult"	1	—	1	2
Total	36	25	82	143

a higher mean age than tumours of the right colon. Tumours are most commonly seen in the age group 55—64. Age-specific incidence rates show a steady rise throughout life, except in the very old when statistics are unreliable.

Histological grading of adenocarcinomas was possible in 127 cases and the distribution of cases is shown in Table 20. Tumours of the left colon and rectum appeared to be somewhat less well differentiated than those of the right colon. A striking feature in all parts of the bowel was the very small number of poorly differentiated tumours.

Table 20. Showing grading of adenocarcinomas of the colon and rectum

	Right colon	Left colon	Rectum	Total
Grade 1	14	7	21	42
Grade 2	11	14	50	75
Grade 3	5	2	3	10
Total	30	23	74	127

The histological appearance of tumours varied in different parts of the bowel (Table 21). Colloid (mucoid) carcinomas were found quite frequently, 26 of 73 cases in males had a colloid appearance whereas among females the figure was only 6 out of 42 tumours. The proportion of colloid carcinoma was very similar in different parts of he colon (Table 21). Seven out of 30 tumours in the right colon, 6, out of 23

Table 21. Showing the distribution of different histological types of adenocarcinomas in the left and right colon

Site	Histological type	Cases	Mean age	Range Age
Right colon	Colloid	7	41	(20—50)
	Caecal type	17	46	(16—79)
	Sigmoid type	4	63	(48—70)
	Scirrhous	3	41	(35—50)
Left colon	Sigmoid type	13	55	(38—70)
	Colloid	6	46	(25—58)
	Caecal type	4	34	(20—45)
Rectum	Colloid	16	50	(26—80)
	Not colloid	57	68	(28—85)

in the left colon and 16 out of 74 in the rectum had this appearance. Coloid carcinomas have been noted to be more common in Bantu than in white patients, to occur more frequently in men than in women, to be located in the caecum or rectum and to occur at a younger age than other histological types (OETTLÉ, 1967).

Almost all caecal tumours showed a pattern easily distinguishable from tumours of the left colon. The nuclei were small and round and tended to lie at the periphery of each tubule. Tubules were rather tightly constructed with very narrow lumina (Fig. 5). The cells were slender and columnar in shape, and the cytoplasm did not stain positively with P.A.S.; extracellular mucin was often detectable. Such tumours frequently contained areas in which the cells were arranged in solid clumps or islands very much reminiscent of carcinoid tumours; however, Diazo and Fontana stains were negative. Poorly differentiated caecal tumours quite frequently showed a signet-ring appearance. Close correlation has been found between carcinoid tumours and signet-ring cells in animal transplantation experiments (GOLDENBERG and FISHER, 1970). In

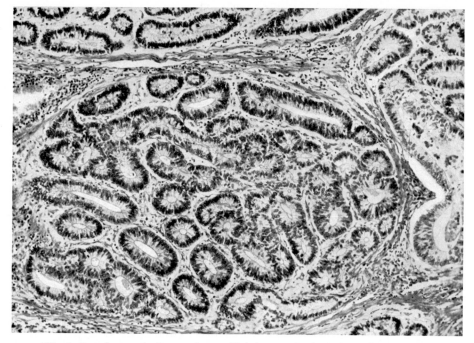

Fig. 5. Caecal type of adenocarcinoma. Tightly organized tubules with round nuclei

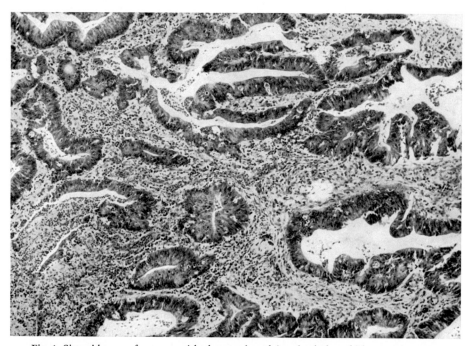

Fig. 6. Sigmoid type of tumour with elongated nuclei and tubules which are not compact

caecal tumours such areas were often closely apposed but in all cells the nuclei were small and dark and mitoses were seldom numerous. Such tumours are referred to as the caecal type. The close relation of adenocarcinomatous with carcinoid-like portions of tumours has been noted in other countries. Toker (1969) noted this association in 3 cases, 2 of which occurred in the right colon. Tumours of the sigmoid region were also made up of columnar cells but in this region the nuclei were usually elongated and often large and rather paler-staining than those of the caecal type (Fig. 6). Lumina of tubules were not so tightly organized and strips of cells lying within considerable quantities of mucus were regularly seen. P.A.S. staining showed rather greater amounts of positive material intracellularly. Poorly differentiated sigmoid tumours showed many more mitoses, a lesser tendency to clumping of cells, and much greater cellular pleomorphism than caecal neoplasms. Signet-ring forms were seen less commonly than in the right colon.

The mean age at diagnosis of these different types of tumours varied markedly. Colloid tumours and "caecal pattern" occurred in younger patients than the "sigmoid type" of tumour, whether they occurred in the right or left colon. Four tumours of the left colon have been classified as caecal type and 2 of these tumours contained schistosome eggs. These occurred at a younger age than the more typical tumours of the region (Table 20). There were 6 cases in which there was evidence of adenoma as well as carcinoma in the bowel. One occurred in the caecum, 1 in the left colon and 2 in the rectum but all these patients had a sigmoid pattern of tumour.

Tumours of the rectum showed the same appearances as the typical sigmoid pattern in 50 of the 74 cases. These cases were indistinguishable from tumours of European subjects except that 20 (40%) were well differentiated and only 2 (4%) were poorly differentiated.

The remaining 24 cases appeared rather different. These were made up of rather plumper cells with rounder nuclei. Often the appearance was reminiscent of an adenoid cystic carcinoma but more frequently there was very marked mucus secretion. The age and sex distribution was very similar to the other rectal tumours but clinically there were considerable differences. There was a history of perianal ulceration in 16 out of 24 cases and 4 patients had had an ischiorectal fistula for some years. In 6 patients there was no evidence of involvement of the rectal mucosa. There is therefore a strong presumption that these tumours arose either from anal glands or from the lining of a fistula track rather than from rectal mucosa. Tumours of the anal canal itself were predominantly composed of poorly differentiated squamous cells. Frequently there was a well marked basloid appearance sometimes described as a transitional cell carcinoma. Perianal carcinomata, on the other hand, were most frequently well differentiated squamous cell tumours, and most showed keratin formation.

Associated Conditions

During the period of this survey note was taken of the number of polyps of the large bowel seen at autopsy and in the biopsy material since many authorities believe that malignant tumours develop in pre-existing benign lesions in at least a proportion of cases. A total of 27 patients with adenomas of the colon was found, including 16 cases of juvenile hamartomatous "retention" polyps, all under the age of 14 years.

Only one adenomatous polyp was seen in the surgical material (41,719 specimens) and only one metaplastic polyp in a 60-year-old man was biopsied. Inspection of operative and postmortem specimens of malignant tumours of the bowel revealed 6 cases with a co-existent adenomatous polyp in the specimen. Two of these patients had been educated in England and had adopted a rather western style of life. In a further 2 cases carcinoma of the colon had developed in a colon bearing multiple polypi; these were assumed to be of the familial variety even though no family history of bowel disturbance was obtained. Microscopic examination revealed the remains of villous papilloma in 2 cases, both males over the age of 65 years. No adenomas were

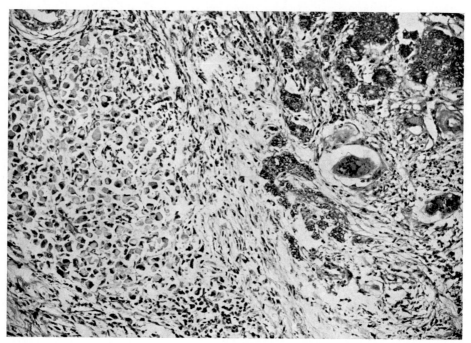

Fig. 7. Tumour with schistosomiasis. Note the dimorphic structure of the tumour with clumps of cells on the right, reminiscent of a carcinoid tumour, and signet ring formation on the left

found in the colon in 2,000 post mortems in adults carried out at Mulago Hospital during this five-year period. It may be that some tumours were overlooked, but more recently an active search for polypi has been made in the colon and rectum in a personal series of 343 post mortems on Africans over the age of 25 years, and no case of adenomatous polyp, villous papilloma or hyperplastic polyp has been found (HUTT and TEMPLETON, 1971).

Ulcerative colitis is a condition involving an increased risk of the development of malignancy of the colon. Only 4 examples of this condition were seen in the surgical material of this five-year period and 2 of these occurred in Asian patients. Diagnosis is more difficult in a country where amoebiasis, bacillary dysentery and schistosomiasis may give rise to diffuse ulceration of the bowel, but nonetheless it appears certain that idiopathic ulcerative colitis is a rare disease in Africans (BILLINGHURST and WELCHMAN, 1966).

Schistosoma mansoni is common in the north of the country around the Nile
valley but is relatively unusual elsewhere (BRADLEY, 1968). There appears to be no
excess of cases from this area, which is consistent with the findings of the majority
of workers in Egypt (NASR, 1967). However, in the few cases seen at Kampala the
histopathology of colonic tumours in which schistosome eggs were found is rather
different from those without evidence of schistosomiasis. The patients were younger
than the mean for patients with tumours at the site. The cells appeared cuboidal and
had round nuclei, being arranged in sheets in which lumina were formed rather than
in tubules (Fig. 7). Mucus secretion by such tumours was minimal except where signet-
ring cells were found. The general pattern was suggestive in some ways of carcinoid
tumour, but the diazo reaction was negative.

Discussion

It has been estimated that about 80% of human cancer is environmentally induced. The environment of the colon is largely dependent upon the volume, content
and consistency of the faeces. The content of the diet, bacterial flora and speed of
faecal transit through the bowel will obviously have a bearing on the presence and
concentration of any carcinogenic material applied to the gut wall. Preliminary
studies have shown that Africans have a much quicker bowel transit time than Europeans (BURKITT, 1971) and that the faecal flora in these two groups of people is very
different (ARIES, CROWTHER, DRASAR, HILL and WILLIAMS, 1969). If the faeces do
indeed contain carcinogenic substances it seems most likely that they are manufactured by bacterial breakdown of dietary material (WYNDER, KAJITANI and ISHI-
KAWA, 1969) or of bile salts (HILL, CROWTHER and DRASAR, 1971). The predominant
site of colonic cancer should be in the more distal portions of the bowel where any
material would have had time to accumulate and would be most concentrated. In
those areas where faecal content is most static the mucosa would be constantly exposed to such materials and the frequency should be higher. It might be expected,
therefore, that any tumours induced by such a mechanism would occur most frequently
in the sigmoid colon. It would also be predicted that the higher the incidence of
tumours of the colon the greater the proportion which would occur at the sigmoid.
Tumours of the sigmoid colon occur very frequently in Europeans where in Africans,
Indians and Colombians this is an area of the bowel peculiarly immune from neoplasia (HAENZEL and CORREA, 1971). Tumours of the caecum and rectum, though
infrequent in Africans, are proportionally more common. It seems likely that tumours
of the sigmoid colon are induced by rather different factors than are operative
elsewhere in the large bowel. In experimental situations various chemicals may induce tumours in one area and not the other (STEWART, 1967). In Europeans the sigmoid colon is the site of maximal occurrence of diverticular disease and a common
site for the development of adenomatous polyps. In Africans no diverticular or polypi
were found in the colon during a post-mortem survey of 343 adult cases. In contrast,
the incidence of sigmoid volvulus is many times higher (SHEPHERD, 1968). These facts
suggest that there are considerable differences between the faecal content, neuro-
muscular action, occurrence of various diseases and tumour incidence between two
populations, and it is suggested that these factors may be related in cause and effect.
All may be influenced by faecal consistency, content and speed of flow.

Epidemiological differences indicate that different aetiological factors are active in different parts of the bowel. The histological differences between tumours of the caecum and sigmoid suggest that they may have a different cell of origin. Tumours of the caecum frequently showed areas which had some resemblance to carcinoid tumours though the diazo reaction was always negative. The majority of such tumours secreted relatively smaller amounts of mucus than those of the sigmoid region. Tumours of the sigmoid showed an increasing incidence with increasing age whereas those of the caecum occurred in younger patients. It is postulated that the majority of tumours of the caecum arise from cells in the crypts which they strongly resemble histologically, whereas sigmoid tumours are predominantly derived from surface cells. It is suggested that tumours of surface epithelium probably result from the continued application of some carcinogenic material in the faeces which has its highest concentration in the sigmoid colon. Most tumours of the caecum and some tumours of the sigmoid seem to arise from the depths of the crypts and are less likely to be the result of application of a faecal carcinogen to the surface of the bowel.

In contrast to the findings in other parts of Africa (MORSON and PANG, 1967) the majority of tumours of the colon in Uganda are well differentiated. In fact tumours of the caecum characteristically reached a huge size without evidence of metastasis to nodes or liver. Occasional cases were encountered of poorly differentiated signet-ring cancers in young people, but these were exceptional.

There has been considerable debate as to the relationship of adenomatous polypi, villous papillomas and adenocarcinoma. Some have suggested that carcinoma frequently arises within such polypi (MORSON, 1971). Others have pointed out that the distribution of polypi and carcinoma vary and suggest that cancer usually arises direct from normal epithelium. HORN (1971) has re-emphasized the malignant potential of villous adenomas. In this series adenomas and carcinomata are both unusual. In only two cases, both occurring in old people, was there evidence of a villous papilloma in the neighbourhood of adenocarcinoma. One further case showed a pedunculated appearance but there was no residual benign adenoma. The frequency of adenomata and carcinoma are usually related in different populations (BREMNER and ACKERMAN, 1970). This association does not necessarily argue a causal relationship though it is compatible with this interpretation. It may be that both are produced by similar stimuli but remain sharply separate.

Tumours of the Anus

The anal canal, the anal margin and the glands of the region give rise to a number of different tumour types. Many bear a strong relation to tumours of the skin but it seems more logical to discuss them here rather than under the heading of skin, as suggested by the I.C.D. (World Health Organization, 1957). Eighteen primary epithelial tumours were diagnosed. Ten cases arose in the anal canal and 8 at the anal margin. The age and sex distribution of tumours at these different sites are shown in Table 22. In addition, 4 cases of rhabdomyosarcoma occurring in the perineal area were diagnosed. One patient with a malignant melanoma of the anal canal was seen.

Five of the 8 tumours of the anal margin were well differentiated squamous carcinomas. Two patients, a 62-year-old male and a 60-year-old female, had basal

Table 22. Showing the age and sex distribution of tumours in the anal region

| | Margin | | Canal | |
	Male	Female	Male	Female
15—24	—	1	—	—
25—34	1	1	—	2
35—44	—	1	1	1
45—54	—	—	2	3
55—64	1	3	—	—
65—74	—	—	1	—
All ages	2	6	4	6

cell carcinomas. The female patient had numerous vulval and perianal condyloma accuminata in addition. The eighth patient was a 60-year-old female Muganda who had an anaplastic carcinoma with a structure suggesting origin from sebaceous gland.

Tumours of the anal canal were less well differentiated than those on the margin and usually contained an extensive basaloid rim around the islands of tumour cells. One case showed an undifferentiated appearance and another contained pools of mucus in the islands of squamous tumour cells. This tumour type has been called muco-epidermoid (HAMPERL and HELLWEG, 1957). Though descriptively correct this tumour does not resemble the muco-epidermoid of salivary tumours in behaviour or structure, and the use of the term is therefore misleading. A term such as squamous carcinoma with mucoid areas is preferred. Eight of the 10 tumours showed areas of keratinization. This is a rather greater proportion than that found in other countries, and may indicate some pre-existing metaplasia of the epithelium.

Differential diagnosis from amoebic ulceration and condyloma accuminata some-times posed problems. Perianal ulceration by amoebae is not common but it gives rise to complete disruption of the squamous epithelium and the remaining islands of dys-plastic cells can closely resemble squamous carcinoma. Condylomata are usually easy to distinguish unless they have become secondarily infected and ulcerated when diagnosis is more problematic. In both cases treatment of infection usually resolves the problem and a further biopsy is not often required.

Tumours of both anal canal and anal margin were more common in females. In other parts of the world tumours of the anal canal occur more commonly in females but males predominate in tumours of the anal margin (MORSON, 1960).

The geographical distribution of cases around Uganda showed some anomalies. The majority of cases were reported from Buganda but this is probably only an effect of greater efficiency of registration in this region.

Patients were aged 24—65 (mean age 45.5 years). There was no significant dif-ference between the mean age of patients with tumours of the anal canal and anal margin but 9 out of 10 patients with neoplasms of the anal canal were under the age of 55, compared with 4 out of 8 patients with tumours at the anal margin.

Carcinoma of the anal region appears to be relatively more common than colonic neoplasms. If it is accepted that the 24 cases in which carcinoma appeared to arise in the ischiorectal fossa derived from anal glands then the total number of histologically proven cases of anal carcinoma seen was 42 compared with 54 in the rectum, 32 in the right colon and 25 in the left. This proportion is very different from that reported from other countries. Neoplasms of the anal canal and margin are probably no more frequent than in other areas but appear to be more common because of the low incidence of colonic and rectal neoplasms. Granuloma inguinale has been fairly common in Uganda. More recently rather fewer cases have been diagnosed but condylomata accuminata are common. Schistosomiasis was not found in any of these cases. Any of these diseases might have influenced the incidence of tumours of this region but their effect is entirely unknown. Adenocarcinomas arising in the pararectal region may arise from congenital or acquired fistulae or from anal glands. The incidence of such tumours seems to be considerably higher than in other parts of the world. The paucity of reports of this entity underestimates its true frequency. Cases are seen from time to time in many countries but are seldom recorded. They are usually assumed to arise in fistulae and usually appear as locally infiltrating tumours with a low metastatic potential. Fistulae and haemorrhoids are both uncommon in Uganda and it seems more logical to suggest that these growths arise from anal glands than from unproven pre-existing fistulae.

Chapter 3

Tumours of Liver, Biliary System and Pancreas

M. S. R. HUTT and P. P. ANTHONY

With 13 Figures

Hepatocellular carcinoma is probably the commonest cancer in Uganda. Under diagnosis is probable in a tumour which produces symptoms late and kills rapidly. The relationship to cirrhosis, Australia antigen and aflatoxin is examined. Biliary duct cancer by contrast is not particularly common and cancer of the pancreas is probably also uncommon. Diagnosis of hepatocellular carcinoma on needle biopsy is relatively straight forward if the pathologist is familiar with the various patterns of tumour growth.

The great majority of tumours of the liver and biliary system are malignant and arise either from the liver parenchymal cells or from the cells lining the intra- or extrahepatic ducts. The clinical, pathological and epidemiological features of these two groups of tumours suggest that they have a different aetiology and should be regarded as separate entities.

In this chapter the term liver-cell carcinoma is used to describe tumours arising from the liver cells and tumours of the intra- or extrahepatic biliary tree are called bile duct carcinomas. The term hepatoma, which is often used to describe malignant tumours of liver cells, has been abandoned because of the confusion surrounding its use, particularly in the field of experimental animal tumours (I.A.R.C. publication 1971).

Although liver-cell carcinomas similar to those seen in adults may occur in childhood, the tumour of embryonic liver cells designated hepatoblastoma is a separate entity in terms of histogenesis and aetiology.

During the period of this survey 573 primary malignant tumours of the liver and biliary system were seen. This represents 7.9% of all malignant tumours, an incidence of 2.0 cases per year per 100,000 of the population. During the period of this survey the annual incidence figures for liver-cell carcinoma in Kyadondo County were 5.1 cases per 100,000 women and 11.1 cases per 100,000 men per year (figures corrected for African standard population). In the country as a whole the figures were 0.86 and 2.6 respectively. This suggests that outside Kyadondo County only about one in five tumours is diagnosed. Primary liver-cell carcinoma was diagnosed histologically in 528 of these tumours (Table 1). There were 27 cases of bile duct

carcinoma, 19 of which were intrahepatic and 8 extrahepatic and there were 9 primary carcinomas of the gallbladder. Four cases were diagnosed as hepatoblastomas and
5 primary intrahepatic malignant mesenchymal tumours were seen. Benign tumours
of the liver were very rare apart from haemangiomas found incidentally at post
mortem. Only two cases thought to be examples of benign liver-cell adenoma were
found.

Table 1. Primary malignant tumours of the liver and biliary system 1964—1968

Liver-cell carcinoma	528
Intrahepatic bile-duct carcinoma	19
Hepatoblastoma	4
Other intrahepatic tumours	5
Extrahepatic bile duct carcinoma	8
Carcinoma of the gall bladder	9
Total	573

Primary Liver-Cell Carcinoma

The final diagnosis of liver-cell carcinoma was made on needle biopsy material in
331 cases, surgical biopsy of the liver in 91, at post mortem in 89 and from biopsy of
a secondary tumour in 17 cases. In the following description of the pathology the information on the macroscopic features, methods of spread and relation to cirrhosis are
based mainly on the post mortem analysis.

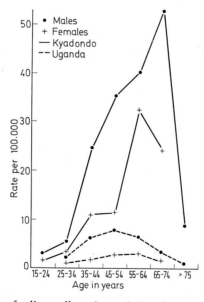

Fig. 1. Incidence rates for liver cell carcinoma in Kyadondo County and in Uganda

Age: The age range of patients with liver-cell carcinoma was from 8 to 90 years with a mean of 42.5 years. The diagnosis was most frequently made in the third and fourth decades but the overall age-specific incidence rates for the Kyadondo area show a steady rise except in old age (Fig. 1). 15.8% of the cases were, however, under the age of 30 and occurrence in the first decade is reported in most African series. Seventy-seven tumours (86%) seen at post mortem were associated with cirrhosis and all but one of the non-cirrhotics were under the age of 40.

Sex: There were 435 cases in men and 143 in women in this series, giving a male : female ratio of 3 : 1. A prospective clinical analysis of liver-cell carcinoma cases admitted to the Mulago Hospital in 1966—67 showed a male : female ratio of 2 : 1 (ALPERT, HUTT and DAVIDSON, 1969) and a similar ratio was found by VOGEL et al. (1970) in a recent clinico-pathological study. The ratio of clinical admissions to the Mulago Hospital is the same as that found for all non-obstetric admissions. The higher male predominance in the whole series is probably due to the fact that women in the more rural areas are less likely to seek advice or to be admitted to a hospital. This applies more particularly to old women and this may account for the earlier decline in age-specific rates in women. In the autopsy series there were only six women (a male : female ratio of 14 : 1) and only 3 of these cases had associated cirrhosis. However, in a prospective clinico-pathological study with confirmation of the diagnoses by laparotomy the association of cirrhosis and carcinoma is similar in both sexes (VOGEL et al., 1970 and 1972 a).

Pathology

Macroscopic Appearances

Eighty-nine cases of liver-cell carcinoma were seen at post mortem at Mulago Hospital, Kampala. In 77 cases (86%) the tumour occurred in a cirrhotic liver. The majority of liver carcinomas occurred in macronodular types of cirrhosis (posthepatitic or postnecrotic, according to Gall's classification) and the micronodular (fatty or nutritional) type was rarely seen. Many liver-cell carcinomas are massive and replace much of the liver. In such cases it may be difficult to be certain whether the changes in the residual liver tissue are due to cirrhosis or to the effects of the tumour. The term "diffuse", sometimes used as a macroscopic description (EDMONDSON, 1958), refers to the surface appearances, and the cut surface of such tumours usually shows an almost complete replacement of the liver by either massive or nodular growth. The tumour was of the massive type in 22 cases (Fig. 2) and nodular in 67 (Fig. 3). The liver weights in this series varied from 810 to 5,300 with an average of 2,950 g. There was a tendency for younger subjects with no cirrhosis to have larger tumours than older subjects with cirrhosis but the differences were not significant. The right lobe was more frequently involved than the left, but in many tumours both lobes were involved.

Ascites was present in nearly all cases and was grossly haemorrhagic in 22 cases; bleeding in such cases was from the tumour surface and the exact bleeding spot was usually seen. In 11 cases a needle biopsy had been performed and in 2 this was evidently the cause of haemorrhage and death. Haemorrhage from oesophageal varices

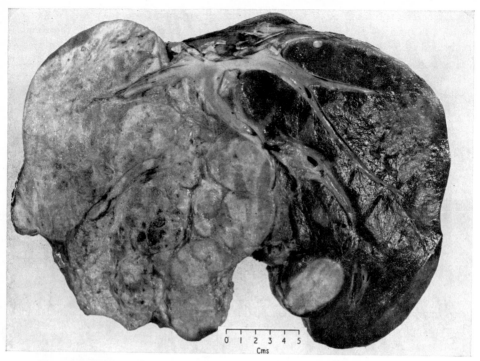

Fig. 2. Massive type of primary liver-cell carcinoma (By permission of W. G. Spector)

was present in 20 cases, 17 of whom had an accompanying cirrhosis; in 3 there was
portal vein thrombosis without cirrhosis.

In the majority of cases the tumour had spread into the radicles of the portal vein
and/or the hepatic veins, but despite this 41 cases (46%) had no distant macroscopic
or microscopic metastases on routine post mortem examination. Spread by lymphatics
to the regional lymph nodes around the hilum, free margin of the lesser sac and head
of the pancreas was noted in 20 cases. The commonest site of blood-borne metastasis
was the lungs, followed by bone, adrenals, heart and stomach (Table 2). Involvement
of the peritoneum is extremely rare in liver-cell carcinoma and was only seen in three
cases in this group. This may explain why cytological examination of the ascitic fluid
in patients with liver-cell carcinoma is usually negative. Direct involvement of the

Table 2. Distribution of Metastases in 89 autopsies

Local lymph nodes	20
Blood-borne	
Lungs	33
Bone	7
Adrenals	6
Heart	4
Stomach	3

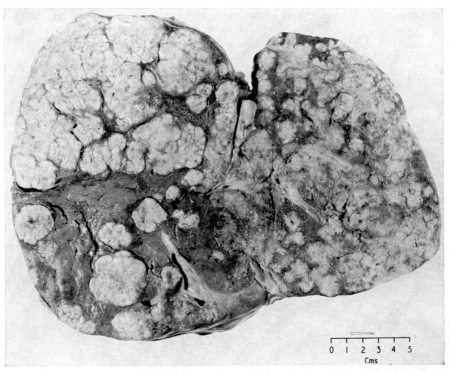

Fig. 3. Multinodular type of primary liver-cell carcinoma (By permission of W. G. Spector)

stomach, usually in the region of the cardia, may sometimes lead to an erroneous diagnosis of primary stomach carcinoma with liver secondaries.

The exact cause of death is often difficult to assess in these cases on purely pathological grounds, but intraperitoneal or intragastric haemorrhage was an important factor in 43 cases. A combination of carcinomatous cachexia and liver failure accounted for most of the remaining cases and death resulting from metastases was not seen.

Microscopic Features

An analysis of the histopathological types of liver-cell carcinoma is shown in Table 3. The classification chosen evolved in the course of this study and is based on simple descriptive criteria (ANTHONY, 1972). It is possible to make many subdivisions on histological type but we have limited these to five (Table 3). When more than one histological type is present in a tumour the predominant pattern is chosen. The stromal component of liver-cell carcinoma is usually minimal, but there are exceptions to this and occasional liver-cell carcinomas have a stromal reaction, though this is often present in only part of the tumour. The commonest form is the *trabecular* type which grows in cords or in cylindrical masses with accompanying sinusoids. This may be classified as well, moderately or poorly differentiated (Fig. 4 a, b). The main features are a well marked trabecular pattern, the presence of sinusoids and the absence of connective tissue stroma. Individual tumour cells have abundant eosinophilic cyto-

Table 3. Histopathological type of liver cell carcinoma. Based on examination of 200 biopsy specimens and 89 post mortem examinations

	Biopsy	PM
Trabecular	66%	70%
Pleomorphic	12%	15%
Adenoid	10%	10%
Clear cell	5%	2%
Others	7%	3%

plasm and the nuclei usually contain prominent nucleoli. Even the poorly differentiated group which may have a more basophilic cytoplasm and larger or more hyperchromatic nuclei are usually easily distinguished from other tumours in the liver, whether primary, intrahepatic bile duct carcinoma, or secondary carcinoma. In the well differentiated group the resemblance to normal liver-cell structure and arrangement is striking, often with well developed sinusoids. Although the accumulation of bile is a diagnostic feature it is rarely seen; it is of course not a feature of normal liver cells. The glycogen content of tumour cells is generally less than that of the surrounding liver.

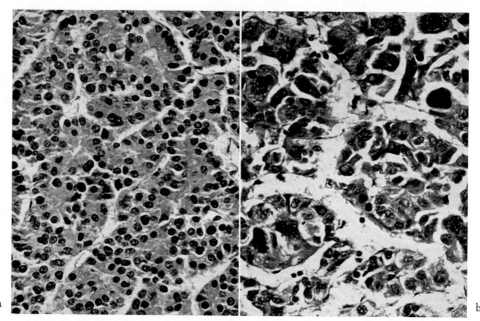

Fig. 4 a. Well differentiated trabecular (hepatic) type of primary liver-cell carcinoma. H and E
Fig. 4 b. Poorly differentiated trabecular (hepatic) type of primary liver-cell carcinoma. H and E

The second group have been termed *pleomorphic* and these merge with the poorly differentiated variants of hepatic cell type. The characteristic feature of these tumours is the extreme pleomorphism of nuclei and cytoplasm, often with giant cell forms, resembling some of the cells seen in neonatal hepatitis (Fig. 5). Although very arypi-

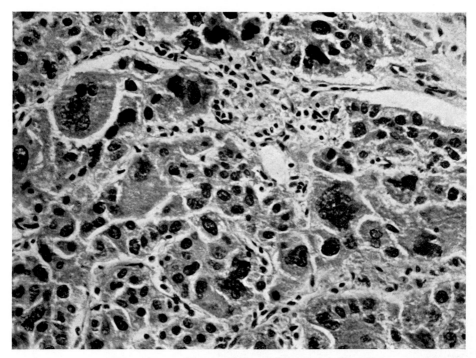

Fig. 5. Pleomorphic type of liver-cell carcinoma. H and E

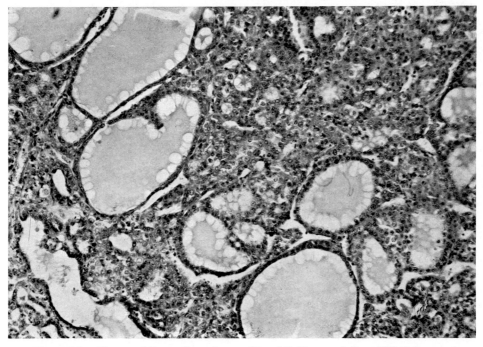

Fig. 6. Adenoid type of liver-cell carcinoma. H and E (By permission of W. G. SPECTOR)

cal cells are seen, mitoses are infrequent. Some resemblance to hepatic cells is usually apparent somewhere in the tumour.

The third group presents the most difficult problem for the diagnostic histopathologist. This is the *adenoid,* acinar or glandular type. This category really conceals three varieties: tumours of obvious hepatic cytology which have a glandular or pseudo-glandular pattern (Fig. 6), tumours with an adenocarcinomatous appear-

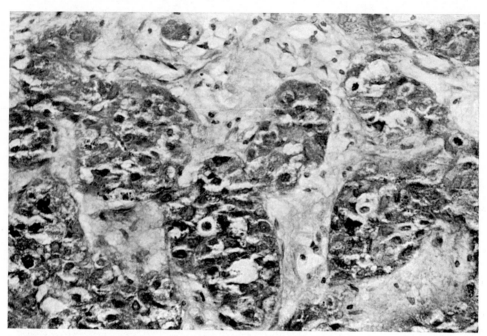

Fig. 7. Liver-cell carcinoma with stromal reaction. Granules of glycogen are seen in the liver cells. PAS (By permission of W. G. SPECTOR)

ance, often with some connective tissue stromal response but with areas of cellular differentiation towards hepatic cells (Fig. 7) and, lastly, tumours with adenocarcinomatous pattern but with minimal hepatic-cell differentiation (Fig. 8). The distinction of the latter two groups from bile duct or secondary adenocarcinomas is obviously more difficult in biopsy material. In these circumstances one is influenced by experience from post mortems and surgical biopsies. As others have shown (EDMONDSON, 1958) careful scrutiny of many so-called bile duct carcinomas will reveal areas of hepatic-cell differentiation—these have all been included in this series as primary liver-cell carcinomas. Periodic acid Schiff stain before and after diastase digestion helps to distinguish adenoid liver-cell carcinoma from bile duct carcinoma. The former may contain glycogen in their cells and never secrete mucus, while the latter are always negative for glycogen and frequently secrete mucus.

The fourth type, *clear-cell carcinoma,* has not received much attention in the literature. The tumours histologically resemble hypernephromas in many ways and have been misdiagnosed as such on several occasions, particularly when they present as a bone secondary (Fig. 9). Tumours of the trabecular type quite often show clear cell areas that are due to hydropic change in their cytoplasm but only those tumours with a uniform clear cell type have been included. The intense staining of the cytoplasm by P.A.S. in clear-cell carcinomas is completely abolished by diastase, indicating the presence of glycogen. Clear cells of this type can be distinguished by this technique from tumour cells containing fat; however, this is usually possible in ordinary sections as fat in tumour cells forms discrete vacuoles rather than a clear cytoplasm.

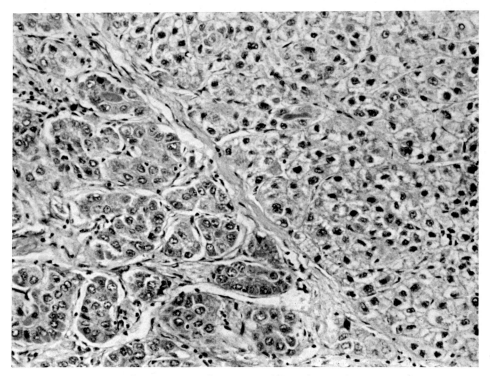

Fig. 8. Liver-cell carcinoma with areas resembling adenocarcinoma. H and E

There remains a *miscellaneous* group of tumours of epithelial origin which cannot be classified with the above. Some are characterized by small cells with rather uniform nuclei resembling a carcinoid tumour. Others are composed of large cells with abundant cytoplasm and an alveolar pattern; these tumours are often squamoid in appearance and the possibility of a secondary tumour has to be excluded. Other tumours have a spindle cell component which may be difficult to distinguish from a sarcoma but a trabecular pattern, the contiguous arrangement of cells, their relation to blood vessels, and the finding of areas with a cuboidal structure, suggest that they originate from hepatic cells.

In addition to assessment of histological type, the tumours in the post-mortem series were graded according to three characteristics; resemblance to original tissue, nuclear pleomorphism and the number of mitoses were each given scores from 1—3.

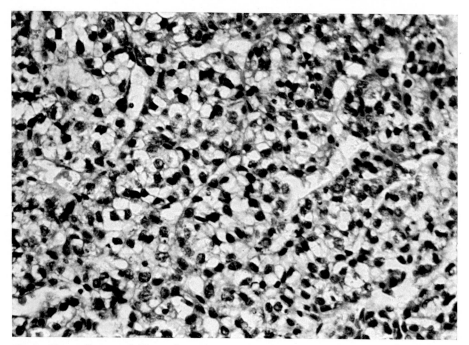

Fig. 9. Clear-cell type of liver-cell carcinoma. H and E (By permission of W. G. Spector)

Thus, the best differentiated tumour would have an aggregate score of three and the worst of nine. The results are given below.

Grade 1 (well differentiated)   19 cases
Grade 2 (moderately differentiated)   45 cases
Grade 3 (poorly differentiated)   16 cases

The natural history of liver-cell carcinoma in Uganda is invariably that of a rapidly progressive disease and no significant differences were noted between the histological grade and the survival of the patient.

Differential Diagnosis

In the majority of cases in this series, only needle biopsy material was available. Some of the problems encountered in histological diagnosis have already been discussed, the most difficult being the differentiation of the predominantly adenoid liver-cell carcinoma from a bile duct carcinoma or from a secondary carcinoma from gastrointestinal tract, breast or lung. Many have emphasized that a marked scirrhous reaction is a characteristic of primary or secondary adenocarcinomas, but this may also be seen around liver-cell tumours; moreover, the intense atypical bile duct proliferation that may be seen in cases with cirrhosis can be confused with adenocarcinoma. Sometimes the differential diagnosis on biopsy material is almost impossible, and occasional false allocations of tumour origin may occur. In the East African context, the low incidence of cancer at these sites and the very high incidence of liver-cell carcinoma make it a strong probability that a tumour presenting in the liver is a primary liver-cell carcinoma (Davies and Owor, 1960).

Secondaries from Primary Liver-Cell Carcinoma

In Uganda the second commonest tumour presenting clinically as a skeletal deposit is liver-cell carcinoma (TEMPLETON, HUTT and DODGE, 1972). This reflects the high incidence of the tumour rather than a special tendency for African liver-cell cancer to metastasize. The most common sites of such secondaries are the bones of the axial skeleton, particularly the skull. The tumours are of varying differentiation and, like thyroid, some of the best differentiated tumours may metastasize early. In most cases the primary had not been diagnosed at the time of the biopsy. Bile was more frequently seen in secondary deposits of liver cell carcinoma than in the primary site. This may be due to a lack of bile ducts in tissue adjoining secondaries.

Alpha-Fetoprotein (A.F.P.)

In 1963 ABELEV and his co-workers reported the presence of an embryo-specific alpha globulin in the sera of mice with chemically induced liver-cell carcinoma. TATARINOV (1965) found a similar protein in human sera from patients with liver-cell carcinoma. The transitory liver-cell antigens are normal biosynthetic products of the cellular genome and the activity of the genes that direct their synthesis is restricted to a transient period of the overall process of cell differentiation; they are normally absent in fully differentiated cells (URIEL, 1968). For routine testing a modified Ouchterlony double-diffusion technique is used (URIEL, 1971) though more sensitive techniques such as a radio-immune assays are available. ABELEV (1971) has demonstrated the presence of alpha-fetoprotein in cells from cases of liver carcinoma using the indirect immunofluorescent technique. Preliminary results from cases of liver-cell carcinoma in Africa indicated that the test was frequently positive (URIEL et al., 1968; ALPERT, URIEL and DE NECHAUD, 1968).

In a worldwide collaborative study conducted by the I.A.R.C. (O'CONOR et al., 1970) 813 sera were examined for alpha-fetoprotein (A.F.P.). In histologically proven cases of liver-cell carcinoma, A.F.P. was found in 75%, closely paralleling earlier studies in Dakar and Johannesburg (MASSEYEFF et al., 1969; PURVES et al., 1970). The test is negative in all unequivocal cases of bile duct carcinoma, in secondary carcinoma of the liver and in other types of liver disease. Embryonal or teratomatous tumours are the only other malignancies which give a false positive test. The incidence of positive A.F.P. tests in cases of liver-cell carcinoma is higher in the tropics than in non-tropical areas. This may be related to the occurrence of the tumour in younger patients in the tropics, for VOGEL et al. (1970, 1972 a) and BAGSHAWE and PARKER (1970) have shown that a positive A.F.P. test is more common in young patients. There appears to be no correlation between A.F.P. positivity and the histological features of tumour (O'CONOR et al., 1970). The specificity of the test makes it a valuable tool for epidemiological studies in populations, for following high risk groups such as those with cirrhosis and for monitoring the effect of treatment in positive cases.

VOGEL et al. (1970, 1972 b) have demonstrated a positive correlation between A.F.P. and hepatitis-associated antigen (H.A.A.) in patients with liver-cell carcinoma in Uganda and they report that there is a tendency for younger patients to be both

A.F.P.- and H.A.A.-positive, while older patients are generally A.F.P.- and H.A.A.-negative.

Epidemiology of Liver Cancer

Primary liver-cell carcinoma is a tumour with a very variable incidence rate in different geographical areas (Table 4). High incidence rates have been reported from all the cancer registries set up in Africa (Higginson and Oettlé, 1960; Davies et al., 1965; Prates and Torres, 1965; Edington and Maclean, 1965). High rates are also recorded in Hong Kong (Gibson, 1971), Singapore (Simons et al., 1971) and in the Japanese population of Hawaii (Doll, Payne and Waterhouse, 1966). Low rates are recorded throughout Europe, North America, Australia, in many parts of South America (Doll, Payne and Waterhouse, 1966; Doll, Muir and Waterhouse, 1970) and in Bombay, India (Jussawalla et al., 1970). Proportional rates suggest that there is a high incidence in New Guinea (Booth et al., 1968) and in China (Liang and Tung, 1959; Gibson, 1971).

Table 4. Malignant liver tumours. Average annual incidence per 100,000 all ages, males (Doll et al., 1966 and 1970)

North and South America	
Chile	2.6
Jamaica, Kingston and St. Andrew	2.2
U.S.A. New York State	1.8
Canada, Manitoba	1.3
Europe and Middle East	
U.K., England, South-Western Region	2.5
Norway, Urban	2.3
Yugoslavia, Slovenia	1.8
Israel: All Jews	1.7
Asia and Far East	
Hawaii: Hawaiian	7.4
Hawaii: Japanese	6.6
Japan, Miyagi Prefecture	1.0
India, Bombay	0.3
Africa	
Mozambique, Lourenco Marques	98.2
Rhodesia, Bulawayo: African	20.9
South Africa, Natal, African	20.1
South Africa, Johannesburg, Bantu	14.2
Nigeria, Ibadan	5.9
Uganda, Kyadondo	5.5
South Africa, Cape Province, White	1.1

Analysis of incidence and proportional rates from many parts of Africa suggests that the high incidence occurs generally throughout subsaharan Africa, though there appear to be regions with a particularly high incidence such as Mozambique (Prates and Torres, 1965), Rhodesia (Skinner, 1967), Senegal (Payet, 1957) and Ethiopia (Pavlica and Samuel, 1970). The tendency to under-diagnose deep-seated malignancies in rural parts of Africa makes it difficult to compare many of these regions.

Analysis of the admissions to the Mengo Hospital in Kampala established in 1897 suggests that liver-cell carcinoma has always had a high incidence in rural Africa (DAVIES et al., 1964). Moreover, recent figures from Johannesburg indicate a declining incidence with urbanization (ROBERTSON et al., 1971).

Previous analyses of clinical admissions and post mortem results at the Mulago Hospital, Kampala, have shown that liver-cell carcinoma has a higher frequency in immigrants from Rwanda (SHAPER and SHAPER, 1958; ALPERT, HUTT and DAVIDSON, 1968 a and 1969; SHAPER, 1970). In this study the proportional rate in Rwandan men was 16.3% as compared with 6.2% among Baganda males and this distribution is also evident in both the Kyadondo rate surveys (DAVIES et al., 1965; TEMPLETON et al., 1972). The 1968—1970 study showed that the rate was also high among non-Rwandan immigrants (TEMPLETON et al., 1972). Baganda men have a lower proportional rate than any other tribe and one could therefore interpret these findings in terms of a protective factor for the Baganda.

ALPERT, HUTT and DAVIDSON (1968 and 1971) found that the highest incidence per 100,000 cases per year occurred in the Karamajong living in the North-West of Uganda, and this is confirmed in the present analysis.

Associated Conditions and Aetiology

Cirrhosis of the Liver

An association between cirrhosis of the liver and primary liver-cell carcinoma has long been established in areas of both high and low tumour incidence (STEINER, 1957). BERMAN (1951) reviewed the literature and found that 67.2% of 893 patients with primary liver cell carcinoma were associated with cirrhosis, and EDMONDSON and STEINER (1954) in a series of 75 cases of liver-cell carcinoma from the U.S.A. found associated cirrhosis in 89.2%. While some authors have reported lower figures, most references from all parts of the world quote figures in the range 60—90%. In Uganda, DAVIES and STEINER (1957) record the association in 79% of cases and in the autopsied cases of this present review the figure is 86%.

The frequency with which carcinoma of the liver is found at autopsy in patients with cirrhosis is more variable. For example, in cases of cirrhosis in Chicago, liver-cell carcinoma was present in 15% (STEWART, 1965); while in Mozambique and other parts of Africa it has been stated to be as high as 40% (BRAS, 1961). DAVIES and STEINER (1957) estimated that about 17% of cirrhotics in Uganda develop liver-cell carcinoma and SHAPER (1970) has shown that the percentage of cirrhotics with liver-cell carcinoma at autopsy in Kampala is similar in the indigenous Baganda (14%) and the immigrant Rwanda (15%). He has also shown, however, that both cirrhosis and liver-cell carcinoma occur significantly more frequently in Rwandans and that liver-cell carcinoma unassociated with cirrhosis of the liver is also slightly more frequent in Rwandans (SHAPER, 1970).

These apparent differences in the liability of a cirrhotic liver to develop liver cell carcinoma probably depend both on the macroscopic type of cirrhosis and its aetiology. Liver-cell carcinoma is more frequently seen in cirrhosis of the macronodular (postnecrotic and posthepatitic) types than in the micronodular (nutritional) form

(Scheuer, 1971). There is however evidence to suggest that the type of cirrhosis in patients with alcoholic cirrhosis may change from a micronodular to a macronodular type and that this is associated with an increased incidence of liver-cell carcinoma (Lee, 1966). In South Africa, Becker and Chatgidakis (1961) have shown that liver-cell carcinoma is present in 44% of cirrhotic livers in Africans, but only in 6% of cases of cirrhosis in Europeans. This probably reflects differences in the type of cirrhosis which is dominantly macronodular in the Africans and micronodular in Europeans. Anthony et al. (1972) have shown the predominance of macronodular forms of cirrhosis in Ugandan Africans and their association with H.A.A.

In terms of pathogenesis it would seem logical to assume that liver-cell carcinomas in a cirrhotic liver arise from foci of nodular hyperplasia and that the change is more likely to occur in the larger, more hyperplastic nodules. In some cirrhotic livers carcinoma appears to arise in multiple sites, though it is not easy to discount a intra-hepatic vascular spread with secondary nodule formation. Elias (1960) supports the multicentric origin of liver-cell carcinoma in cirrhotic livers and describes discrete

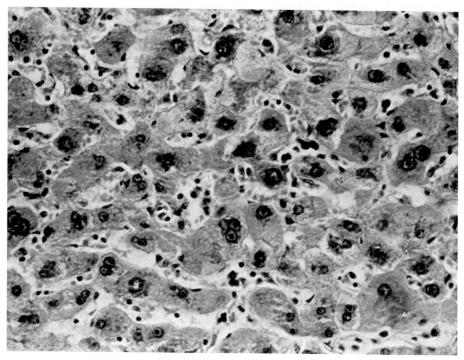

Fig. 10. Liver-cell dysplasia. H and E

foci of transformation of normal liver cells into malignant cells. Examination of many cirrhotic nodules in Ugandan livers not infrequently reveals one or more nodules in which there are marked cellular abnormalities, characterized by large cells which are often multinucleate with grossly pleomorphic nuclei, prominent nucleoli and occasionally mitoses (Fig. 10). These changes, which may be described as liver-cell dysplasia, are sometimes difficult to distinguish from a small carcinomatous nodule except that the latter usually lack the normal reticulin framework. In the present post mortem series liver-cell dysplasia was present in some nodules in 62% of 56 cases with cirrhosis but was not seen in any of the 11 cases without cirrhosis. The presence of dysplasia was, in itself, associated with H.A.A. (ANTHONY, VOGEL and BATZER, 1973). STEINER (1957) suggests that carcinoma originating in non-cirrhotic livers are unicentric and do not have a recognizable precarcinomatous phase.

STEINER (1957) has reviewed the possible relationship between cirrhosis and carcinoma and suggests either that the presence of cirrhosis provides a more favourable environment for the action of a carcinogen or that there is a common cause. The evidence from Africa suggests that one or more factors in the environment act as carcinogenic and cirrhogenic agents and that dose, duration of action, and the presence of other environmental or host factors determine whether liver-cell carcinoma develops alone or is associated with cirrhosis. It is of interest that many patients with liver-cell carcinoma associated with cirrhosis die of their tumour without having had clinical manifestations of the latter. This suggests that the causative agents may produce both lesions almost simultaneously (GIBSON, 1971).

It is evident that no consideration of the causal factors of liver-cell carcinoma can be undertaken in isolation from the causation of cirrhosis.

Viral Hepatitis

Viral hepatitis is endemic in Africa, usually manifesting itself as sporadic cases but with occasional epidemics (SOOD et al., 1966; MORROW et al., 1968). The latter are probably due to infective hepatitis (common source, epidemic or type A) while many of the sporadic cases are due to serum hepatitis (type B—long incubation period), though this virus is now known to be transmissible by the oral route as well as by injection (KRUGMAN and GILES, 1970).

Although it is generally accepted that cases of acute viral hepatitis of both types may ultimately give rise to cirrhosis, and individual cases have been followed by repeat liver biopsies, the frequency with which this occurs is not known. NEFZGER and CHALMERS (1963), for example, examined 96 cases for a period of over 10 years and found none with serious evidence of liver disease, and CHUTTARI et al. (1966). who followed up many cases during the Delhi epidemic in 1955—56, did not find histological or biochemical evidence of permanent liver damage. On morphological grounds GALL (1960) suggested that there was a distinct post-hepatitic form of cirrhosis, and STEINER (1960) emphasized its frequency in Africa.

The discovery of the Australia antigen by BLUMBERG et al. (1965) and of the serum hepatitis antigen (H.A.A.) by PRINCE (1968), and their association with long incubation period, or serum hepatitis, opened the way for a more direct approach to the relation of this type of viral hepatitis to cirrhosis (PRINCE, 1971). Australia and S.H. antigen are now known to be identical and will be referred to as H.A.A. (Hepatitis-associated antigen).

Studies from many tropical countries have shown that H.A.A. is more commonly found there than in Europe or the U.S.A. PRINCE (1970) found the antigen with frequencies of 1—6% in Africa, 0—10% in tropical America and 0—2.5% in the Indian subcontinent; these percentages are on the whole higher than in countries of the temperate zones. The presence of H.A.A. in some cases of chronic liver disease (Wright et al., 1969) suggests that the virus may be responsible for cirrhosis. In Uganda, Maynard et al. (1970) found the antigen in 15 of 20 patients with hepatitis, in 15 of 49 with cirrhosis, but in only 3 of 142 controls. In Kenya, Bagshawe et al. (1971) found H.A.A. in 51% of cases of acute hepatitis and in 20% with cirrhosis, and similar results have been reported from other parts of Africa. In two Ugandan studies Vogel et al. (1970 and 1972 b) found a significant association between hepatocellular carcinoma and the hepatitis-associated antigen. These authors also noted that there was a tendency for H.A.A.-positivity to be associated with the presence of alpha-fetoprotein in the younger age groups (Vogel et al., 1972). The data recorded at different centres are not strictly comparable owing to the use of different techniques for the detection of antigen and variability in the composition of control groups.

The overall evidence, however, suggests that viral hepatitis of type B is an important cause of liver disease in Uganda and middle Africa and that it probably plays a role in the aetiology of cirrhosis and possibly of liver-cell carcinoma, though the low incidence of liver-cell carcinoma in places like India suggests that other factors are involved.

Mycotoxins

The discovery of aflatoxin and the description of its chemistry and biological activities have been the subject of several reviews (Wogan, 1968; Schoental, 1968; Newberne and Butler, 1969; Magee, 1971). Since the first isolation from *Aspergillus flavus* several closely related substances have been defined, of which aflatoxin B_1 has been most extensively studied. It has also been shown that Aspergillus grows on a variety of different foodstuffs and that the microenvironment of food-storage areas is a major determining factor in the degree of mould growth (Alpert et al., 1971). Other fungi such as *Aspergillus versicolor* (Wogan, 1966) also produce a toxin, sterigmatocystin.

Aflatoxin is one of the most powerful hepatoxins isolated though there is considerable variation in species response. Carcinogenic activity has been demonstrated in many species but to date no tumours have been produced in monkeys (Magee, 1971). Deo et al. (1970) have produced a variety of hepatic lesions in monkeys but only a limited number of long-term experiments have been carried out. Serck-Hanssen (1970) has reported one case of acute hepatic necrosis in a Ugandan, where circumstantial evidence suggested aflatoxin ingestion.

In Uganda, Lopez and Crawford (1967) found that groundnuts sold in the markets contained 10 p.p.m. of aflatoxin and noted seasonal variation. Widespread contamination of foodstuffs was reported by Alpert, Hutt and Davidson (1968 a) and Alpert, Hutt, Wogan and Davidson (1971). In the latter survey 29.6% of food samples contained detectable levels of aflatoxins and 3.7% contained more than 1 mg per kg. The frequency of aflatoxin contamination was particularly high in districts with a high incidence of liver-cell carcinoma or where cultural and economic factors favoured the ingestion of mouldy foods; this might explain the high incidence in the Rwandans. In Kenya, Linsell and Peers (personal communication, 1972) have shown a positive correlation between the amount of aflatoxin contamination and the incidence of liver-cell carcinoma in the Murranga district of Kenya. Torres et al.

(1970) draw attention to the presence of toxic liver damage in liver biopsies from Africans in Mozambique and suggest that this would support the hypothesis that primary liver carcinoma is produced by a food-borne toxin, possibly a mycotoxin such as aflatoxin or sterigmatocystin (PURCHASE and VAN DER WATT, 1968).

The importance of other naturally occurring carcinogens in the African environment, such as the pyrrolizidine alkaloids, the aliphatic azoxy compounds (cycads and cyasins) and nitrosamines have been reviewed by MAGEE (1971). While none of these can be excluded as factors in the causation of liver disease and liver-cell carcinoma, the very varied ecology in areas of high incidence makes it unlikely that a specific plant or group of plants can explain the epidemiological incidence.

Despite the high incidence of malnutrition in children there is no evidence that nutritional deficiency plays a direct role in the aetiology of liver cirrhosis in Africa (HUTT, 1971 a). It is quite possible, however, that the nutritional state may play a part in determining the effects of carcinogens or viruses.

Other factors which may play a role in the aetiology of cirrhosis and of liver-cell carcinoma in the tropics have been reviewed by SCHEUER (1971), HUTT (1971 b), GIBSON (1971) and MAGEE (1971). None of these explains the curious epidemiological pattern and some interaction of H.A.A. and a mycotoxin on the liver seems to provide the best hypothesis for further work.

Hepatoblastoma and Other Embryonal Tumours

There were four cases diagnosed as hepatoblastoma. The youngest patient was a two-month-old infant and the eldest a child of four. There were three females and one male.

KEELING (1971) reported a series of 46 tumours in infancy and childhood and classified them into 4 groups: hepatoblastoma, rhabdomyoblastic tumours, hamartoma and liver-cell carcinoma. In her series there were 32 cases of hepatoblastoma with an age range of 2 weeks to 2 years 9 months on presentation, whereas the youngest of the four patients with liver-cell carcinoma was nearly 7 years. The youngest patient with liver-cell carcinoma in the Uganda series was 8 years old. One case of teratoma of the liver was included in our material. This has been reported elsewhere (KIRYAB-WIRE and MUGERWA, 1967).

Haemangioendothelial Sarcoma

The diagnosis of haemangioendothelial sarcoma was made in three cases. There were two men, aged 43 and 56 and one woman, aged 55. A full post mortem was carried out on one of these cases. The liver contained multiple haemorrhagic nodules with occasional cavernous areas, a picture similar to that described by EDMONDSON (1958). The debate as to the origin of these tumours, either from vascular endothelium or Kupffer cells, is still not settled. The intense stimulation to Kupffer cells by parasitic diseases in Africa might be excepted to give a higher incidence of these tumours if they were of Kupffer cell origin. The high incidence of histiocytic medullary reticulosis in Ugandans, which is characterized by the presence of malignant histiocytes in the hepatic sinusoids (SERCK-HANSSEN and PUROHIT, 1968), suggests that malignancy of Kupffer cells should be regarded as part of these lymphoreticular neoplasms and that haemangio-endothelial sarcomas are of vascular endothelial origin.

Intrahepatic Bile Duct Carcinoma (Cholangiocarcinoma)

There were 19 cases diagnosed as intrahepatic bile duct carcinoma, with an age range of 28 to 70 years and a male : female ratio of 1 : 2. The symptoms and signs in these cases were indistinguishable from those seen in liver-cell carcinoma, though in one case a small tumour produced early obstructive jaundice by virtue of its origin near the entrance of the main ducts into the liver substance. EDMONDSON (1958) noted that icterus was less common and less severe in cases of bile-duct carcinoma than in liver-cell carcinoma. In view of the selective factors in favour of male registration in Uganda, the sex ratio suggests that this condition is significantly more common in women than in men in Uganda which is a marked contrast to liver-cell carcinoma in which the male : female ratio is 4.1 : 1.

Intrahepatic bile-duct carcinoma, or cholangiocarcinoma as it is sometimes called, has a high incidence in parts of the Far East, where it is associated with infection by *C. sinensis* (GIBSON, 1971). In an autopsy series from Hong Kong active clonorchiasis was found in 29% of 83 cases of liver-cell carcinoma, a lower rate than that found in the general autopsy population of the same age and sex; whereas in cholangio-carcinoma the frequency of active clonorchiasis was nearly twice that found in controls. Similar findings have been reported from Canton (LIANG and TUNG, 1959) and Bangkok (BHAMARAPRAVATI and VIRANUVATTI, 1966). More recent reports refer particularly to the association between mucin-secretory adenocarcinomas of the intra-hepatic bile ducts and clonorchiasis (CHOU and GIBSON, 1970). Carcinoma of the extrahepatic bile ducts does not have such a clear association with *C. sinensis* (GIBSON, 1971). The proportion of cholangiocarcinomas out of all primary liver-cell carcinomas was 1 : 5 in Hong Kong and 1 : 4 in Canton (LIANG and TUNG, 1959). As GIBSON (1971) points out, this is very similar to the ratio seen in Europe or America. By contrast, in areas where there is a very high incidence of liver-cell carcinoma, such as in Africa, the ratio is 1 : 38 (STEINER, 1960) or 1 : 20 in Johannesburg. In this series from Uganda the ratio is just over 1 : 24. Overall analysis suggests that in Hong Kong the incidence of both liver-cell carcinoma and cholangiocarcinoma is high; in Uganda and other parts of Africa there is a very high incidence of liver-cell carcinoma with no significant increase in cholangiocarcinoma and in Europe and America both have a low incidence.

Pathology

Only one of the 19 cases diagnosed as intrahepatic bile-duct carcinoma was known to have cirrhosis, though it is difficult to exclude when only needle biopsy material is available. In those cases coming to autopsy the tumours varied consider-ably in size but when situated near the porta hepatis a small growth can cause ob-

struction with deep jaundice leading to biliary cirrhosis (Fig. 11). Bile duct carcinomas are usually grey or grey-white in colour and are hard in consistency. If they
cause obstruction, the tumour as well as the liver may be deeply bile-stained. Intrahepatic metastases are not common and in those cases coming to autopsy the regional
lymph nodes and peritoneum were frequently involved.

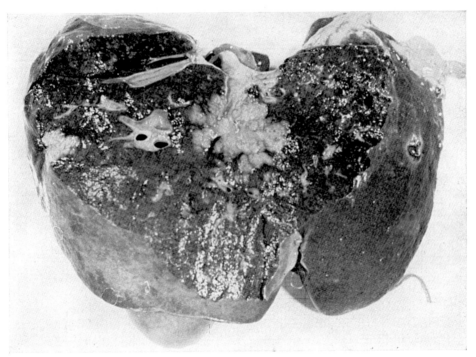

Fig. 11. Primary carcinoma of the bile duct arising near the hilum (By permission of W. G.
Spector)

The diagnosis of intrahepatic bile duct carcinoma was only made when tumours
had a ductular structure and no evidence of differentiation towards hepatic cells
(Fig. 12). In some an intra-acinar papillary pattern was evident. Nearly all had a
marked stromal response and occasionally this led to a trabecular pattern with an
ill-defined tubular arrangement, compressed by fibrous tissue. Mucus secretion was
evident in most tumours but not all bile duct carcinomas produce mucin.

Extrahepatic Bile Duct Carcinoma

There were eight cases of extrahepatic bile duct carcinoma with an age range of
23 to 70 and a male : female ratio of 1 : 1. In one of these cases the tumour originated
in the Ampulla of Vater. All presented with persistent obstructive jaundice.

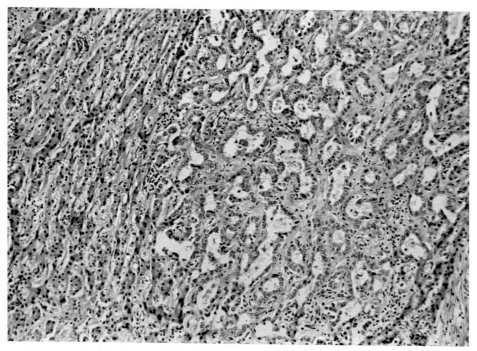

Fig. 12. Moderately differentiated bile duct carcinoma infiltrating the liver. H and E (By permission of W. G. Spector)

The proportion of extrahepatic bile duct carcinomas to carcinomas of the head of the pancreas is higher in Uganda than in series from Europe and North America.

None of these cases was associated with gallstones or showed clinical evidence of previous gallbladder disease. The histopathological features of the tumours were similar to those reported elsewhere (Edmondson, 1958).

Carcinoma of the Gall Bladder

There were nine cases of carcinoma of the gallbladder with an age range of 30 to 70 and a male : female ratio of 1 : 2.3. This is a significant female predominance when when allowance is made for the selective sex factors that determine hospital admissions and cancer registration. The female predominance is also noted in series from Europe and North America, where it is related to the higher incidence of cholecystitis and cholelithiasis in women.

Only one of these cases was associated with gallstones, which are rare in Ugandans of both sexes (Owor, 1964). Cholecystitis is also uncommon in Uganda (Shaper and Patel, 1964) and therefore the aetiology of carcinoma of the gallbladder in Uganda may be different, though the sex ratio is similar.

The histopathological features of these cases were similar to other reported series (Edmondson, 1958).

Carcinoma of the Pancreas

A. C. Templeton

The pancreas must be about the most difficult organ in the body to examine by clinical methods and undoubtedly many neoplasms of the pancreas in Uganda are never diagnosed, particularly those in the tail. Many patients with obstructive jaundice will undergo an exploratory laparotomy, however, so that variations in the site of origin of tumours are likely to be due to the different symptoms produced. A review of the diagnostic problems posed by carcinoma of the pancreas in Uganda has recently been published (James and Templeton, 1971). No case of either Zollinger-Ellison syndrome or insulin-secreting islet-cell tumour has been diagnosed in Uganda up to the present time though two apparently funtionless islet-cell tumours have been found in the pancreas.

Thirty cases were seen during the period under review. This represents 0.4% of tumours overall. Five of these cases were not confirmed by histology. These figures probably represent only a small fraction of the true incidence.

The mean age at presentation was 53 years with a range of 35 to 80. The two patients with islet-cell tumours were aged 22 and 36. There were 20 males and 10 females.

Of the cases recorded, 65% were first seen at Mulago Hospital and 9 were diagnosed only at necropsy, so that tribal distribution is certain to be biased. Twenty patients were Muganda, 3 came from northern tribes and 7 from western districts. No cases were seen from eastern region.

Only one tumour was found in the tail of the pancreas and 8 involved the body. The remaining 21 patients had tumours in the head of the pancreas and all had obstructive jaundice.

Twenty-five cases were confirmed by histology and virtually all cases were average-grade adenocarcinomas, though a few poorly differentiated tumours were seen. Sclerotic reaction around the tumour cells was common and afforded a useful differential diagnostic point from tumours of the bowel which very rarely showed this response. A few tumours were seen with signet-ring cell forms and one was noted to produce copious extracellular mucin. In general the tubules formed in the tumours were wide and lined with flattened cells allowing fairly easy differentiation from adenocarcinomas arising in the bowel.

At operation the only condition which is likely to be confused with carcinoma of the pancreas is chronic pancreatic disease. This latter disease is very common in Uganda and the aetiology is unknown (Owor, 1970). Some cases possibly have their origins in the pancreatic degeneration that accompanies kwashiorkor. In this type the pancreas shows a fine diffuse fibrosis with grossly dilated ducts. Acute pancreatitis is rare and this may relate to the rarity of cholelithiasis. Recurrent episodes of inflammation leading to scarring and destruction of pancreatic parenchyma do occur and this results in rather broad bands of fibrous tissue separating small islands of relatively normal pancreatic glands. It is this latter type which mimics carcinoma macroscopically.

Six cases were seen during the period under review, in which laparotomy for obstructive jaundice had been undertaken resulting in an operative diagnosis of carcinoma of the pancreas. Biopsy, however, showed only chronic pancreatitis. It is possible that some of these biopsies were not representative and that the pancreas contained a small carcinoma. But even if only half these cases were in fact due to non-malignant conditions this means that 10% of patients with obstruction due to lesions of the head of the pancreas have no malignant condition. Bypass operations should therefore be carried out in all cases except those obviously due to huge tumours.

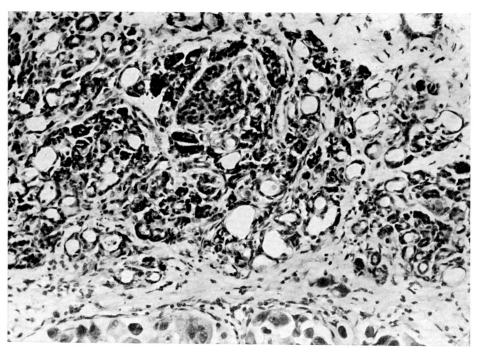

Fig. 13. Tumour cells (along the lower edge of the picture) may be difficult to distinguish from islets and distended acini buried in fibrous tissue

Histologically it may be very difficult indeed to differentiate scirrhous carcinoma from fibrosis and disruption of the pancreatic architecture (Fig. 13). The resemblance to carcinoma is heightened by the survival of clumps of islet cells and the regenerative activity of ducts. This differentiation is particularly difficult in small biopsy specimens.

Clinically, the syndromes produced are exactly similar to those seen in other parts of the world. Tumours at the head of the pancreas present with obstructive jaundice, the differentiated diagnosis of which is rather easier than in Caucasians because of the rarity of gallstones. The only tumour in the tail of the pancreas was found in a woman who had had a series of thrombotic episodes without evidence of metastases culminating in portal venous thrombosis which had resulted in fatal bleeding from varices.

Chapter 4

Tumours of the Respiratory Tract

G. T. O'Conor and A. C. Templeton

With 6 Figures

The frequency of tumours of the respiratory tract show well marked differences from other countries. Nasopharyngeal tumours and carcinoma of the maxillary antrum are commonly seen, whereas tumours of the larynx and lung are rare. Nasopharyngeal carcinoma is poorly differentiated, occurs at a young age and is found more commonly in patients from the north of the country. Tumours of the nasal sinuses occur in older people and do not appear to be related to snuff taking. Adenocarcinoma of the bronchus accounts for a slightly greater proportion of cases than where tumours of the bronchus are more common. There is as yet no indication of a rise in the incidence of bronchial cancer.

The respiratory tract, as defined in this chapter, comprises the nose and accessory sinuses, the nasopharynx, larynx, trachea, bronchi and lungs. Inclusion of the nasopharynx is a departure from the standard scheme employed in the International Classification of Disease where nasopharynx is classified under the alimentary canal. However, the function and the histology of the nasopharynx, as well as the type of exposure and response to presumed carcinogenic influences, are more logically related to the nose and accessory sinuses than to the oral cavity.

During the period under review 429 tumors arising in the respiratory tract were recorded. These are grouped by site and listed by histological type in Table 1. Burkitt's tumour and other lymphomas accounted for 25% of all cases. These and the various sarcomas are considered in detail in other chapters but are listed here along with a number of frequently occurring benign tumours simply to indicate the variety and relative frequency of tumour types seen in the respiratory tract. This chapter is principally concerned with the histological characteristics, distribution, and relative frequency of malignant epithelial tumours.

Malignant epithelial tumours of the respiratory tract as a whole are less common in Uganda than in many other countries. The relative frequencies of these tumours in several different population groups are shown in Table 2. In Uganda and in Nigeria the percentages are much lower than in the three Asian populations and in the United States. However, the significant differences, which must reflect environmental influences, are only appreciated when percentages are compared in specific segments of the respiratory tract (Table 3). There seems to be an independent variability between sites in population groups. Tumours of the nose and sinuses are common in Africa and uncommon elsewhere. Tumours of the nasopharynx occur relatively frequently in

Table 1. Site and histological type of tumours of the respiratory tract

Nose and sinuses	240
98 Burkitt lymphoma	
45 Squamous carcinoma	
12 Adenocarcinoma	
21 Undifferentiated carcinoma	
12 Sarcoma	
8 Other lymphomas	
4 Plasmacytoma	
5 Anaplastic malignant tumours	
3 Melanoma	
2 Aesthesioneuroblastoma	
6 Pleomorphic adenoma	
15 Transitional cell papilloma	
7 "Cancer" not biopsied	
2 Mid line granuloma	
Nasopharynx	95
85 Anaplastic carcinoma	
3 Sarcoma	
3 "Cancer" not biopsied	
2 Myeloma	
1 Histiocytic lymphoma	
1 Unclassified malignant tumour	
Larynx	45
16 Squamous carcinomas	
28 Papilloma	
1 Granular cell myoblastoma	
Lung	49
7 Squamous carcinoma	
12 Adenocarcinoma	
2 Combined adeno and squamous	
6 Oat-cell carcinoma	
12 Large cell undifferentiated	
2 "Carcinoid" adenoma	
7 "Cancer" not biopsied	
1 Mucoepidermoid	
	429

Table 2. Malignant epithelial tumours of the respiratory tract expressed as percentages of all malignant tumours

Place	Year	Percentage
Uganda	1964—1968	3.5
Ibadan [a]	1960—1965	4
Okoyama (Japan) [a]	1966	9.5
Connecticut [a]	1963—1965	12.5
Bombay [a]	1964—1966	14
Hawaii (Chinese) [a]	1960—1964	16

[a] Figures taken from Doll, Muir, Waterhouse, 1970.

Uganda and among Chinese in Hawaii, but are less frequent in Ibadan and unusual in India, Japan, and the United States. Tumours of the larynx are very frequent in Bombay, but much less common in other countries, particularly in the Hawaiian-Chinese. Tumours of the bronchus account for an over-whelming portion of the cases in Connecticut and are also very frequent among Hawaiian-Chinese and in Japan. They are less common in Bombay, even less frequent in Ibadan, and relatively uncommon in Uganda. Thus, tumours of one site bear no regular relationship to tumours of another site, either direct or reciprocal.

Table 3. The relative frequency of carcinoma in different parts of the respiratory tract

ICD (7th)	Site	Hawaiian Chinese	Uganda	Ibadan (Nigeria)	Bombay (India)	Okoyama (Japan)	Conn. (U.S.A.)
		%	%	%	%	%	%
160	Nose and Sinuses	8	37	30	7	17	5.5
146	Nasopharynx	26	36	15	3	1	1
161	Larynx	1.5	7	20	47	13	12
162	Lung Bronchus	64	20	35	43	69	81.5
	Total cases	63	243	58	1372	280	3071

It may be postulated that different aetiological factors are concerned in the development of tumours at these different sites. For example, whatever factors are involved in the relative increase in tumours of the nose and sinus in both Uganda and Ibadan do not appear to influence the tumour frequency in the nasopharynx or larynx. Likewise, whatever factors are responsible for the high frequency of carcinoma of the bronchus among Hawaiian-Chinese do not equally affect the larynx.

Tumours of the Nose and Sinuses

The most common tumour which produces a mass in the nose or maxilla is Burkitt's lymphoma. These tumours occur predominately in children and are therefore unlikely to be mistaken clinically for carcinoma, which is found in the older age groups. Other types of lymphoma including plasmacytomas, sarcomas, neurogenic tumours, and melanomas, however, may occur at any age and do pose a problem in differential diagnosis.

The twelve sarcomas recorded during this survey included two myxomata of the maxilla, three rhabdomyosarcomas, two Kaposi sarcomas, one chondrosarcoma, one fibrosarcoma, and four undifferentiated sarcomas that were otherwise unclassifiable.

Histological examination is mandatory not only for tumour classification but also for the exclusion of a number of benign tumours and inflammatory conditions which may mimic malignant neoplastic processes. Rhinoscleroma is frequent in Uganda and during the period of this survey there were 136 histologically documented cases. Even with microscopic study, this condition may be difficult to distinguish from plasmacytoma or lymphoma. Adamantinomas, fibrous dysplasia and other benign jaw tumours are common and must be considered in the differential diagnosis. Rhinosporidiosis, phycomycosis, other fungus diseases, tuberculosis, and leprosy are among the infectious diseases which can be misdiagnosed as cancer. As stated earlier, the lymphomas and mesenchymal tumours will be discussed in other chapters. There is one type of lymphoma, however, which is peculiar to the nose or nasopharynx and which should be mentioned here. The term pleomorphic reticulosis has been used for a tumour composed of mixed lymphoreticular elements which arises primarily in the nose or nasopharynx and is locally invasive (DE FAVIA et al., 1956; KASSEL et al., 1969). Regional or distant spread is either absent or late and atypical in distribution. One of the three tumours of this type found in the Uganda material is illustrated in Fig. 1. This is a relatively rare tumour but has been particularly observed in certain Latin America countries and may show some increased frequency in developing societies (ROMERO and METH, 1970).

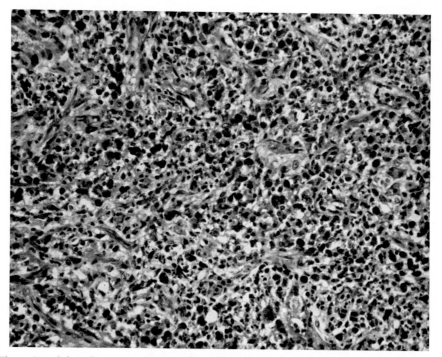

Fig. 1. *Nasal lymphoma*. The pleomorphic cellular infiltrate in a fibroreticular stroma are characteristic features. Extensive necrosis and nuclear pyknosis distorts cytological detail. H and E ×180

Frequency of Carcinoma

Carcinomas of the nose and sinuses are common in Uganda and represent 37% of the epithelial tumours of the entire respiratory tract. This increased frequency has been reported previously from Uganda (DODGE, 1965) and from other parts of the

African continent (KEEN et al., 1955; SINGH and MARTINSON, 1969) and is probably indicative of a significant difference in incidence rates compared with most western countries.

Site

It is well known that in developing countries with limited medical facilities cancer patients often present with advanced disease. This is particularly true of cancers of the upper respiratory tract and identification of the exact site of origin for large destructive lesions is often difficult. Based on the best clinical, radiological and histological criteria available for each case, 63 out of the 78 carcinomas (80%) in the nose and sinuses were thought to be of antral origin. This was true of tumours of all histological types. Most of the remaining cancers arose in the nose; the frontal and ethmoid sinuses accounted for only a few cases.

Age, Sex, and Tribal Distribution

There was a 2 to 1 male predominance in epithelial tumours of the nose and paranasal sinuses. Age-specific rates show a steadily rising curve. However, the majority of patients present at around the age of 40 years and there is a rapid fall-off in younger and older age groups. This had led to the suggestion that these tumours occur at a younger age in Africa than in Europe (SHAPIRO et al., 1955), but it is probably only an effect of the youthful population at risk. Carcinomas are occasionally seen in very young patients and both the neuroepithelial tumours occurred in children. No significant tribal variation was noted in this group of tumours. A preponderance of cases were diagnosed in Kampala but this probably reflects the access to better diagnostic facilities at Mulago hospital than elsewhere in the country, rather than a true rise in incidence in this area.

Histological Characteristics

Variability in classification, nomenclature, and histological criteria sometimes make international and regional comparisons difficult. It is therefore important to clarify these points in the simplest and most objective terms possible. In this section, as well as in the other sections of the respiratory tract, a diagnosis of squamous cell carcinoma is made only when there is keratin formation, including individual cell keratinization, and/or intercellular bridges can be seen. A diagnosis of adenocarcinoma implies recognizable gland formation, and the term undifferentiated or anaplastic is used when there is neither keratin production nor glandular differentiation in an epithelial tumour. We have chosen not to employ the terms transitional cell carcinoma, cylindromatous carcinoma, Schneiderian tumour, or Schmincke tumour. Many of the tumours we have classified as undifferentiated might be called epidermoid or transitional cell by other authors.

It will be seen in Table 1 that there were a few tumours—5 in the nose and sinuses and 1 in the nasopharynx—which were so undifferentiated that they could not be confidently classified as either epithelial or mesenchymal.

The majority of carcinomas in the nose and sinuses, 45 of 78, were of the poorly differentiated squamous cell type. These often have a wide basiloid rim around islands, sheets or cords of tumour cells, in contrast to oral tumours in which keratinization is more pronounced and diffuse (Fig. 2). This is perhaps an indication of origin

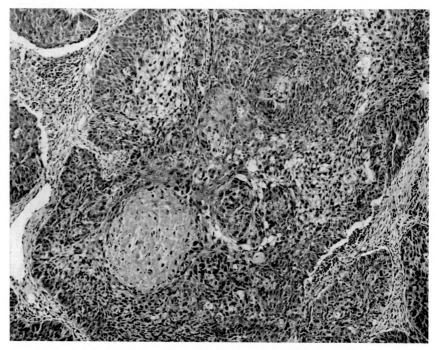

Fig. 2. *Squamous cell carcinoma of the maxillary antrum.* The tumour is poorly differentiated with only focal keratinization. H and E ×70

from respiratory tract epithelium and may be useful in suggesting a primary site when biopsy material from a cervical node is examined. There were 21 undifferentiated carcinomas in this group and 12 adenocarcinomas. Five of the latter were of the adenoid cystic type, all arose in the maxillary sinus, and four of the five occurred in males. This is in contrast to six tumours of the adenoid cystic type occurring in the palate, all of which were in males. These and the other mucous gland tumours are discussed further in chapter 2.

Discussion

Chronic irritation by a variety of agents is believed to be an important factor associated with the aetiology of carcinoma of the paranasal sinuses. Chronic infections have been implicated both in Europe (Ringentz, 1938) and in Africa (Clifford, 1967) and it has also been suggested that vasomotor rhinitis might predispose the mucous membrane to damage by other factors.

In western countries and particularly in the United States, nose and sinus cancer has been associated with use of snuff and more specifically to industrial exposure to nickel, chromium, arsenic, isopropyl alcohol, and radioactive materials (HUEPER, 1964). In Africa the latter are not factors for serious consideration at the present time. Snuff taking is not widely practiced in Uganda but has been implicated as a possible factor of importance in South Africa where the incidence of antral cancer is also high (KEEN, 1967).

Inhalation of smoke from cooking fires in poorly ventilated huts was believed to bear a logical relationship to the increased frequency of both sinus and nasopharyngeal cancer in Kenya, and benzpyrine was recovered from soot deposited in some abodes (CLIFFORD and BEECHER, 1964). This hypothesis, however, is not entirely consistent with the sex ratio or with documented habits in many areas of East Africa. Such exposure may be one of several factors in some but not all groups.

Carcinoma of the Nasopharynx

Frequency

Nasopharyngeal cancer is known to be very common among Chinese living in many countries and in Africans from certain regions within Africa (LINSELL and MARTYN, 1962; CLIFFORD, 1970). In the early reports from Kampala (DAVIES et al., 1965) it was infrequently recorded but more recent studies in Uganda have shown that it is, in fact, fairly common in certain parts of the country (MARTIN, 1967; SCHMAUZ and TEMPLETON, 1972). The earlier under-diagnosis in Uganda was the result of four factors: (1) the lack of skilled personnel required to visualize the tumour; (2) unawareness that patients with this tumour often present with cervical lymphadenopathy without local symptoms; (3) an important tribal variation in incidence; and (4) the failure of pathologists to recognize the distinctive histological appearance of this tumour in cervical nodes. Many cases were previously called histiocytic lymphoma or atypical Hodgkin's disease.

Ninety-five cases of malignant tumour arising in the post-nasal space were recorded in the period of this review (Table 1). These included 85 poorly differentiated carcinomas, 3 cases which were not biopsied but were assumed to be carcinomas, and one malignant tumour not otherwise classified. The remaining 6 nonepithelial tumours are discussed elsewhere. 36% of carcinomas of the respiratory tract were located in the nasopharynx, a proportion which is considerably higher than in most countries (Table 3).

Age, Sex, and Tribal Distribution

The age at diagnosis ranged from 10 to 80 years, but nearly 25% of all patients were under the age of 20 years. This age distribution is unique among epithelial neoplasms in Uganda. Tumours which develop as a result of accumulative carcinogens usually show an expotential rise with age, whereas nasopharyngeal carcinoma is as common in young adults as in older people.

There were 61 males and 27 females. This male preponderance is slightly exaggerated by a tendency towards under-recording in females which occurs in most districts of Uganda. The histological patterns and age distribution of tumours in each sex are similar.

Table 4. Annual crude incidence of carcinoma of the nasopharynx per 100,000 population for 1964—1968 analysed by region, ethnic group and tribe (The scale shows the incidence rate. No. of cases in brackets.)

	South	North-west	North	
	Bantu	Sudanic	Nilotic	Para-Nilotic
1.8				Pokot (2)
0.9			Acholi (14)	
	Samia (2)			
				Sebei (1)
0.5				Kakwa(1)
				Karamojong (3)
			Lango (6)	
0.3				Teso (8)
	Ankole (8)			
		Madi (1)		
0.2	Kiga (5)			
	Gwere (1)			
	Ganda (7)			
0.1	Nyoro (1)			
	Toro (1)			
		Lugbara (1)		
0.05	Gisu (1)			
	Soga (1)			

The incidence of nasopharyngeal carcinoma varies greatly in different tribes but all Nilotic and para-Nilotic tribes, regardless of the part of the country in which they live, appear to be at higher risk than any Bantu tribe (Table 4). The highest incidence among tribes classified as Bantu was in the Munyankole. However, about 30% of the Ankole tribesman are Bahima people who are of para-Nilotic derivation and 5 of the 8 patients from Ankole had Bahima surnames. This suggests that the incidence among para-Nilotic Ankole people is about 3 times that of the Bantu living in the same area. In former times, the way of life of these different peoples was very distinct. The Bahima were cattle-herding nomads while the Bantu society was agricultural and more sedentary. In recent years these distinctions have been progressively obscured and it is difficult to be certain why there should be this apparent ethnically determined variation in tumour incidence.

Histological, Characteristics

Carcinomas of the nasopharynx arise in a region where there are respiratory, squamous, and transitional types of epithelium (Ali, 1967). The tumours have thus been designated as transitional and squamous carcinomas or lymphoepitheliomas, but there is no clear line of distinction between these entities. Electron microscopic studies have shown that all the types are merely variants of a basic squamous pattern (Svoboda et al., 1967). Some cases are so poorly differentiated as to mimic histiocytic lymphomas and are quite frequently misdiagnosed. In Uganda nasopharyngeal

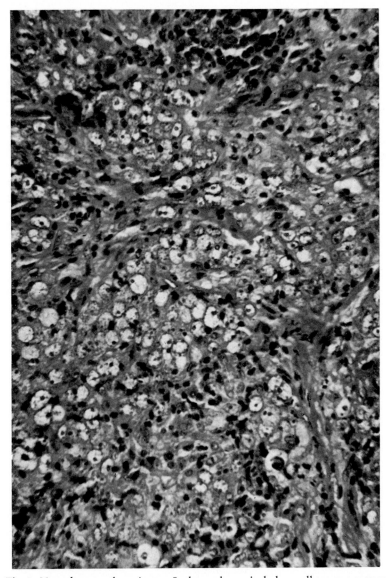

Fig. 3. *Nasopharyngeal carcinoma*. It shows the typical clear-cell tumour pattern

tumours are always poorly differentiated. They are composed of large, pale-staining cells, usually arranged in small clumps (Fig. 3). Lymphocytes are often found in large numbers between the clumps but these do not comprise an integral part of the tumour and simply represent remaining lymphatic tissue from the adenoid or a lymph node. In some cases the groups of epithelial cells are extremely small, comprising only a few cells or even separate single cells (Schmincke type). It is in such cases that the term lymphoepithelioma has been applied and in tumours with this pattern the diagnosis of secondary deposits in a lymph node is the most difficult. The cells themselves are often poorly demarcated and appear as syncytial masses. The nuclei are large, pale and oval and contain one or two very prominent nucleoli. These large cells are present in virtually all cases but are sometimes associated with smaller, more elongated cells. These latter occur more frequently in biopsies from the primary tumour than in the metastases. The smaller cell type shows a greater degree of regimentation and is often found arranged in a radial fashion around vessels or at the periphery of clumps of tumour cells, reminiscent of the pattern seen with transitional epithelium. Exfoliative touch preparations confirmed the distinction between these two cell types (SCHMAUZ and TEMPLETON, 1972).

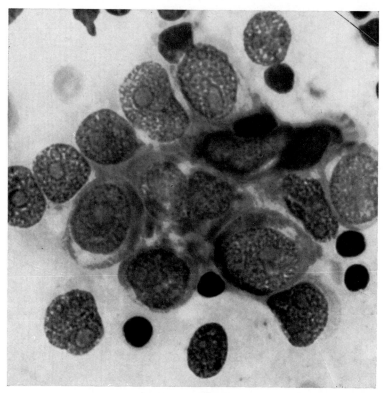

Fig. 4. *Nasopharyngeal carcinoma.* Touch preparation of an enlarged node showing exfoliated tumour cells

Examination of all lymph-node biopsies in Uganda over a five-year period showed that the distinctive cytology described above was found only in cervical nodes with metastatic carcinoma of the nasopharynx. Metastatic tumours of the bronchus present the major difficulties in differential diagnosis but in Uganda these are uncommon and are usually found in an older age group. Metastatic tumours from the sinuses, pharynx or oesophagus usually contain obvious areas of keratinization whereas nasopharyngeal tumours in our series did not. Histiocytic lymphoma is distinguished by the clumped pattern of invasion; the architecture of the node is usually preserved in cases of metastatic nasopharyngeal carcinoma but not in lymphomas.

The complete absence of demonstrable keratin in the Uganda cases is surprising. Chinese (YEH, 1967) and Caucasians (SHEDD et al., 1967) show a significant proportion of cases with keratinization. In the Sudan only 4 of 34 cases showed any evidence of keratin and then only in small quantities (EL HASSAN et al., 1967), and the findings in Kenya are similar (LINSELL, 1964). The effect is possibly a result of the lower average age of patients since in Chinese patients the degree of differentiation is greater in older people (YEH, 1962).

Discussion

The high incidence of nasopharyngeal carcinoma in many parts of the world but particularly among Chinese has evoked much speculation about aetiology and investigation of environmental factors. CLIFFORD and BEECHER (1964) on the basis of work in KENYA, thought that this disease, as well as sinus cancer might be a result of smoke inhaled in the huts, particularly in cold mountainous areas. Experience in Uganda and Sudan would suggest that this is unlikely to be of major importance. In Uganda this tumour is not common at higher altitudes; in fact the general tendency is for it to occur in the drier, lower lying areas. In Sudan virtually no cooking is done indoors and men particularly have almost no contact with smoke and yet the disease is common (EL HASSAN et al., 1967). In Uganda the increased frequency in Nilotic tribes has been mentioned but it is unlikely that the disease is genetically determined since in Kenya, Bantu tribes seem to be as frequently affected as para-Nilotics (CLIFFORD, 1970).

Serological studies in Asia and in Kenya have shown an association of the Epstein-Barr virus with nasopharyngeal carcinoma (HENLE et al., 1970), but it is quite unclear as yet whether this virus plays a significant aetiological role or is simply a passenger. The age distribution of nasopharyngeal cancer in Uganda, characterized by early onset and the very slow rise of age-specific incidence, is consistent with a tumour induced by a single episode and with a viral etiology.

Carcinoma of the Larynx

Frequency

This is a rarely diagnosed tumour in Uganda; only sixteen cases were recorded during the 1964—1968 period. It is axiomatic that in Africa all tumours are rare until the arrival of a specialist capable of making a diagnosis. Twelve of the sixteen cases of laryngeal carcinoma were observed at Mulago hospital in Kampala and three others at a single mission hospital in Acholi district. Although one suspects that this tumour is greatly underdiagnosed its true incidence is nevertheless probably much lower than in industrialized societies (Table 3). As the age structure of the population in Uganda changes and rapid development of the country brings expanded medical facilities as well as potential increased exposure to environmental carcinogens a sharp increase in the frequency of this cancer may be expected.

Age and Sex Distribution

Most cases of laryngeal carcinoma occurred in males and in the older age groups. These data are shown in Table 5.

Table 5. Age and sex distribution of carcinoma of the larynx

Sex	30—34	35—44	45—54	55—64	65—74	Total
Females	1	1	1			3
Males	1	2	3	5	2	13
Total	2	3	4	5	2	16

Histological Characteristics

All carcinomas were of the squamous cell type and most were poorly differentiated. The disease was usually far advanced at the time of diagnosis and in most instances the patients refused radical surgery.

Carcinoma of the Lung and Bronchus

Frequency

In this series pulmonary cancers accounted for 0.7% of all tumours and 13% of tumours of the respiratory tract. The incidence was 0.1 cases per 100,000 per year in women and 0.18 in men (both figures corrected for an African standard population). The equivalent figure reported from Bulawayo for Africans is 25 and 2.5 in males and females respectively (Skinner, 1970). The frequency of this tumour in Uganda is probably underestimated since any rare tumour tends to be underdiagnosed as a result of the rigid criteria usually applied. Bronchogenic carcinoma may be easily confused with tuberculosis which is widespread and the diagnosis of a double lesion is difficult. In this series a large portion of cases were first diagnosed in Mulago hospital where are found the only facilities for thoracic surgery in the country, and most of these were first diagnosed at necropsy. Raper et al. (1952), reporting six cases of lung cancer in Africans from Kampala, found only one patient who had been diagnosed prior to death. Many cases throughout the country are certainly being missed; nonetheless, the incidence of this tumour is believed to be significantly low compared to most western countries.

Age and Sex Distribution

The age and sex distribution of cases is shown in Table 6, and both parameters differ significantly from observations in countries with a high incidence of the disease. The excess of patients under 45 years is remarkable, but correction for the population at risk shows a steadily rising incidence in each succeeding decade except in the very old.

Of particular interest is the male-to-female ratio. KREYBERG (1961) has shown that in the period which antedates the rise of bronchogenic carcinoma in a population secondary to introduction of an environmental aetiological factor, the sex distribution tends to be equal. In Great Britain there was a male excess of 5.7 to 1 in 1951 whereas in 1915, before the incidence began to rise, the sex ratio was only 1.5 to 1 (DOLL, 1953). In Uganda the male excess of 1.7 to 1 is probably a result only of social factors (TEMPLETON and BIANCHI, 1972 a), and in reality the sex incidence is probably equal. This is in contrast to the male-to-female ratio of 5 to 1 in high-incidence countries.

Table 6. Age and sex distribution of pulmonary cancers [a]

Sex	< 25	25—34	35—44	45—54	55—64	Unknown	Total
Female	0	2	4	2	0	1	13
Male	1 [b]	6	6	2	4	2	28
Total	1	8	10	4	4	3	41

[a] Histologically unconfirmed cases not included.
[b] Mucoepidermoid carcinoma in 6-year-old male.

Histological Characteristics

Cases are listed according to histological type and sex in Table 7. In Table 8 the histological type of tumour in Buganda patients is compared with that in other tribes. Nearly a third of the tumours are adenocarcinomas and three of these are of bronchiolar type (Fig. 5). This predominance of glandular tumours is in marked contrast to experience in those countries where bronchogenic carcinoma is frequent and where

Table 7. Histologic types of pulmonary cancers

	Male	Female	Total
Squamous carcinoma	5	2	7
Adeno carcinoma	7	4	11
Large cell undifferentiated	7	5	12
Small cell undifferentiated	6	0	6
Combined squamous-adeno	0	2	2
Carcinoid tumour	2	0	2
Bronchial-gland tumour (mucoepidermoid)	1	0	1
Total	28	13	41

adenocarcinomas account for only 5 to 10% of the total. There is regrettably little information as to the exact site of origin of these tumours so that we are unable to state whether they arose in major bronchi or more peripherally. Three tumours of the bronchial glands and two carcinoid tumours (Fig. 6) in this group represents a remarkable relative frequency and emphasizes the low incidence of squamous and undifferentiated carcinomas. Although the numbers are too small to be of any

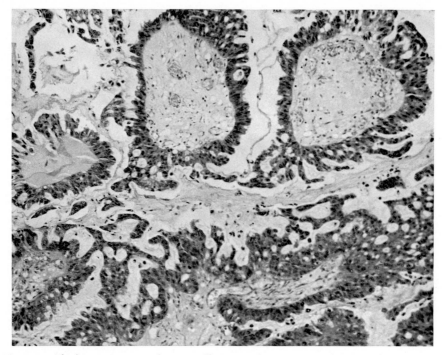

Fig. 5. *Bronchiolar carcinoma*. It has a papillary growth pattern and there is abundant mucous secretion. H and E ×70

Table 8. Tribal distribution of pulmonary cancers

	Baganda	Others	Total
Squamous carcinoma	4	3	7
Adeno carcinoma	7	4	11
Large cell undifferentiated	3	9	12
Small cell undifferentiated	3	3	6
Combined squamous-adeno	2	0	2
Carcinoid tumour	1	1	2
Bronchial-gland tumour (mucoepidermoid)	0	1	1
Total	20	21	41

significance the proportion of large cell undifferentiated tumours in the non-Buganda suggests the possibility of an environmental influence. Oat-cell carcinomas are unusual and were diagnosed in six cases only.

The pattern of spread of bronchogenic carcinoma in Uganda is similar to that found in other countries. Secondary tumours in bones are frequent (Templeton, Hutt and Dodge, 1972). Tumour metastases in the brain are rare in Uganda but carcinoma of the bronchus accounts for a significant proportion of such cases, in both East and West Africa (Adeloye and Odeku, 1969).

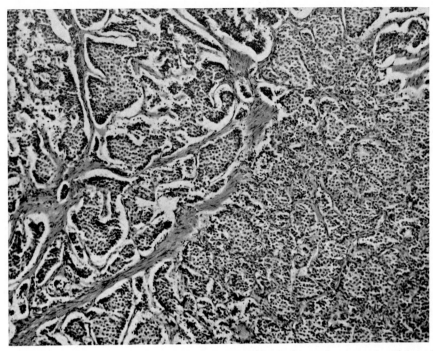

Fig. 6. *Typical carcinoid tumour of the lung.* It is composed of irregular nests of uniform cells bounded by trabeculae

Discussion

Carcinoma of the bronchus was probably rare in all countries 100 years ago. During the twentieth century there has been a dramatic rise in incidence, particularly in the industrial countries. This has been ascribed to atmospheric pollution by various chemicals and by smoking (DOLL and HILL, 1954; United States Public Health Service, 1964). The histological types of tumour which predominate vary with the incidence of the disease. In high-risk areas there is a greater proportion of squamous and oat-cell tumours than in low-risk countries and a preponderance of males (KREYBERG and SAXEN, 1961). In Uganda the sex distribution and the relative proportion of histological types are typical features of a low-risk area and are as might be predicted in a community prior to the onset of industrialization.

The low incidence of pulmonary cancer in Uganda is clearly due to environmental rather than to genetic factors. Bantu Africans resident in Bulawayo, Rhodesia, for example, have a high incidence (SKINNER, 1970), probably a result of industrial exposure and a higher rate of smoking in this city. Similar findings are reported from other major cities of South Africa (SCHONLAND and BRADSHAW, 1970).

It has been suggested that vasomotor rhinitis, which is common in Bantu Africans, may be a strong influence on the incidence of cancer in the respiratory tract (CLIFFORD, 1967). It is postulated that atrophy of the mucosa of the nose and sinuses exposes these areas to carcinogens whereas the concomitant secretion of mucus protects the larynx and lungs from these agents.

Chapter 5

Tumours of the Breast

A. C. TEMPLETON

With 1 Figure

Cancer of the breast is the second most frequent malignancy of Ugandan women. It is, however, very much less common than in western Caucasian females. This altered incidence is probably a result of differences in the age of first pregnancy and possibly of dietary differences between the two communities. Histological studies show little difference except that tumours in Uganda are less well differentiated. Ugandan women present at hospital late in the course of the disease.

Cancer of the male breast appears to be relatively more frequent but its incidence is probably similar to that found in other countries.

Epithelial and mixed tumours of the breast are considered here. Other tumours such as lymphomata and sarcomata are briefly mentioned but are further considered in other chapters. The number of biopsies from the breast and the diagnoses made in sheets of tumour cells. There was no significant difference in the age distribution of patients with medullary and fibrotic tumours, whereas mucous secreting carcinomas occurred slightly more frequently in the older age groups. Papillary carcinoma was

Table 1. Showing the histological diagnosis on 554 breast conditions

	Females	Males	
Benign mammary dysplasia	41	6	(gynaecomastia)
Breast abscess	58		
Chronic mastitis	7	2	
Tuberculosis	2		
Fat necrosis	3		
Fibroadenoma	56		
Intraduct papilloma	1		
Adenocarcinoma	279	41	
Carcinosarcoma	1		
Lymphoma, Burkitt's tumour	9	1	
other lymphoma	1		
Soft-tissue sarcomas	9	1	
Clinical cancer (presumed			
adenocarcinoma)	35	1	
	502	52	

the period 1964 to 1968 are shown in Table 1. This total is a considerable under-estimate of the diseases which occur in Uganda. Women seem to be particularly reluctant to come to hospital with breast lesions; painless non-ulcerating tumours are likely to be ignored. Carcinomas are very frequently in stage III or IV at presentation and almost always ulcerated. Small fibroadenomas are seldom reported from rural Africans and the majority of such nodules have been found in nuns, nurses or private patients, all of whom appear to be more likely to come to hospital earlier than a rural dweller.

Benign mammary dysplasia (fibroadenosis) was diagnosed histologically in 41 African patients. In the same period 15 biopsies were received from European patients and 19 from Asian patients. A rough calculation of the population at risk suggests that mammary dysplasia is about 500 times more common in Europeans and 70 times in Asian women than in Africans. Although these figures are biased by a socially induced exaggeration it remains an impression that benign mammary dysplasia is much less common in Ugandan women than in Europe. Some surveys, for example, by Ellis (1937) in West Africa suggest that this is not true in Nigeria where the incidence of "mastitis" in Africans was thought to be twice that found in England. A recent survey in Uganda succeeded in finding only one benign lump in 400 normal adult female breasts examined clinically (Omaswa and Luyombya, 1971, unpublished). Infective lesions in lactating breasts are very common and only a few are biopsied.

Benign Tumours

1. Fibroadenoma

Fifty-six examples were seen in African women. In the same period specimens from 24 fibroadenomata in Asians and 10 in Europeans were received in the Department. The presentation of fibroadenomata is calculated as being 200 times more frequent in Europeans than in Africans. This figure is probably a considerable falsification of the true position. Africans appear to be unwilling to submit to surgery unless a breast mass is huge, painful or ulcerated. For example, one histologically benign fibroadenoma in an African girl measured 15 cm in diameter and 30% of the masses seen were larger than 6 cm. Fibroadenomata were seen regularly among nursing personnel who are more aware of the desirability of investigation of breast masses. In American negroes fibroadenomata are considered to be somewhat more frequent than in whites. Many patients were lactating at the time of biopsy and it was usual to see quite marked proliferation of the ductular element of these nodules. Apart from this the histological appearance of tumours was not different from that seen elsewhere. The age distribution was exactly similar to that found in other countries (mean 20.6 years, range 7—38 years).

2. Duct Papilloma

Only one example was seen.

Malignant Tumours

Adenocarcinoma accounted for the vast majority of malignant tumours of the breast. Burkitt's tumour, the next most common histological type, was fairly easily distinguishable in that it presented as bilateral enlargement of the breast in pregnancy, at a much younger age than that at which carcinoma is common (SHEPHERD and WRIGHT, 1967). Soft tissue sarcomas were found quite frequently and were virtually impossible to differentiate from carcinoma prior to biopsy. Tumours of the skin of the breast were rare but skin accessory tumours arising in the axilla were very difficult to distinguish from tumours of the axillary tail.

Carcinoma of the Male Breast

Forty-two cases were seen, that is 12% of adenocarcinoma of the breast in Ugandans. This proportion is considerably higher than that reported from other countries. Theoretically this alteration in the ratio might be a result of reduction in the incidence of female cases, an increase in the incidence among males or both. Two surveys of cancer of the breast in males have both estimated that the incidence in Ugandan Africans was 0.2 cases per year per hundred thousand males (DAVIES et al., 1965; KAYABUKI et al., 1968). This figure closely approximates to the incidence in other parts of the world. This is in spite of the fact that many conditions thought to predispose to male breast cancer are very common in Uganda. For example, gynaecomastia and cirrhosis are common, malnutrition at some period of life is almost universal and Africans excrete larger quantities of oestrogenic adrenocortical hormones than age-matched Caucasian males (WANG, BULBROOK and CLIFFORD, 1966).

Histological study shows that all the different types of tumour (except lobular carcinoma) found in the female occur in males. The proportion of histological types in this series is similar to that seen in Ugandan females except for a possible greater proportion of mucous and papillary patterns.

Tumours were usually advanced at the time of presentation at hospital. Half the patients had ulceration of the lesion and a mass had been present for an average of one year. Metastases to the axillary nodes were frequently noted and a few patients were found to have skeletal metastases.

The mean age was higher in male patients (49 years) than in female patients (42 years). The age-specific incidence rates among females rises sharply and falls in older age groups (Fig. 1), while the peak in male patients shows a later apogee before falling. In other countries the age-specific incidence in males increases in older age groups whereas in Uganda it tends to fall (PELLAKALLIO and KALIMA, 1969).

Carcinoma of the Female Breast

Breast cancer accounts for 9.3% of malignant tumours in Ugandan females, a crude incidence of 147 cases per million females per year. Incidence surveys in different parts of the world have shown that African negro females are much less frequently affected than Caucasian women resident in industrial western countries. On average the difference is about five-fold (see DOLL, MUIR and WATERHOUSE, 1970). These variations may possibly be influenced by genetic factors, for in both

South Africa and California the incidence in black women is much lower than in whites. However, it is likely that environmental factors are at least as important in determining the incidence in a given community. The incidence in genetically similar people varies widely in different parts of the world (Table 2). Thus women in Nigeria have a low incidence, whereas their cousins in Jamaica and California show a progressive increase. Similarly, the variation in Semitic and Northern European people

Table 2. The incidence of breast cancer in women in different countries

Low risk		Moderate risk		High risk	
Poland (rural)	10.9	Norway (rural)	24.2	Norway (urban)	30.4
Arabs in Israel	5.5	Jews from Africa	17.1	Jews from U.S.	38.9
Ibadan	9.4	Jamaica	22.2	California negro	28.2
Kyadondo	10.8	Bombay Indians	13.9	South Africa white	39.6
Natal Bantu	8.0	Natal Indians	13.5	California white	42.8
Japan	9.7	Japanese in Hawaii	19.1		

all figures quoted are cases per 100,000 women per year.

is also wide. Japanese in Japan show a lower incidence than Japanese in Hawaii. It appears, therefore, that increasing affluence correlates well with increasing incidence. The age at first pregnancy (LOWE and MacMAHON, 1970) and dietary factors (HEMS, 1970) are both thought to be important in determining the incidence. In Uganda the young age at first pregnancy and the low fat content of the rural African diet might be expected to contribute to the low incidence. Studies on the hormonal status of African patients with carcinoma of the breast similar to those carried out elsewhere (MacMAHON et al., 1971) might prove of interest. A finding which is at variance with the above suggestions is the apparently high incidence of breast cancer in Khartoum (DAOUD et al., 1968) where the age at first pregnancy and length of lactation are on a par with those in Uganda.

The mean age of patients was 42 years (range 22—80) and 40% of patients were under the age of 45. A considerable proportion of the younger patients were pregnant or lactating at the time of presentation (SHEPHERD, 1964). The age-specific incidence rates of breast cancer in Caucasians tend to show a fairly rapid rise to the age of 45, with a post-menopausal plateau or dip preceding a sharp rise in older age groups. In Ugandan women the incidence rises to a peak at the age of 50 and then falls away rapidly. Fig. 1 shows the age-specific incidence rates of carcinoma of the breast and colon in females in Connecticut (EISENBERG, 1966). If the figures for colon are subtracted from the breast a third curve is derived. The general shape of this curve is very similar to the fourth curve, which is the age-specific incidence rate found in Ugandan women. Carcinoma of the colon is most probably due to a long-continued accumulative dietary factor and it is suggested that the older woman with breast cancer is suffering from a disease with a similar aetiology (HEMS, 1970). The additional component in the breast-cancer curve is possibly a hormonally dependent fraction rising to a peak at the age of the menopause and falling thereafter.

The proportional rate of cancer of the breast is very similar in most districts. There was no marked tribal difference except in the north of the country (which abuts on Sudan) where the proportional rate was somewhat lower, particularly in the Lango tribe. The reason for this reduction might well be due to social factors rather than a true reduction of incidence.

Histologically the vast majority of tumours were relatively poorly differentiated adenocarcinomas with a fibrotic stromal response. The distribution of the histological types is shown in Table 3. Medullary carcinoma was commonly diagnosed but only

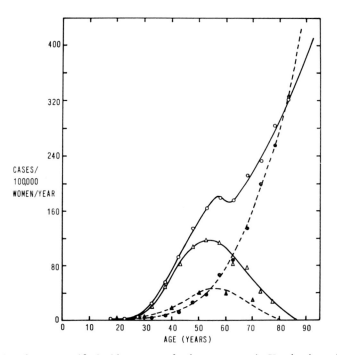

Fig. 1. Showing the age-specific incidence rates for breast cancer in Kyadondo and Connecticut. See text p. 97 for further explanation.

Code: ◯—◯ Connecticut females Ca. Breast
       ●—● Connecticut females Ca. Colon
       △—△ Curve 2 subtracted from curve 1
       ▲—▲ Ugandan females Ca. Breast

in 5 out of the 34 cases was there a well-marked lymphocytic response around the diagnosed in 3 patients, none of whom had involvement of axillary nodes or evidence of distant spread. Intraduct carcinoma was seldom seen without invasive tumour. Two of these patients had Paget's disease of the nipple and one was pregnant. Lobular carcinoma in situ was found in addition to invasive tumour in three cases. Attempts to identify invasive lobular carcinoma as distinct from ductular cancer was not successful. Six patients had Paget's disease of the nipple.

Tumours were graded according to the scheme originally propounded by PATEY and SCARFF (1928). This system was also used to grade a series in Scotland (TOUGH et al., 1969) which is used for comparison (Table 4). The age of patients in Uganda was much younger than in the Scottish series (47% under 45 as compared with 20%

Table 3. Histological types of adenocarcinoma of the breast in Uganda

	Females	Males
Adenocarcinom with fibrous reaction	223	32
Medullary	34	3
Mucous	10	3
Papillary	3	2
Intraduct	3	
Other patterns (cribriform, squamous, carcinosarcoma)	3	
Unclassified	3	
No histology	35	1
	314	41

in Scotland). There was no significant difference in grade in Ugandan patients of different ages. Scottish patients under the age of 45 showed a larger proportion of grade 3 tumours than in older patients but still had a greater proportion of grade 1 tumours than Ugandan patients of the same age. The stage of presentation is also related to grade and Ugandan patients presented much later than in Scotland

Table 4. Histological grading of adenocarcinoma of the breast in females

	Cases	Grade 1 %	Grade 2 %	Grade 3 %
Scotland	687	11	52	37
Uganda	270	3.5	52	44.5

Table 5. Staging of carcinoma of the breast at presentation in Scotland and Uganda

	Cases	Stage 1 %	Stage 2 %	Stage 3 %	Stage 4 %
Scotland	687	39	27	10	23
Uganda	269	4	22.5	52	21.5

(Table 5). Information for staging in Uganda was deficient and in many cases the stated stage represents a minimum, i. e. many of the patients tabulated as being stage 2 would probably be found to be in stage 3 if more information on the state of axillary glands had been available. Medullary tumours were found to involve the draining lymph nodes rather less frequently than scirrhous tumours in spite of the lack of reactive lymphocytes in the primary tumour. Only a tiny minority of Ugandan patients were found to have stage 1 tumours. Out of these 11 patients, 3 had intraduct carcinoma, 3 had papillar carcinomas, 1 cribriform pattern, 2 medullary and only 2 scirrhous tumours. The distribution of grading of all tumours in Uganda was very similar to that found among stage 4 tumours in Scotland. It is usually considered that the grade of tumour may determine the stage of presentation but it seems just as likely on this evidence that the stage determines the grade.

Other tumour types were seen much less frequently. One pure squamous carcinoma of the breast was diagnosed but extensive squamous metaplasia was seen in 2 others. Only one carcinosarcoma was diagnosed but pure connective tissue sarcomas were seen more frequently (9 cases). This latter group comprised two haemangiosarcomas, three fibrosarcomas and four undiagnosed soft tissue sarcomas. Lymphoma of the breast is unusual except for the occasional bilateral involvement of the breast in Burkitt's lymphoma. Such involvement is seen in pregnancy or lactation in young girls. It is invariably bilateral and may resolve spontaneously on cessation of lactation (Shepherd and Wright, 1968). Synchronous bilateral adenocarcinoma was not seen in any Ugandan patients, but 4 patients are known to have developed tumour later in the contralateral breast.

Chapter 6

Tumours of the Female Genitalia

P. D. James, C. W. Taylor, and A. C. Templeton

With 9 Figures

Cancer of the cervix is by far the commonest tumour of Ugandan women. The incidence is high in all parts of Uganda. Patients present late in the course of the disease and therapy is often impossible at this stage. Carcinoma of the corpus uteri is an uncommon tumour and often shows unusual histological patterns. Tumours of the ovary are common but mucinous cystadenomas appear to be relatively infrequent. Tumours of the vulva are unusual and are not often associated with obvious leukoplakia. Those tribes showing a high incidence of penile carcinoma also appear to have a higher incidence of vulval tumours. Choriocarcinoma and hydatidiform mole are probably no more common than in Caucasians. However, fertility statistics are difficult to obtain and incidence figures are therefore only approximate.

All tumours occurring in the female genital organs will be mentioned here, but tumours of soft tissues and lymphomata are discussed in greater detail under the relevant chapter headings. Benign tumours are markedly under-represented since the majority are probably not submitted for histological examination. The sample included 1387 benign tumours and tumour-like conditions, the majority of these (943 cases) being leiomyomata of the uterus. The site of origin of the different tumour types is shown in Table 1. The substance of this chapter is therefore concerned with malignant epithelial tumours of the female genital tract.

During the five-year period of this survey there was a total of 3,359 cases of cancer in females, and 1,209 (36%) of these malignant tumours arose in the genital tract. The lowest proportion in various registries around the world (DOLL, MUIR and WATERHOUSE, 1970) was 14.5% in Jewish females in Israel (STEINITZ, 1970). Most white populations in Europe and American had rations of about 20%. Negro populations in Africa, America and Jamaica all recorded high proportional rates varying between 31 and 35.5%. The highest recorded figure (48%) was found among the African population of Natal, South Africa(SCHONLAND, 1970); however the figures in this particular series were very small. Only one small series from Africa showed a relatively low incidence of 18% in the Bantu population of Cape Province, South Africa (MUIR, GRIEVE, 1970). The proportion of genital cancer in Indian females living in India or Africa is also high, accounting for 33% of cancer in Indian females in Natal (SCHONLAND, 1970) and 32% of cancer in females in Bombay (JUSSAWALLA, 1970).

Table 1. Primary gynaecological tumours seen in Uganda

	No. of cases	% gynaeco- logical malignancies	% of all female malignancy
Malignant			
171 Carcinoma of the cervix	751	62.5	22.3
175 Malignant ovarian tumours	223	18	7.1
173 Choriocarcinoma	68	6	2.0
172 Carcinoma of uterine body	49	4	1.5
176 Carcinoma of vulva	44	4	1.4
174 Uterine sarcomas	39	3	1.2
176 Carcinoma of vagina	19	2	0.6
176 Carcinoma of Fallopian tube	9	1	
Other gynaecological malignancies	7	1	
Sarcoma of cervix	(4)		
Malignant melanoma of vulva	(1)		
Fibrosarcoma of vulva	(1)		
Fibrosarcoma of Fallopian tube	(1)		
Total	1,209		
Benign			
Uterine Leiomyomata	943		
Hydatidiform mole	224		
Ovarian tumours	173		
Condyloma accuminata	42		
Vulval tumours	5		
Total	1,387		

Comparison of the relative proportions of tumours at other sites is difficult because of the different systems of classification of tumour types used. However, generally speaking, the incidence of tumours classified under rubrics 173 and 174 (chorio carcinoma and other tumours of the uterus) was higher in African series than in those from America or Europe. There was no significant racial difference between tumours classified under rubric 176 (other female genitalia) from various cancer registries.

The influence of non-neoplastic disease of the genital tract on the development of cancer is largely unknown. There is an association between cervical cancer and herpes simplex infection (Rawls et al., 1969) but whether this is causal or casual is undecided. The pattern of fertility will obviously influence the incidence of chorio-carcinoma. A brief review of infections of the genital tract and information on fertility patterns in Uganda is therefore germane to the present chapter.

Kibukamusoke (1965) stated that attendance at the Venereal Disease clinic at Mulago Hospital accounted for 10% of all out-patients. He studied 1000 consecutive cases of venereal disease and found that acute gonorrhoea was responsible for 54% of cases and syphilis for 4%. Any hospital-based series is likely to underestimate the true incidence, for example, it was only in 1969 that the first venereal disease clinic in Uganda exclusively for females was opened at Mulago. In addition, these figures derive from an urban population and therefore do not necessarily reflect the country-wide problem. Table 2 shows the incidence of venereal disease in government hospital out-patient departments recorded in two annual reports in which venereal diseases represented 3.7% and 5.1% of all out-patient attendances. The importance of gonococcal infections lies not only in the acute manifestations which are produced

Table 2. Out-patient visits to government hospitals

		1962—1963 [a]		1968—1969 [b]	
		No. of cases	% of total O.P.'s	No. of cases	% of total O.P.'s
Total male out-patients		756,902	47.3	1,647,119	49.8
Total female out-patients		842,720	52.7	1,630,486	50.2
All out-patients		1,599,622		3,277,605	
Cases of	Male	3,193		3,371	
syphilis:	Female	4,441		2,631	
	Total	7,634	0.5	6,002	0.2
Cases of	Male	24,542		85,442	
gonorrhoea:	Female	17,752		42,222	
	Total	42,294	2.6	127,667	3.9
Cases of	Male	147		746	
ophthalmia	Female	117		581	
neonatorum:	Total	264	0.01	1,327	0.04
Other	Male	5,634		17,721	
venereal	Female	4,404		13,582	
diseases:	Total	10,038	0.6	31,303	0.9
All	Male	33,516		107,280	
venereal	Female	26,714		59,016	
diseases:	Total	60,230	3.7	166,296	5.1

[a] Annual report of the Ministry of Health, Uganda, 1st July, 1962 to 30th June, 1963.
[b] Medical Services Statistical Records, Ministry of Health, Uganda, 1st July, 1968 to 30th June, 1969.

but also in the complications which may result. A strong correlation between gonorrhoea, sterility and urethral stricture, particularly among the Teso and Baganda, has been shown (GRIFFITH, 1963). The social determinants of gonorrhoea in an East African town (BENNETT, 1962) and the rural pattern of transmission (BENNETT, 1964) have been described. Venereal diseases are also an important predisposing factor in pelvic inflammatory diseases and trichomonas vaginalis infections were found in 40% of 10,000 exfoliative cytology specimens obtained from out-patients in Kampala (TRUSSELL, 1968). Chancroid, lymphogranuloma venereum and granuloma inguinale are all seen regularly. Syphilis was probably introduced in the middle of the 19th century and rapidly reached epidemic proportions (DAVIES, 1956).

The population of Uganda is rising rapidly. Fertility rates are high but show considerable variation in different parts of the country. Rates, expressed as live births per year per 1000 women aged between 16 and 45 years were 169 in Eastern Region, 170 in Buganda, 207 in Western Region and 215 in Northern Region (Uganda Census, 1959). The peak fertility rate was found in the age group 20—24 years in most tribes and rates fall rapidly among older women. In the peak group the fertility rates exceeded 400 in all but two tribes, the Basoga and the Teso. The reduction of fertility among women over the age of 25 has been ascribed to the high incidence of gonorrhoea. Griffith (1963) estimated that half the women of the Baganda tribe were sterile as a result of gonorrhoea by the age of 30. In most tribes fertility rates are already quite high in the 15—19 years age group, reflecting an early age of first intercourse and first pregnancy. Both these factors are significant in the pathogenesis of cervical cancer (Malhotra, 1971). There are a number of reasons why this might be so but among them are included the possible influence of smegma (see Chapter 7) or spermatozoa (Coppleson and Reid, 1967). There is some evidence to suggest that women using barrier contraceptives are less likely to develop cervical cancer (Melamed et al., 1969). Bennett (1962) has pointed out that the use of contraceptive sheaths is considered an insult by Baganda women. The procreative aspect of sexual intercourse is of no deterrent to most Uganda women, as a high proportion are either sterile or actively trying not to be proved so.

Carcinoma of the Vulva

The histological diagnoses of tumours of the vulva and vagina seen in this period are shown in Table 3. Benign tumours are not further discussed.

Table 3. To show the histological types of tumours of the vulva and vagina

Carcinoma of vulva (+1 without biopsy)	44 (+1)
Carcinoma of vagina	19
Adenoma of Bartholin's gland	2
Granular cell myoblastoma	2
Other tumours of vulva:	
In situ carcinoma	
Fibrosarcoma	1 case each
Malignant melanoma	
Fibroma	
Total	72

Forty-four carcinomas were seen, that is 4% of female genital malignancies and 1.4% of all malignant tumours in females. The age ranged from 26—70 years (mean 43 years). The age distribution is shown in Table 4. Twenty-three patients (58%) were under 45 years of age at presentation.

The Ganda and Teso tribes accounted for nearly half the cases. The Baganda account for one-third of cancer overall, a proportion resulting from their numerical superiority and proximity to Mulago Hospital (see Chapter 1). The relatively large proportion of Teso is unexplained but it is of interest that this tribe records a high incidence of acute gonococcal infections (GRIFFITH, 1963). The tribes with the highest incidence of vulval cancer (Toro, Teso, Ganda) also have a high rate of penile carcinoma (see Chapter 7).

Table 4. Age distribution of carcinoma of the vulva and vagina

Age	Ca. vulva	Ca. vagina	Combined
0—14	0	0	0
15—24	0	1	1
25—34	10	1	11
35—44	13	3	16
45—54	9	4	13
55—64	6	7	13
65—74	3	2	5
75+	0	0	0
"Adult"	3	1	4
Total	44	19	63

The majority of tumours were well differentiated keratinizing squamous cell carcinomas (Table 5). One basal cell carcinoma was seen. Two cases were not histologically classifiable because of lack of satisfactory material. A prominent infiltration by eosinophils was seen around the tumour in some cases; this was also found in some squamous cell carcinomas of the cervix. No parasites were identified histologically to explain this finding and it may possibly represent some immunological reaction against the tumour. No distinctive tribal or geographical distribution was found which distinguished tumours with eosinophils from those that did not show this feature.

Table 5. Histological grading of carcinoma of the vulva and vagina

	Ca. vulva	Ca. vagina
Well differentiated	24	8
Average differentiation	10	3
Poorly differentiated	7	8
Basal cell carcinoma	1	—
Not classifiable	2	—
Total	44	19

Discussion

The proportion of histologically proven cases relative to other gynaecological malignancies is similar to that seen outside Africa (PALMER, SADUGOR and REINHARD, 1949; HARTNETT, 1952; CHARLES, 1972). Previous studies from Uganda (DAVIES and

Wilson, 1954; Davies, Knowelden and Wilson, 1965) and other parts of Africa (Prates, 1958; Higginson and Oettlé, 1960; Lynch, Verzin and Hassan, 1963; Edington and Maclean, 1965) record proportional rates essentially similar to our own.

Fourteen of the 44 cases (35%) were seen at Mulago Hospital, which gives some indication of the extent of under-diagnosis in other parts of the country.

Carcinoma of the vulva has been described as a disease of post-menopausal and elderly females (Hertig and Gore, 1960). In Uganda the mean age of onset is nearly 20 years younger than in series from outside Africa (Palmer et al., 1949; Charles, 1972) and about two-thirds of all patients were under 50 years of age at the time of diagnosis. This distribution is partly explained by the population structure of Uganda but the mean age of onset is nearly ten years earlier than that in Sudanese women (Lynch et al., 1963) where the age structure of the population is similar. We have no explanation for this early onset. Gonococcal or other venereal infections and poor standards of hygiene are possible influences but no direct evidence is available to incriminate these factors. In clinical practice it is most unusual to find leukoplakia of the vulva, and biopsies from only two such cases were seen during this five-year period. Condyloma accuminata occur extremely frequently and some grow to enormous size. Some controversy surrounds the possible precancerous nature of giant condylomata but in none of the cases of carcinoma did the history suggest transition from one of these entities to the other. There was no history of lymphogranuloma venereum infection in any of our cases.

Carcinoma of the Vagina

Nineteen cases were seen during the five-year period, that is, 1.7% of neoplasms of the female genitalia and 0.6% of all malignant tumours in females. Carcinoma of the vulva was approximately twice as common as carcinoma of the vagina.

The age at diagnosis ranged from 21—70 years, mean 50.9 years (Table 4). Six patients were under 50 at presentation and 12 were less than 60 years old. Tribal distribution showed no predominance in any group. All the malignant tumours were squamous cell carcinomas. The histological grading of these cases is shown in Table 5. Nearly half the tumours in the present series were poorly differentiated. In Uganda, as in other countries, squamous cell carcinoma of the vagina is less well differentiated than carcinoma of the vulva, most tumours being of intermediate or poor differentiation (Livingstone, 1950).

Discussion

The age of presentation is earlier than that seen outside Africa (Livingstone, 1950) but the difference is not so marked as with carcinoma of the vulva. The proportion of carcinoma of the vagina relative to other tumours of the genitalia is similar to that seen in America (Frick, Jacox and Taylor, 1968). Direct comparison with other African countries is difficult because of the small numbers and because most registries combine the returns for carcinoma of the vulva and vagina. However, the incidence and pattern of disease among Sudanese (Lynch et al., 1963) and the

South Africa Bantu (HIGGINSON et al., 1960) are essentially similar to our findings in Uganda.

Carcinoma of the Cervix

Carcinoma of the cervix is by far the commonest cancer of women in Uganda, accounting for 22.3% of cases overall. The incidence in Kyadondo County was 24.3 cases per year per 100,000 women (corrected for a standard African population). The figure for Uganda as a whole was 4.7 cases. This lower figure is largely a result of under-diagnosis in rural districts, but there is some evidence to suggest that the incidence in some tribes is in fact lower than in the Baganda who constitute the majority of people living in Kyadondo County.

Table 6. Age distribution in cases of carcinoma of the uterine body and cervix. Cases in which the age was not stated have been distributed in proportion with patients of known age

Age	Ca. cervix	Ca. corpus uteri
0—14	0	0
15—24	16	0
25—34	163	5
35—44	253	13
45—54	174	14
55—64	107	10
65—74	30	7
75+	8	0
Total	751	49

The age at diagnosis ranged from 15—90 years (mean 42 years) (Table 6). The age-specific incidence rate shows a rapid rise up to the age of 50 years and a fall thereafter (Fig. 1). The fall in older age groups is probably at least partly a result of factors governing appearance at hospital rather than a true fall in incidence. The figures for the country as a whole are much lower and rise to a plateau between the ages of 40 and 60 years before falling away in older age groups.

Histologically tumours were classified as follows:—

1. Keratinizing squamous carcinomas — 153 cases. These tumours showed prominent areas of keratinization in islands of easily recognizable squamous cells.

2. Poorly differentiated squamous carcinoma — 55 cases. The cells were large and pleiomorphic, usually rounded but sometimes spindle-shaped. Small areas of more differentiated tumour were present.

3. Undifferentiated — 406 cases. The tumour usually consisted of a monotonous sheet of cells with large nuclei and prominent nucleoli. Less frequently the cells were small and uniform, an appearance described as basaloid or transitional.

4. Adenocarcinoma — 36 cases. These were usually of average-grade malignancy.

5. Unclassifiable — in 13 cases the amount of material available for study was not sufficient to classify the tumours satisfactorily.

The diagnosis in a further 88 cases was made on cytological evidence only. There was no significant difference in the age or tribal distribution of each histological type of tumour.

A moderate to marked infiltration by eosinophils was seen in and around tumour deposits in about a quarter of cases overall. The intensity of the infiltrate did not vary significantly between the various histological groups outlined previously. However, in the undifferentiated variety the infiltrate was more marked in tumours composed of large cells than in the transitional or basaloid tumours, and occurred in about one-third of cases in the former group.

An exfoliative cytology service opened in 1964 on a limited experimental basis [1]. The service was originally available to women attending the Gynaecological Clinic at Mulago Hospital but has recently been extended to include all the larger towns in Uganda. During the study period 24,760 cervical smears were examined and on the basis of the cytological findings 119 cone biopsies were performed. This figure underestimates the true incidence of severe cytological abnormality, as only about 60% of women for whom biopsy is recommended consent to operation and have a histological diagnosis. The biopsy findings are shown in Table 7.

Table 7. Histological findings in 119 cone biopsies recommended following abnormal smear (1964—1968)

	No. of cases
Normal	10
Chronic cervicitis	12
Squamous metaplasia	12
Squamous hyperplasia	3
Mild dysplasia	10
Moderate dysplasia	12
Severe dysplasia	8
Carcinoma in situ	43
Microinvasive carcinoma	3
Invasive squamous cell carcinoma	4
Adenocarcinoma	2
Total	119

Monilia and Trichomonas vaginalis infections were a frequent finding in the smears examined, the latter occurring in about one-third of cases; the filarial worm *Dipetolenema perstants* was also occasionally seen (Sharma, Zeigler and Trussell, 1971). The incidence rate of abnormal smears in women attending Family Planning Association clinics was much lower than those from gynaecological outpatients, a fact probably explained by the higher social class of the former group. A more detailed account of exfoliative cervical cytology in Uganda will be published (Leighton, Zeigler, Trussell and Sharma, 1972).

---

1 Funded by the Cancer Research Campaign.

The majority of patients presented late in the course of the disease and in many cases the diagnosis was all too obvious and no biopsy was taken. Treatment by radical surgery was carried out in a few cases but in the majority little could be done. No facilities exist for radiotherapy in Uganda at present though it is hoped to introduce a service in the near future. Local perfusion with cytotoxic agents intra-arterially has been used with some good short-term responses (TRUSSELL, 1962).

Cancer of the cervix is common in all parts of Uganda but there are considerable variations in different tribes. It accounts for 30% of all cancer among the Acholi but only 10% among the Lugbara. These two tribes are equally well served with medical facilities and there is little reason to suppose that this variation in proportion is due to diagnostic bias. The incidence of carcinoma of the penis is higher in the Acholi than in the Lugbara and there is some broad correlation between the percentages of these two tumours in the different tribes of Uganda (see Chapter 7). This would suggest that some factors are involved in the development of both tumours. An association between the two diseases occurring in married partners has been noted in Puerto Rico (MARTINEZ, 1969). Fertility rates vary in different parts of the country, being highest in Northern Region and lowest in Eastern Region. There is no sustained relationship between fertility and proportional rates of cervical carcinoma in different tribes.

Discussion

Except in orthodox Jewish communities carcinoma of the cervix is a common cancer of women in all countries of the world. The highest rates are to be found in Africa and South America (DOLL, MUIR and WATERHOUSE, 1970). These communities in which cervical cancer is common are characterized by a low standard of living,

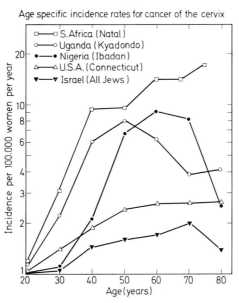

Fig. 1. Graph showing the age specific incidence rates of carcinoma of the cervix in different communities

high fertility and an early age at first intercourse (Stern and Dixon, 1961; Eliott, 1964). The frequency of intercourse is also related to the incidence of cervical carcinoma (Malhotra, 1971). Within communities the disease occurs more frequently in the lower social groups than the higher. Age-specific incidence rates of carcinoma of the cervix from different countries are shown in Fig. 1. African series show a much higher rate among young adults than is found in Connecticut. In Africa the fall in older women is probably at least in part due to failure of diagnosis due to social factors. The curve of incidence in Ibadan, Nigeria, is very similar to that in Kyadondo but delayed by a decade. We have no explanation as to why this might be unless the younger women in Ibadan are destined to have a lower incidence than the present population, thus introducing a cohort effect.

Factors thought to be important in the causation of cervical cancer include viruses such as herpes genitalis (British Medical Journal, 1970), spermatozoa (Coppleson and Reid, 1967), chemicals such as smegma (Heins, Dennis, Pratt-Thomas and Charleston, 1958), and a low standard of genital hygiene (British Medical Journal, 1964). The apparent variation in incidence among the different tribes of Uganda affords a natural experiment where the effect of these factors might be measured.

Carcinoma of the Uterine Body

Forty-nine cases of endometrial carcinoma were seen, which represents 4.4% of female genital cancers and 1.5% of all cancers in females. In Kyadondo County the incidence rate was 1.5 cases per 100,000 women per year (corrected for an African standard population), but this calculation is based on only eight cases. The incidence is similar to that found in Nigeria and Rhodesia, Japan and India, and is significantly lower than that reported in Jews or Caucasians (Doll, Muir and Waterhouse, 1970). There were 751 cases of cervical carcinoma seen during the same period, that is a cervix-to-body ratio of 15.3 to 1.

The age at presentation ranged from 27 to 70 years with a mean of 49.2 years (Table 6). Six patients were under 40 and almost half were under 50 at the time of presentation. Sixteen patients were seen at Mulago Hospital and the clinical notes were available for study, but apart from these cases little clinical information was recorded. Information as to parity was available in only 13 cases. Three married patients were infertile, five had had no normal full-term deliveries and six had had more than two pregnancies. Blood pressure recordings were noted in 12 patients and in only one case was there an isolated diastolic blood pressure exceeding 100 mm Hg. This returned to normal limits following hysterectomy. The mean diastolic blood pressure was 80 mm Hg in the remaining patients. In the above group one woman was a known diabetic and in another case glycosuria was reported post-operatively. No further details were available. Body weights were not recorded but generally speaking obesity is relatively uncommon in Uganda.

Histological Classification

It was difficult to classify the tumours under study as many of them were unlike uterine carcinomas seen outside Uganda and a mixture of histological patterns was a frequent finding. A simple classification was adopted as outlined below.

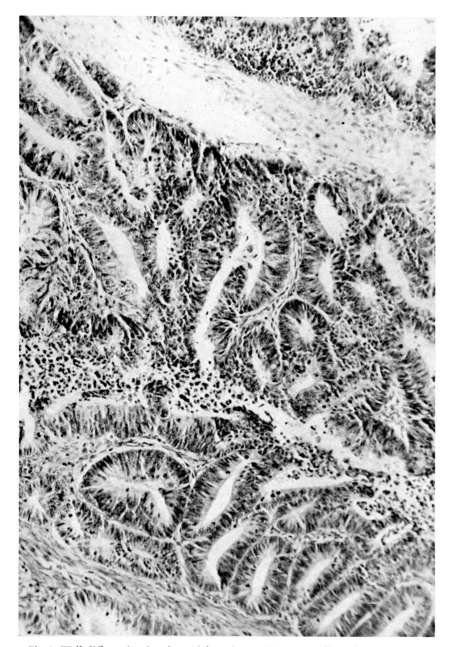

Fig. 2. Well differentiated endometrial carcinoma (Haematoxylin and Eosin) ×125

1. Well differentiated endometrial carcinoma (Fig. 2). The bulk of the tumour consisted of well formed glandular spaces of regular size, mitoses were variable but were usually less than 3 per H.P.F.

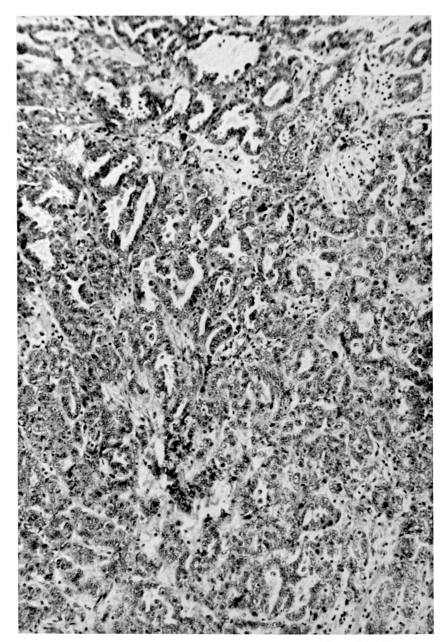

Fig. 3. Poorly differentiated endometrial carcinoma (Haematoxylin and Eosin) ×125

2. Poorly differentiated endometrial carcinoma (Fig. 3). The major part of the tumour consisted of sheets of cells but a few recognizable glandular spaces were present.

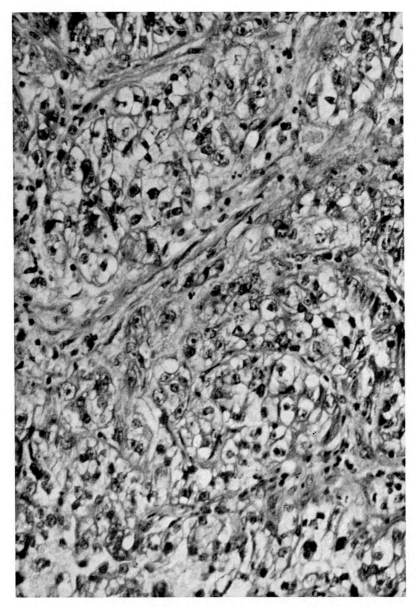

Fig. 4. Anaplastic Adenocarcinoma (Haematoxylin and Eosin) ×300

3. Anaplastic adenocarcinoma (Fig. 4). Solid sheets of cells with no recognizable glandular elements.

4. Papillary adenocarcinoma. The well differentiated papillary adenocarcinoma had a connective tissue stroma covered by regular epithelium with few mitoses; this was the predominant pattern in four cases. A further subgroup of tumours was noted in which the epithelial cells had hyperchromatic nuclei situated away from the

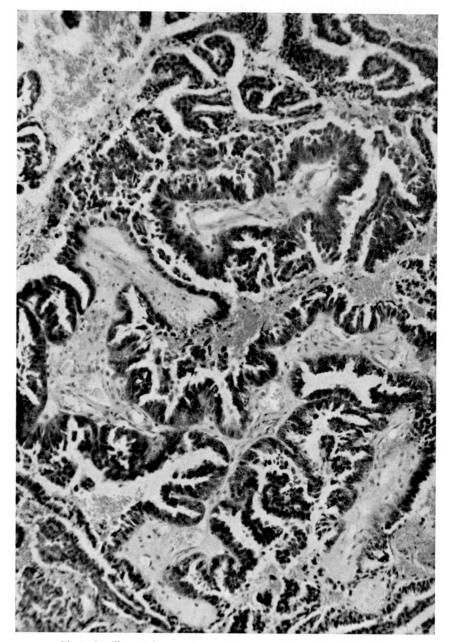

Fig. 5. Papillary Adenocarcinoma (Haematoxylin and Eosin) ×125

basement membrane of the cell, producing a "peg shaped" appearance. Five such cases were seen (Fig. 5). The remaining tumours showed a mixture of papillary and solid areas and some had a prominent clear-cell component (Fig. 6).

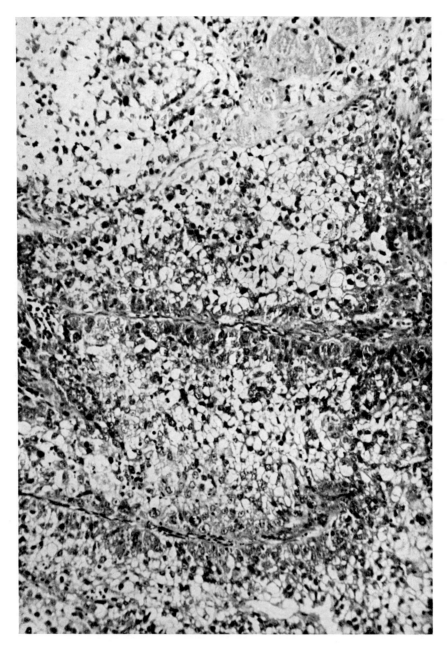

Fig. 6. Clear-cell areas in an Endometrial Carcinoma (Haematoxylin and Eosin) ×125

Two cases were histologically unclassifiable because of the small amounts of material available for study. The number of cases in each group is shown in Table 8. Squamous metaplasia was seen in tumours in most of the tumour groups (Table 8)

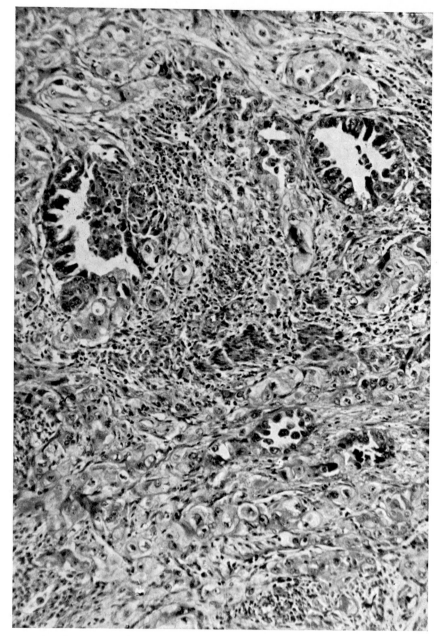

Fig. 7. Areas of Squamous Metaplasia in an Endometrial Carcinoma
(Haematoxylin and Eosin) ×125

but was a marked feature in only two cases (Fig. 7). No significant age differences
were noted in the various groups (Table 8) although the only three patients under
30 had well differentiated endometrial carcinomas.

Table 8. Histological types of endometrial carcinoma

	No.	Age range (years)	Mean	No. of cases with squamous metaplasia
Endometrial carcinoma (well differentiated)	12	27—70	48	5
Endometrial carcinoma (poorly differentiated)	15	39—68	52	3
Anaplastic carcinoma	7	31—65	49	3
Papillary adenocarcinoma	13	40—70	50	4
Unclassifiable	2	30 and 40	35	—

Discussion

Endometrial cancer is an uncommon tumour in African women. The comparison of age-standardized incidence rates may be misleading with such a small series, but the figure from Uganda is lower than that from other countries (DOLL, MUIR and WATERHOUSE, 1970). Table 9 shows carcinoma of the cervix as a proportion of cancer overall and cervix-to-body ratios in various parts of the world. Since the mean age at onset for cervical carcinoma is lower than for carcinoma of the body, cervix/body ratios have been calculated after age standardization. Cervix/body ratios from white populations are close to unity and endometrial carcinoma represents from one quarter to one third of gynaecological cancer. In African populations, on the other hand, ratios range from 7.5 to 20 to 1, that is endometrial cancer accounts for 4.1 to 7.6% of gynaecological cancer. The incidence of cancer of the corpus in the negro population of Alameida County, California is very similar to that in white populations

Table 9. Showing the proportional rates of cancer of the uterine body and cervix together with the ratio between them (compiled from DOLL, MUIR and WATERHOUSE, 1970)

Country	Proportion of gynaecological cancer represented by cancer of the		Cervix to body ratio
	Cervix	Body	
Nigeria:	52.6	4.1	12.2 : 1
Rhodesia:	66.6	4.8	13.0 : 1
South Africa (Cape Province):			
White	47.6	29.4	1.6 : 1
Coloured	66.6	14.7	4.4 : 1
Bantu	58.8	7.6	7.5 : 1
U.S.A. California: White	35.7	35.7	1.0 : 1
Black	52.6	25.6	2.0 : 1
Israel: Jews	18.1	33.3	0.6 : 1
U.K.: Birmingham	34.4	25.6	1.3 : 1
Uganda: Kampala	50.3	4.3	13.5 : 1

(Linden, 1970), suggesting that environmental factors play an important part in the pathogenesis of uterine cancer.

In Western communities the proportion of endometrial cancer relative to cervical carcinoma is changing. Twenty years ago cervical carcinoma was six to eight times as common as cancer of the corpus but more recently the proportions have become closer to unity. This change is probably influenced by the better prophylaxis of cervical cancer and by the greater longevity enjoyed by women in the modern world. Sall, Sonnenblick and Stone (1970) reported that in the U.S.A. endometrial cancer represented 31% of gynaecological malignancy, a percentage figure 7 times greater than that found in Uganda. Carcinoma of the uterine body is usually considered as a disease of the elderly female, the mean age at presentation is generally in the late fifties (Novak and Woodruff, 1962; Payling Wright and Symmers, 1966). Numerous studies have drawn attention to the association of endometrial cancer with diabetes, hypertension, obesity, infertility and other metabolic disorders (Lewis, 1965). Early marriage and multiple pregnancies are commonplace in Uganda and the life expectancy in women is lower than in Western countries. The elderly, pyknic, infertile, hypertensive and diabetic female who is the archetypal candidate for endometrial carcinoma is only rarely to be found in Uganda.

In Uganda only a quarter of the uterine carcinomas seen were histologically well differentiated adenocarcinomas and a similar number were papillary in type. Nearly half the cases in the latter group displayed the unusual histological pattern already described (Fig. 5). Although papillary formation is often seen in endometrial carcinoma (Haines and Taylor, 1962), predominantly papillary tumours seem to be an unusual variant in series from countries where the disease is common.

Woodruff, Julian and Novak (1970) argue that the similar embryological origins of the female genital tract and the normal responsiveness of the endometrium to various stimuli could lead to a confusing array of tumours. The majority of studies on endometrial cancer emphasize the typical histological pattern of tumour seen, and mention is only rarely made of less typical pictures. In many series well differentiated adenocarcinomas account for about half the histological patterns seen (Dobbie, Taylor and Waterhouse, 1965; Yahia, Benirschke and Sturgis, 1963). The distribution of uterine malignancy in Jamaica is similar to that in Uganda. Endometrial carcinoma accounts for only 2% of cancer in Jamaican females (Persaud and Knight, 1968) and 14% of these tumours were papillary adenocarcinomas.

It is possible that where endometrial cancer is common the unusual patterns of malignancy are overshadowed by the more typical types and that where it is rare these types assume a greater proportion. The corollary of this finding is that the endocrine anomalies which appear to influence the frequency of endometrial carcinoma are not the pathogenetic factors involved in the papillary types of tumour. Statistics are difficult to obtain but it is probable that the incidence of papillary tumours is much more stable across the world than endometrial carcinoma of the more usual type.

Uterine Sarcomas

The classification adopted for this study is shown in Table 10. Carcinosarcomas and mixed mesodermal tumours are dealt with separately although many authors

consider that they differ only in histological pattern (CHUANG, VAN VELDEN and
GRAHAM, 1970). Rhabdomyosarcomas have also been separated although some may
be examples of mixed mesodermal tumours.

Sarcomas of the uterine body accounted for 3.4% of gynaecological malignancies
and 1.2% of all female malignant tumours.

Table 10. Showing the distribution of histological types of sarcomas of the uterus

	No. of cases	% of sarcomas	Age range (years)	Mean age (years)
Mixed mesodermal tumours	11	28.2	40—70	54.0
Carcinosarcomas	4	10.3	36—60	48.2
Stromal sarcomas	2	5.1	50—60	55.0
Leiomyosarcomas	16	41.0	23—60	40.0
Rhabdomyosarcomas	3	7.7	$1^1/_2$—60	38.2
Sarcomas N.O.S.	3	7.7	48—70	56.0
Total	39	100.0	$1^1/_2$—70	47.3

The mean age at presentation for all sarcomas was 47.3 years which is similar to
that of endometrial carcinoma. Leiomyosarcomas and rhabdomyosarcomas presented
at a younger age than other sarcomas.

There was no significant tribal preponderance.

Histological Features

A diagnosis of carcinosarcoma was made when a tumour consisted of a mixture
of glandular epithelium and connective tissue elements but showed no differentiation
towards heterologous tissue. By contrast, all mixed mesodermal tumours contained
heterologous elements, most commonly cartilage and striated muscle (Figs. 8 and 9).
In five cases either cartilage or striated muscle was seen and one tumour contained
both. The glandular element was usually poorly differentiated and nuclei were often
terminally situated producing a "peg cell" appearance; papillary and clear cell areas
were occasionally seen. The histological features of the other tumours were essentially
similar to those described from other countries.

Discussion

Carcinoma and sarcoma of the uterine body are uncommon tumours in Uganda
and account for 10.2% of uterine malignancies. Endometrial carcinoma is much less
frequent in Uganda than elsewhere and uterine sarcomas therefore appear relatively
more common (Table 11), and there are also small differences in the relative
frequencies of individual tumours (Table 12). In the present series leiomyosarcomas
accounted for 41% of sarcomas and were the commonest histological type; this
proportion is rather lower than in some series. Mixed mesodermal tumours, on the
other hand, account for a slightly higher proportion of sarcomas in Uganda, but this

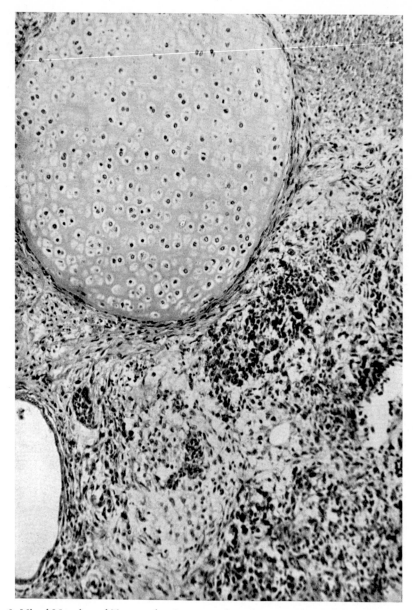

Fig. 8. Mixed Mesodermal Tumour showing areas of cartilage (Haematoxylin and Eosin) ×125

is probably due to varying criteria in differentiating such tumours from carcino-sarcomas since the combined percentages are very similar in different series. During the period of study 943 benign uterine leiomyomas and 16 leiomyosarcomas were seen. Malignant tumours are much more likely to be sent to the laboratory and this suggests that malignant transformation occurs in considerably less than 2% of uterine

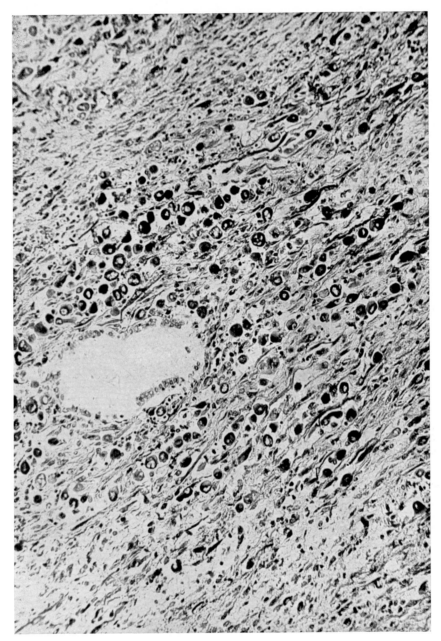

Fig. 9. Mixed Mesodermal Tumour showing Rhabdomyosarcomatous areas
(Haematoxylin and Eosin) ×125

fibroids. In no case was there incontrovertible evidence of a pre-existing benign tumour in which a malignant tumour was found. This situation would be expected to occur more commonly if sarcomas always arose in pre-existing benign tumours.

Table 11. Relative proportions of different uterine tumours (excluding choriocarcinoma) in various series compared with Uganda

	Canada 1950 [a]	New York 1952 [b]	Louisiana 1959 [c]	Ohio 1962 [d]	New York 1970 [e]	Uganda 1964— 1968
Carcinoma of cervix	74.1	57.8	88.6	83.0	73.8	89.4
Carcinoma of body	23.4	36.0	8.8	14.9	17.4	5.7
Uterine sarcomas	2.5	5.5	2.6	2.1	3.5	4.5
Others		0.7				0.4
Carcinoma of body and cervix					5.3	
Total cases in each series	1696	464	1301	1790	1946	839

[a] MacFarlane, 1950
[b] Fenton and Burke, 1952
[c] Crawford and Tucker, 1959
[d] Boutselis and Ullery, 1962
[e] Chuang, Van Velden and Graham, 1970

Table 12. The proportions of different types of uterine sarcoma in various series

	Louisiana 1959 [a]	Ohio 1962 [b]	Los Angeles 1963 [c]	New York 1967 [d]	New York 1968 [e]	New York 1970 [f]	Uganda 1964— 1968
Leiomyosarcoma	76.5	39	60.5	44.8	48.7	40.6	41.0
Stromal sarcoma	8.8	14	6.1	9.6	10.4	11.8	5.1
Mixed mesodermal	14.7	41	21.2	20.0	21.7	16.9	28.2
Carcinosarcoma	—	5	3.1	25.6	19.2	23.6	10.3
Rhabdomyosarcoma	—	—	9.1	—	—	2.6	7.7
Others	—	—	—	—	—	0.9	—
Unclassifiable	—	—	—	—	—	2.6	7.7
Total number	34	36	33	125	115	118	39

[a] Crawford and Tucker, 1959
[b] Boutselis and Ullery, 1962
[c] Edwards, Sterling, Keller and Nolan, 1963
[d] Bartsich, O'Leary and Moore, 1967
[e] Bartsich, Bowe and Moore, 1968
[f] Chuang, Van Velden and Graham, 1970

Rhabdomyosarcoma is a rare tumour of the uterus. Middlebrook and Tennant (1968) found 35 cases recorded in the literature. Four cases of rhabdomyosarcoma were recorded in Uganda during the present five-year study, three of which arose in the uterine body and one in the cervix. The cervical tumour occurred in a 20-year-old woman, and the patients with uterine tumours were $1^1/_2$, 55 and 60 years of age.

Generally speaking the age at presentation of the rhabdomyosarcoma increases as the site of origin moves caudally from vagina to uterus; vaginal rhabdomyosarcomas occurring in children, the uterine varieties in the elderly.

Mixed mesodermal tumours and carcinosarcomas are often associated with previous pelvic irradiation. This factor cannot explain the high incidence of these tumours in Uganda as X-ray facilities are few and limited to diagnostic purposes.

Direct comparison with other studies from Africa is difficult because all uterine tumours are often classified together without any indication as to whether sarcomas are included or not. In the Sudan uterine sarcomas represented 0.2% of female cancer (LYNCH et al., 1963). EDINGTON and MACLEAN (1965) recorded 7 uterine sarcomas in 341 malignancies from the female genital tract, an incidence of 2%. In the West Indies uterine sarcomas account for about 1% of all female malignancies (PERSAUD and KNIGHT, 1968). These figures are similar to those quoted for Caucasian populations in standard textbook. It would seem, therefore, that uterine sarcomas are no more common in African races than in Caucasian and that the incidence in Uganda does not differ significantly from elsewhere.

Sarcomas occur more commonly in the post-menopausal female and the age distribution is similar to that reported for endometrial carcinoma (NOVAK et al., 1962). The mean age at presentation in Uganda (Table 10) was younger than that reported elsewhere. This partly reflects the younger population but is further reduced by the inclusion of a $1^{1}/_{2}$-year-old child with a rhabdomyosarcoma. Rhabdomyosarcomas and the sarcomas of endometrial origin (mixed mesodermal tumours, carcinosarcomas and stromal sarcomas) occurred at a significantly later age than the leiomyosarcomas but this is in keeping with experience outside Uganda (BARTSICH et al., 1968).

Trophoblastic Disease

Histological material from 224 hydatidiform moles, 55 choriocarcinomas and 12 chorioadenoma destruens were seen in the period under review.

Incidence

The incidence of different forms of trophoblastic disease are usually expressed as the number of cases per pregnancy. In Uganda this is problematic since there is no effective birth registration and only about 30% of deliveries are supervised by qualified personnel (TRUSSELL, GRECH and GALEA, 1968). The number of abortions

Table 13. Showing the incidence of hydatidiform mole, chorioadenoma destruens and choriocarinoma in Uganda (expressed as cases per pregnancy)

	In Uganda	In Mulago Hospital
Pregnancies	400,000 per year	12,000 per year
Hydatidiform mole	1 in 9,000	1 in 1,500
Chorioadenoma destruens	1 in 166,000	1 in 60,000
Choriocarcinoma	1 in 36,000	1 in 15,000

occurring in the country, particularly in early pregnancy, is entirely unknown. From the rate of increase in the Ugandan population between 1959 and 1969, it is estimated that there were approximately 400,000 pregnancies each year in the country. Rates calculated on this basis are shown in Table 13. These results are a considerable underestimate and it is probably much more accurate to work from the returns of a single hospital. Mulago Hospital dealt with approximately 12,000 pregnancies annually in the years of this survey (Department of Obstetrics Annual Report, 1966—1967). Calculation of incidence of trophoblastic disease is potentially biased by referral of cases from other hospitals. Only those cases which were first seen at Mulago Hospital, excluding those delivered elsewhere, are considered. The incidence figures so calculated (Table 14) are likely to be reasonably representative for the country as a whole. Table 14 also shows the incidence of hydatidiform mole and malignant trophoblastic disease in different countries.

Table 14. Incidence of trophoblastic disease in different countries expressed as cases per pregnancy

	Hydatidiform mole	Malignant trophoblastic disease
Indonesia (Soejoenoes et al., 1967)	85—300	—
Asia (Joint Project, 1959)		250—3708
Philippines (Acosta Sison, 1967)	173	1,400
Australia (Beescher and Fortune, 1968)	695	—
U.S.A. (Douglas, 1959)	1,000	—
Uganda	1,500	12,000
U.S.A. (Brewer and Gerbie, 1967)	1699 (deliveries) 2093 (pregnancies)	20,000
U.K. (Park, 1967)	2,000	50,000 (fatal cases only)

Table 15. Incidence rates of malignant trophoblastic disease in different countries (expressed as cases per 100,000 females per year, corrected for an African standard population)

South Africa	Natal, African	3.1
Nigeria	Ibadan	2.9
Rhodesia	Bulawayo	2.3
Japan	Miyagi	1.6
U.S.A.	California, Negro	1.5
Uganda	Kyadondo Country	1.2
Jamaica		1.1
Norway		0.4
India	Bombay	0.3
Israel	All Jews	0.2
U.S.A.	Connecticut	0.04

All figures except Uganda taken from "Cancer Incidence in 5 Continents", Vols. 1 and 2 (Doll, Payne and Waterhouse, 1966; Doll, Muir and Waterhouse, 1970).

Another method of expressing the incidence of trophoblastic disease is in terms of the population. This method takes no cognizance of the fertility rates in different communities but figures are available from a wider range of African countries and are shown in Table 15. The Ugandan figure quoted is based on Kyadondo County returns. Ugandan women seem to fall midway between the extremes of Eastern Asia and Western nations.

Tribal Variation

There did not appear to be any significant differences in incidence of trophoblastic disease in the various tribes. Statistics on hydatidiform mole were difficult to interpret since each hospital had its own different practice with regard to sending material from abortion cases for histology. The Baganda accounted for 15 of the 67 cases of trophoblastic disease and 40% of cases of hydatidiform mole; one hospital in Ankole provided 20% of the remainder but this excess was probably only a result of the presence of an enthusiastic gynaecologist. These variations serve to emphasize the probable extent of under-reporting.

Age

The age range and mean age of patients with hydatidiform moles and chorionic malignancy were very similar (Table 16). The average age of pregnant females in Uganda is difficult to compute since hospital cases are a considerably biased sample, but a small survey in Mulago Hospital showed only 5% over the age of 35 years (Smith, 1970). The true proportion in the country as a whole is probably lower than this since older patients are admitted to hospital more readily than younger. The risk

Table 16. Showing the age range and mean age of patients with trophoblastic disease

	Cases	Age range	Mean	% over 35 years
Choriocarcinoma	55	17—46	23.4	36%
Chorioadenoma	12	16—38	24.5	11%
Hydatidiform mole	224	14—47	31.6	30%

of a Ugandan women over the age of 35 developing trophoblastic disease in a given pregnancy may be calculated as being about ten times higher than in a person under that age. In Asia there is a higher fertility among older people and the high incidence may be at least in part a function of this effect. Smallbrook (1957) has calculated that the incidence of hydatidiform mole in pregnancies between the ages of 45 and 50 was 1 in 32. The risk of a given hydatidiform mole giving rise to a malignant tumour seems to be about equal in all age groups.

Parity

Information available in the Cancer Registry as to parity was scanty and is likely to be biased. In a survey of 48 cases seen in Mulago Hospital (Smith, 1970),

37 out of 47 (78%) were para 4 or greater, compared with 21% of random obstetric admissions, suggesting a relative risk about four-fold higher in multiparous patients. These findings are similar to those in Asia where the risk of developing chorio-carcinoma or hydatidiform mole increased with parity (Joint Project, 1959). In the U.S.A. it has been calculated that this risk is greatest in the first fertilization by each different male (Scott, 1963). The finding that choriocarcinoma is more common in multigravid females in Africa and Asia but not in America is as yet unexplained. Reliable information as to whether successive pregnancies were all induced by the same male would obviously be difficult to obtain.

Pathology

The microscopic appearance and mode of spread of choriocarcinoma in Uganda was essentially similar to those recorded in other countries. Hydatidiform mole was classified into three subgroups based upon the volume of trophoblastic tissue seen in many sections. These conformed to minimal, moderate and marked trophoblastic proliferation. Follow-up of these patients to assess the frequency of malignant sequaelae is at present being undertaken.

Chorioadenoma destruens was diagnosed when atypical trophoblast was found invading the myometrium or vagina and villi were still present. Three such cases (out of 12) presented with tumour nodules in the cervix or vagina and in two of these villi were present in the uterus but not in the vaginal growth. Follow-up of these patients was unfortunately not possible. The age of patients with destruens mole was not significantly different from either choriocarcinoma or hydatidiform mole. Fifty-five patients with choriocarcinoma were diagnosed. Information on these patients is scanty and only five patients came to necropsy. Metastases were found in the lung, brain, and vaginal wall in most cases. Other sites were involved much less frequently. Reactive cellular infiltration around the tumour was not marked in any case. Where it did occur, there was usually ulceration and it was probably a result of necrosis. No morphological evidence of an immunological reaction to the tumour cells was seen. The ovaries were usually the site of marked luteal proliferation. This led to an erroneous diagnosis of ovarian carcinoma in one case and choriocarcinoma was only discovered three months after bilateral oophorectomy had been performed.

Predisposing Lesions

The culpable pregnancy was identified in only 29 cases out of the 55 cases with choriocarcinoma. Twelve (42%) followed hydatidiform mole, five followed an apparently normal delivery and 12 followed an abortion, one of which was a tubal pregnancy. Some of the cases of abortion might have been hydatidiform moles but information on some cases was scanty. These proportions are essentially similar to those quoted in standard texts. The interval between pregnancy and presentation was usually less than eight months but in one case was apparently delayed five years. The risk of choriocarcinoma following ectopic pregnancy has been thought to be high (Madden, 1950). In Mulago Hospital 115 cases of tubal pregnancy are seen yearly which suggests that the risk in the Ugandan female is probably quite low.

The very marked variation in incidence of trophoblastic disease in different countries has led to speculation as to the importance of different aetiological factors. Populations in which the incidence is high are usually malnourished and have a high fertility rate. The poorer sections of the community seem to be more likely to develop carcinoma than the richer (SOEJOENOES et al., 1967). However, poorly nourished communities in Africa, South America, and parts of India do not show as high an incidence as in the Far East. DOUGLAS (1959) was unable to find any correlation between mole formation and socioeconomic status in New York. It may be that different diets have an effect or that the variations noted above are genetically induced. Studies on Chinese resident in the U.S.A. have shown a low rate of mole formation so that there is unlikely to be a strong genetic influence. The possibility of a dietary effect on incidence has to be considered seriously. Overall fertility rates and the variation of fertility with age will also influence the incidence of trophoblastic disease. In Uganda family production starts and finishes early in life. It has been estimated that 50% of Ugandan females are sterile by the age of 30 as a result of gonorrhoea and other genital infections (GRIFFITH, 1963). This sharply reduces the incidence of pregnancy in older females and would thereby reduce the incidence of trophoblastic disease.

Before a true assessment of the importance of different aetiological factors can be made it is necessary to know patterns of diet, promiscuity, age of pregnancy, frequency and cause of abortions, nationality and criteria of diagnosis. If information is any less exact than this it is unlikely to enable any factor to be incriminated with certainty. It would require an international prospective trial to ensure homogeneous methods of collection and presentation of data. Such an investigation would yield valuable results such as have been achieved with carcinoma of the breast (MACMAHON et al., 1970).

Ovarian Tumours

Numerous classifications of ovarian tumours have been advanced and none is entirely satisfactory. The classification used here is similar to that adopted at the Johns Hopkins Hospital (NOVAK et al., 1962). This includes the International Federation of Gynaecology and Obstetrics (FIGO) grouping for epithelial tumours. Non-neoplastic lesions are not included in this survey since most would not be submitted for histological examination even when excised. Also excluded are cases diagnosed as simple cysts.

All cases of borderline malignancy have been included in the malignant group.

The incidence, bilaterality, age range and mean for all ovarian tumours seen is shown in Table 17.

Epithelial Tumours

This category included 206 tumours of a total of 394 benign and malignant ovarian tumours, that is 52.3% of ovarian neoplasms. The malignant types accounted for 41.6% and the benign group for 10.7%. The distribution of the epithelial tumours is similar to that reported in an earlier survey of ovarian tumours from Uganda

Table 17. Analysis of 394 ovarian tumours

	Cases (Bilateral)	Age range	Mean	% of benign/ malignant tumours	% of all ovarian tumours
Benign					
Serous cystadenoma	25	23—69	38.1	14.4	6.6
Mucinous cystadenoma	17	24—63	37.1	9.8	4.4
Benign teratoma	83 (8)	2¹/₂—70	32.5	49.6	21.1
Leiomyoma	10	23—50	33.4	5.6	2.2
Fibroma	12	26—50	36.4	7.2	3.3
Brenner	12	30—50	43.5	7.2	3.3
Gyandroblastoma	1	21		0.5	0.2
Thecomas	12	18—50	39.5	7.2	3.3
Unclassifiable	1	10		0.5	0.2
Total	173 (8)	2¹/₂—70	35.8	100	44.6
Malignant					
Serous cystadenocarcinoma	102 (12)	12—70	43.1	46.4	26.8
Mucinous cystadenocarcinoma	15 (2)	25—67	46.5	6.2	3.3
Anaplastic carcinoma	27	5¹/₂—70	45.8	12.5	6.3
Endometrioid carcinoma	3	45—60	51.2	1.7	0.7
Mesonephroid carcinoma	3	12—35	23.1	1.7	0.7
Carcinoma — N.O.S.	14	12—70	49.4	6.7	3.2
Granulosa cell carcinoma	26 (1)	12—70	44.7	11.1	6.2
Dysgerminoma	12	7—40	20.6	5.9	3.3
Malignant teratoma	18	4¹/₂—70	34.3	8.3	4.2
Arrhenoblastoma	1	35		0.1	0.2
Total	221 (15)	4¹/₂—70	42.1	100	54.9

Other ovarian tumours not included in statistics of gynaecological malignancies:—

6 secondary carcinomas	— 5 site not determined
	1 carcinoma of stomach
3 sarcomas	— 1 Leiomyosarcoma
	1 Fibrosarcoma
	1 Histiocytic lymphoma
Burkitt's lymphoma	— about 80 cases

(GRECH and LEWIS, 1967), except that the present series contains a higher proportion of serous cystadenocarcinoma; 26.8% compared with 16.2% in the previous study.

HERTIG and GORE (1961), in an analysis of 1740 ovarian tumours, found that serous cystadenocarcinomas accounted for 60.3% of malignant ovarian tumours and the mucinous variety for 20.4%. Their benign counterparts were responsible for 23.5% and 24.5% of benign tumours respectively. Other series in Caucasian subjects show similar findings (KENT and McKAY, 1960; NOVAK, 1962; BENNINGTON, FERGUSON and HABER, 1968; AURE, HOEG and KOLSTAD, 1971). In Uganda serous and mucous cystic tumours form a much smaller proportion of ovarian neoplasms, the deficiency being most marked with the mucous cystadenomas. Anaplastic carcinomas accounted for 12.5% of malignant ovarian tumours, a similar proportion to that reported elsewhere (MORTON, 1966).

The mean age at onset of malignant epithelial tumours in the present series was 44 years, which is nearly 10 years younger than other reports (WYNDER, DODO and BARBAR, 1969; CONSTABLE, BIRRELL and TRUSKETT, 1969; AURE, HOEG and KOLSTAD, 1971). The age mean for benign tumours was 38 years, which is only 3 years earlier than that found in a series outside Africa (BECK and LATOUR, 1960). The three cases of endometrioid carcinoma occurred in older people (mean age 51 years); this is closer to the age group reported in other countries (LONG and TAYLOR, 1964). Two of the three patients with clear-cell carcinomas of the ovary were aged 12 and 35 years; the age of the third patient was not stated. The mean age of patients presenting with this tumour is usually in the fifties (CZERNOBILSKY, SILVERMAN and ENTERLINE, 1970).

Many of these differences are a result of the structure of the populations at risk. But even after correction for this factor the impression remains that tumours occur in younger subjects in Uganda than in other countries.

Teratomas

Ovarian teratomas accounted for 25.4% of all ovarian tumours and were a narrow second to the serous cystadenocarcinomas as the commonest ovarian neoplasm. The majority of cases were benign and accounted for 21.1% of ovarian tumours, but malignant teratomas were seen quite frequently (4.2% of ovarian tumours). Only one example of malignant change (squamous cell carcinoma) in an otherwise benign teratoma was seen. But since the period of this survey we have seen three examples of such a tumour. Benign cystic teratomas account for between 5 and 25% of all ovarian tumours (PETERSON, PREVOST, EDMUNDS, HUNDLEY and MORRIS, 1955). The proportion in this series is at the upper end of this range. The proportion of the malignant teratomas is much higher than elsewhere. MALKASIAN, DOCKERTY and SYMMONDS (1967) did not encounter a single malignant teratoma in an 18-year period during which 612 benign teratomas were seen. Similar low incidences of malignant teratomas have been recorded by other observers (KENT and McKAY, 1960; MORTON, 1966; WOODRUFF, PROTOS and PETERSON, 1968). Eight benign teratomas (9.6%) were bilateral, this proportion is similar to experience elsewhere.

The mean age at presentation of patients with benign teratomas was 32.5 years and the age at diagnosis varied from $2^1/_2$ to 70 years. This pattern is similar to that found elsewhere (PETERSON et al., 1955). In Uganda the mean age of the 18 patients with malignant teratomas was 34.3 years and the age range was also wide ($4^1/_2$ to 70 years). No more than two cases occurred in any five-year age period, and only one-third of the cases occurred in patients under the age of 26 years. This distribution is in contrast to previously reported series. Malignant teratomas are usually said to occur at a younger age than benign teratomas (HERTIG and GORE, 1961) and in a review of 97 malignant teratomas WOODRUFF et al. (1968) found three-quarters of their patients were under the age of 26.

Tumours of Special Morphology or Function

There may be difficulty in deciding whether tumours of the granulosa theca cell system are benign or malignant. As an arbitrary rule tumours with dominant granulosa-cell component were assessed as malignant whilst spindle-cell thecal tumours were regarded as more probably benign. Together this group represented 9.5% of all ovarian tumours, granulosa-cell carcinoma being nearly twice as common as thecoma. Granulosa-cell tumours accounted for 11.1% of malignant ovarian tumours and theca-cell tumours were responsible for 7.2% of benign tumours. In a previous survey reported from Uganda, Grech and Lewis (1967) recorded that granulosa-theca cell tumours accounted for 11.1% of their cases. Kottmeier (1953) states that these tumours account for 4 to 9% of all ovarian neoplasms. Hertig and Gore (1961) noted a proportion of 6% in their series, and proportions as low as 1.6 to 3% are quoted (Dinnerstein and O'Leary, 1968). The proportion of cases in the Ugandan series is therefore considerably higher than elsewhere.

The age range was wide (Table 17) and cases were seen in adolescents as well as the elderly. The mean ages at presentation with granulosa-cell carcinoma and thecomas were 44.7 and 39.5 respectively, which is similar to other experience (Lyon, Senykin and McKelvey; 1963; Dinnerstein et al., 1968). One granulosa cell tumour was bilateral.

Dysgerminomas accounted for 3.3% of all ovarian tumours or 5.9% of malignant neoplasms; this proportion is higher than in other countries, Mueller, Topkins and Lapp (1950) recorded corresponding figures of 1.1% and 4.7%. Dysgerminoma accounted for between 1 and 3% of malignant ovarian tumours in three other series (Koller and Gjonnaess, 1964; Morton, 1966; Jackson, 1967). The mean age in the present series was 20.6 which is similar to that reported elsewhere (Asadourian and Taylor, 1969). There appears to be an excess of dysgerminomas in childhood. At this age the most common tumour found in the ovary is Burkitt's lymphoma. During the five-year period of this survey ovarian involvement by lymphoma would have occurred in at least 80 children but in many cases biopsy would have been taken from a more accessible site. No case of dysgerminoma was bilateral whereas bilateral involvement is the rule in Burkitt's lymphoma.

In most reports Brenner tumour accounts for between 1 and 2% of all ovarian neoplasms (Jondahl, Dockerty and Randall, 1950; Kent and McKay, 1960; Hertig and Gore, 1961) compared with 3.3% in this series from Uganda. The mean age at presentation in the present series was 43.5. This is ten years younger than that reported by Jorgensen, Dockerty, Wilson and Welch (1970).

Other Tumours

Benign connective tissue tumours accounted for 5.5% of all ovarian tumours and during the study period three ovarian sarcomas were also seen.

Secondary tumours have been reported to account for about 20% of all malignant ovarian tumours. In the present five-year study only six secondary ovarian neoplasms were biopsied, an incidence of less than 1%. The small proportion of secondary tumours reflects the low incidence of tumours occurring at primary sites which commonly metastasize to the ovary, namely the uterus and the gastro-intestinal tract, particularly the colon.

Discussion

Ovarian neoplasms as a group are probably at least as common in Uganda as in other parts of the world. The relative proportion of different entities varies widely. The ovary is probably involved in virtually every case of Burkitt's lymphoma occurring in females though involvement is seldom exclusive. Granulosa-theca cell tumours are also more frequent, which is of interest when this is correlated with the reduced incidence of testicular tumours. Both might be explained by an alteration of the amount of oestrogen hormone production by the adrenal. There are differences in adrenal output between African and Caucasian males but no comparative studies in females are available as yet. The apparent increase in malignant teratomas is unexplained as is the reduction in frequency of mucinous cystadenomas.

Carcinoma of the Fallopian Tube

Several of the cases included in this section presented at a late stage and it was difficult to be absolutely certain of their origin. However, in no case could an obvious primary tumour be found in neighbouring organs.

Nine cases of carcinoma and one fibrosarcoma were seen. The carcinomas represent approximately 1% of neoplasms of female genitalia or 0.3% of cancer in females. The age at presentation ranged from 38 to 50 (mean 44.6 years). Six patients were Baganda and the remaining patients came from Teso, Ankole and Busoga respectively.

Histology

Four cases were well differentiated papillary adenocarcinomas and a further four were poorly differentiated adenocarcinomas with only occasional papillary areas. One case was of intermediate differentiation. The incidence of carcinoma of the Fallopian tube has been reported as varying from 0.03% to 0.3% of gynaecological cancer (FINN and JAVERT, 1949). Although the present series is small the incidence is at the upper limit of these figures. The range of histological patterns compares with that previously reported (LOFGREN and DOCKERTY, 1946). The mean age at presentation in the present series was 44.6, which is younger than that reported by LOFGREN et al. (1960) (50.9 years) and FINN et al. (1949) (52 years). This reduction is merely an effect of the different population at risk.

Chapter 7

Tumours of the Male Genitalia

O. G. DODGE, R. OWOR, and A. C. TEMPLETON

With 5 Figures

Carcinoma of the penis is the most frequently diagnosed cancer in Ugandan men. It usually develops in the coronal sulcus and the incidence is closely correlated with standards of genital hygiene. Circumcision protects against the development of this tumour even if carried out at puberty. Tumours of the testis are uncommon in Africans and tumours of young adults appear to be particularly rare. The correct incidence of prostatic cancer is essentially unknown. The true age of older patients and the true population of older people are both difficult to determine. The high frequency of urethral stricture in many parts of the country may make diagnosis difficult. The histological and clinical features of prostatic tumours appear to be similar to those found in other countries.

Included under this heading are tumours of the testis, epididymis, prostate, seminal vesicles and penis (WHO I.C.D. numbers 177, 178 and 179). Tumours of the scrotum are considered with tumours of the skin. This is in accordance with the I.C.D. classification although a tumour on the biological equivalent of the scrotum, the vulva in females, is considered as a genital tumour. Urethral neoplasms are included under the heading of urinary tract tumours (see Chapter 8). The clinical differentiation of urethral from penile tumours is seldom a problem. Urethral tumours usually arose in the posterior part, while tumours at the tip of the penis were almost all derived from the skin of the corona or prepuce.

Carcinoma of the Prostate

One hundred and forty cases were diagnosed during the period of this survey, 115 of which were histologically confirmed. This constitutes 3.5⁰/o of cancer in males, a crude incidence of 6.5 cases per year per million men. These figures are a considerable underestimate of the true incidence in Uganda. The incidence in Kyadondo County was 35 cases per million compared with 5.7 per million for Uganda (both figures corrected for an African standard population). This suggests that outside Kyadondo County only about 20⁰/o of cases are being diagnosed.

The geographical and tribal distribution is heavily influenced by this bias in diagnosis. Thus prostatic cancer accounts for 8.6⁰/o of cancer in Baganda and less than 3.5% in all other tribes. There is little evidence to suggest that there is a true variation in incidence between the different tribes, since the frequency of recording closely parallels the frequency of diagnosis of cancer overall. In Buganda, cases are found in different counties essentially in proportion to the population at risk.

The age of patients at diagnosis is shown in Table 1. As in other countries, carcinoma of the prostate is a disease of older men. The age-specific incidence rates in Kyadondo and Uganda are shown in Table 2. There is often great uncertainty as to the true age of older Africans and stated figures over the age of 70 should be treated with caution.

Table 1. Age distribution of carcinoma of prostate in Baganda and other tribes

Age	Ganda	Others	Total [a]
25—34	1	1	2.2
35—44	1	2	3.2
45—54	10	3	14.1
55—64	30	17	51.7
65—74	34	9	47.4
75—84	11	4	16.2
85+	5	—	5.4
not known	2	10	
All ages	94	46	140

[a] Cases of unknown age distributed in proportion with patients of known age.

Table 2. Age-specific rates of prostatic carcinoma in Kyadondo and Uganda (cases per 100,000 per year)

	Uganda	Kyadondo	Connecticut [a]
25—34	0.1	—	0.5
35—44	0.1	1.1	3.2
45—54	0.9	4.2	7.5
55—64	5.4	45	30.0
65—74	9.5	36	63.0
75—84	6.5	50	100.0
85+	3.4	—	134.8

[a] Figures adapted from DOLL et al. (1966).

One hundred and fifteen tumours of the prostate were examined histologically. Two cases of rhabdomyosarcoma, both in 6-year-old boys, are not discussed further here (see Chapter 15). The other 113 cases were all adenocarcinomas. These showed a range of appearances from well differentiated tubular formations to poorly differentiated tumours which was exactly similar to that previously reported from Uganda (DODGE, 1963) and to that found in other countries. Latent carcinoma has

not been included in this series but the frequency of this change is currently under
investigation.

Patients were admitted to hospital with symptoms of obstructive prostatic disease,
or with symptoms of bone secondaries at the time of presentation. Twenty-seven
cases were diagnosed as suffering from prostatic cancer without histological proof.
The majority of these patients had symptoms of spinal secondary deposits and had
signs on local palpation suggestive of a primary tumour in the prostate.

Discussion

A detailed study of the epidemiology of prostatic cancer showed that the highest
incidence of the disease occurs in non-whites in the U.S.A., and this holds true for
all regions of the United States (KING et al., 1963; WYNDER et al., 1971). The lowest
incidence figures occur in oriental communities, notably in Singapore. These differences are found in both mortality rates and age-standardized incidence rates (DUNHAM
and BAILAR, 1968). In the case of prostatic carcinoma, the mortality rates are likely
to be misleadingly low, since many elderly patients with the disease will die from
(or will be certified as dying from) unrelated disease. OETTLÉ (1964) gave low mortality figures for both Africans and Asians in South Africa, with a much higher rate
for whites. MOVSAS (1966), using the hospital admission figures for Durban, thought
that the incidence rate for prostatic cancer was likely to be higher in the Africans

Table 3. Carcinoma of prostate. Age-standardized incidence of rates per 100,000 males
in different countries

U.S.A. Alameida County, negro	31.6
U.S.A. " " white	17.9
Connecticut (white and non-white)	16.0
Natal African, 1964—1966	11.1
Lourenco Marques, Mozambique	4.9
Ibadan, Nigeria	4.9
Johannesburg, S. Africa (Bantu)	4.3
Natal Indian, 1964—1966	4.0
Kyadondo, Uganda, 1964—1968	3.5 (present study)
Miyagi, Japan	1.8
Singapore (Chinese)	0.5

All figures standardized for an African population and
taken from DOLL et al., 1966 and 1970.

than in the Indian residents of the city. In a subsequent study from Durban, SCHON-
LAND and BRADSHAW (1968) have shown that there is, in fact, a much higher incidence
of prostatic cancer in Durban Africans than in Durban Indians. Some age-standardized incidence rates are shown in Table 3. It is likely that the Durban figures,
based on close analysis of an urban population, give a more accurate picture of the
true incidence of the disease than the figures from other African registries including
our own. Similarly, the figures from Singapore (DUNHAM and BAILAR, 1968) which

show a low rate in Chinese, Indians and Malays, probably give a true impression of the rarity of prostatic cancer in this urbanized oriental tri-racial population. The lowest incidence of clinical disease in the world seems to be among Japanese, although rates of latent cancer in Japan seem to be as frequent as in other countries (WYNDER et al., 1971).

The numbers of hyperplastic and malignant prostates encountered in various surgical series are shown in Table 4. Carcinoma accounts for a higher proportion of abnormal prostates in both the Durban and the Uganda series. MOVSAS (1966), reporting the high proportion of malignant prostates in Durban Africans, speculated that this might be due either to a relative paucity of hyperplasia, or to a genuinely

Table 4. Relative frequency of hyperplasia and carcinoma in surgically removed prostates

	Total prostates	Hyperplastic	Malignant
Europeans (RICHES, 1962)	2810	2451 (87.3%)	359 (12.7%)
Uganda Africans	524	411 (78.4%)	113 (21.6%)
Durban Africans (MOVSAS, 1966)	130	57 (46%)	73 (54%)
Durban Indians (MOVSAS, 1966)	74	68 (92%)	6 (8%)

high incidence of carcinoma. The studies of SCHONLAND and BRADSHAW (1968) suggest that the latter view may be correct. The infrequency of malignancy in the prostates of Durban Indians further confirms the low incidence of prostatic cancer in populations of Asiatic origin.

Prostatic cancer is strongly associated with the older age-groups in all races. It is known that preinvasive "latent" carcinoma also increases rapidly in frequency in the older age-groups. ASHLEY (1965), who subjected published incidence rates for latent and clinical prostatic carcinoma to mathematical analysis, concluded that latent carcinoma is the end result of three consecutive carcinogenic "events" in the life of the prostatic epithelium, and that invasive carcinoma requires 4—5 further "events" for its induction. It is known that latent carcinoma does occur in African prostates. FRANKS (1962) examined 96 African prostates (89 of which were of Ugandan origin), 10 of which contained foci of latent carcinoma. The number showing tumours at different ages ranged from 0 out of 9 in patients aged 12—29, to 2 out of 7 in patients over 70. A systematic histological survey of the prostates of Uganda Africans of all ages dying from non-prostatic disease would provide a larger series which could be compared with the series published from London by FRANKS (1954) and other series.

Social factors may have an influence on the incidence of disease. Mortality and morbidity from prostatic cancer are higher in the upper social classes in Scotland (RICHARDSON, 1965). In Denmark, CLEMMESEN (1969) gives age-specific incidence rates for prostatic cancer for (a) men ever married, (b) men unmarried, with much lower rates in the second group. It is difficult to apply these findings to the Uganda African population. Breakdown by social class has not been attempted, and indeed European criteria of social-economic status are not applicable. Marriage (following either Christian or tribal custom) is virtually universal among Ugandans. A study on the epidemiology of prostatic cancer in different countries failed to find any constant association with marital status, social class, fertility, height, weight, previous diseases, laboratory data or hair distribution (Wynder et al., 1971).

As a result of studying the incidence of prostatic carcinoma in Sweden and Israel, Apt (1965) claimed that circumcision in itself reduced the risk of developing prostatic cancer by half. This illustrates the pitfalls of taking only one possible factor, and only two countries, into account. The incidence of prostatic cancer is lower among Israeli men (circumcised) than among Swedish men (mostly uncircumcised). But the incidence in uncircumcised Singapore Chinese is lower still. A study confined to Singapore and Israel would have "demonstrated" that circumcision increased the risk of developing the disease. Most Uganda Africans are uncircumcised. The relation between carcinoma of the penis and circumcision is discussed below, but we have no evidence to link prostatic cancer with circumcision status.

Abnormalities of hormone balance in older people have been suggested as causative factors in prostatic cancer. Sommers (1957) showed that many prostatic cancer cases had indirect evidence of pituitary-adreno-cortical hyperfunction, and believe that pituitary and adrenal cortical hormones, and oestrogen of undetermined origin, were important factors in development and growth of these tumours. In a later paper, Sommers (1964), studying the reactions of the male breast in various disease states, found that testicular atrophy, prostate hypertrophy and prostatic carcinoma were all significantly associated with hyperplasia of the breast. The assumption that raised circulating oestrogen levels were responsible for all these conditions is plausible but unproven. High oestrogen levels occur in male Ugandan Africans (Wang et al., 1966) and mammary hyperplasia is not uncommon. The increase in oestrogens may be the result of defective inactivation of the hormone, due to the liver damage which is so frequent in this population. Men with cirrhosis of the liver often show raised oestrogen levels, but Robson (1964), who studied the incidence of prostatic disease as seen at necropsy, found no difference in incidence in those with or without cirrhosis.

Testicular Tumours

During the five-year period 18 testicular and paratesticular tumours were diagnosed histologically. A further 3 cases were considered clinically to be tumours of the testes but histological examination was either not performed or was inconclusive. The age range was between 3 and 62 years. In 9 cases the tumour arose from the right testis, in 5 from the left, and in 4 cases the side was not recorded. There were no tribal differences in this tumour distribution. Thus tumours of the testes represent less than 0.5% of cancer in males.

The interval between recognition of scrotal swelling and seeking of medical care varied between 8 months and 10 years but these time intervals may not be reliable since accurate histories may be difficult to obtain from many patients. It was evident that many patients presented late, and five of them had large ulcerating tumours.

The histological classification used in this survey was based on that of Collins and Pugh (1965). The diagnoses made in 18 cases are shown in Table 5.

Table 5. Testicular and paratesticular tumours seen in Uganda

Seminoma	5
Paratesticular sarcomas	5
Orchioblastoma	3
Teratoma	3
Interstitial cell tumour	1
Embryonal carcinoma	1
Total cases	18

Seminoma

There were four typical seminomas and one spermatocytic seminoma (Fig. 1). Those with typical seminomas were aged between 20 and 40 years and the patient with spermatocytic seminoma was aged 50 years. In two cases there was clinical evidence of metastases affecting inguinal and para-aortic groups of lymph nodes, and in one of these the metastases occurred two years after orchidectomy.

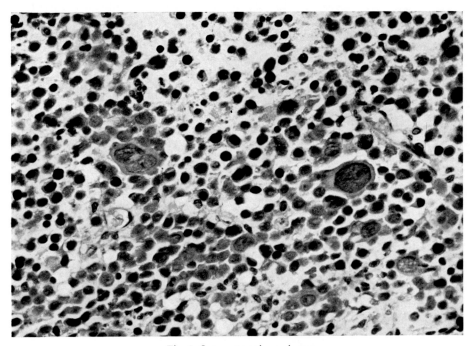

Fig. 1. Spermatocytic seminoma

Teratomas

Three teratomatous tumours were seen. One occurring in a child of 5 years showed well differentiated elements, and 2 adults aged 35 and 50 years had malignant tumours, both of which contained trophoblastic elements. One of these adult patients had a secondary deposit in the femur causing a pathological fracture.

Interstitial Cell Tumour

There was one patient aged 35 years who presented with an ulcerating tumour of two years' duration. There was also a haemorrhagic hydrocele.

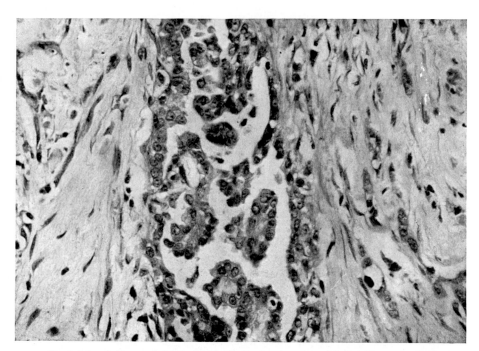

Fig. 2. Mesothelioma of the tunica vaginalis showing the epithelial-like and spindle components of the tumour

Orchioblastoma

Three children, all aged 3 years, had orchioblastoma with typical appearances showing papillary structure with mucin-producing cells. One of these was said to have a history of trauma to the testis. Clinically, one case had secondaries in the liver. There was a fourth case aged 4 years who had poorly differentiated embryonal carcinoma with no papillary structures and no mucin-producing cells.

Paratesticular Tumours

There were 5 cases:— 2 leiomyosarcomas, 2 rhabdomyosarcomas and 1 meso-thelioma. Those with leiomyosarcoma and rhabdomyosarcoma were aged between 15 and 58 years. The 2 with leiomyosarcoma died 2 years after diagnosis. At autopsy examination one had secondary spread in bone and peritoneum while the other had no metastases. One of the cases with rhabdomyosarcoma had clinical evidence of secondaries in the liver and radiological evidence of spread to ribs and vertebrae. Mesothelioma occurred in a 62-year-old man who presented with painless testicular swelling and ascites. The testis was removed and was seen to be covered with typical mesothelial tumour elements (Fig. 2). Six months later a laparotomy showed tumour nodules all over the peritoneum encasing the viscera but with no infiltration of any organ. The histology of the paratesticular and peritoneal tumours was identical and had features of mixed epithelial and fibrous type of mesothelioma.

There were 3 other tumours in the inguinal and pelvic region, which histologically resembled anaplastic testicular teratomas, but these were excluded from this study because there was no certain evidence that these were testicular tumours.

Discussion

The incidence of testicular tumours in Africans is very low. In various cancer registries in all parts of the world the proportion of testicular tumours is smaller than in other races (see DOLL, MUIR, WATERHOUSE, 1970). In Uganda the great reduction in incidence is seen to be largely a result of the infrequency of seminoma and teratoma in young men. Testicular tumours of childhood are not quite so infreqent and accounted for 6 of the cases seen. In America, negro servicemen show an incidence of testicular tumours which is approximately 25% of that seen in whites (DIXON and MOORE, 1952). Why there should be this considerable difference in incidence is unknown, but it is tempting to speculate that it is due to the known differences in hormonal production between Africans and Europeans (WANG et al., 1966). These possibilities are more fully discussed in a survey of ten years of Ugandan tumours (TEMPLETON, 1972 d).

Carcinoma of the Penis

Carcinoma of the penis has long been known to be associated with (a) the uncircumcised state and (b) a low standard of personal and social hygiene, and the disease has been shown to have a relatively high incidence only in communities where these conditions prevail. Cancer of the penis was recognized in Uganda from the early days at Sir Albert Cook's hospital at Mengo and constituted 7.3% of all malignant tumours seen over the years 1897—1956 (DAVIES et al., 1964). By 1958, the results of ten years of cancer registration confirmed an incidence of penile cancer some ten times higher than that expected from Danish rates (DAVIES, WILSON and KNOWELDEN, 1958). By 1963, it was possible to assemble a series of 503 histologically confirmed cases of carcinoma of the penis from Ugandan Africans (DODGE and LINSELL, 1963).

Carcinoma of the penis was diagnosed in 474 cases between 1964 and 1968, and this is the commonest tumour registered in males in Uganda. During this period it accounted for 12% of cancer in males, a crude incidence of 2.2 cases per 100,000 per year. Fifteen cases were diagnosed clinically without histological confirmation. The remaining 459 cases were all squamous carcinomas.

The age at diagnosis ranged from 26 to 90 years. Age-specific incidence rates in Uganda and in Kyadondo County are shown in Table 6.

Clinically the tumour presents as a slowly growing mass situated at the end of the penis. Tumours originating at the base of the penis are almost always derived from

Table 6. Age specific incidence rates of carcinoma of the penis
in Uganda and in Kyadondo county

	Uganda	Kyadondo county
25—34	0.7	1
35—44	3.4	4
45—54	10.2	22
55—64	16.6	27
65—74	12.0	35
75—84	11.1	37
85+	3.4	—

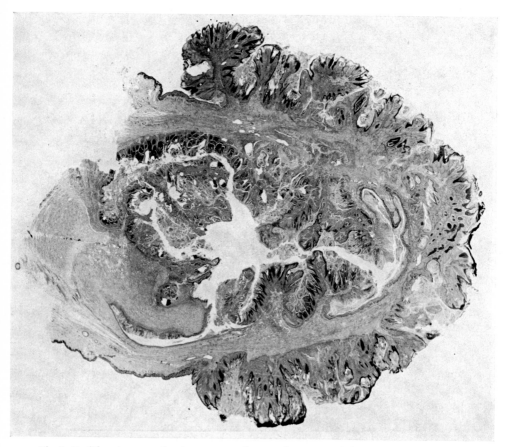

Fig. 3. Proliferative type showing an extensive neoplasm around the prepuce with destruction of the glans penis but with minimal penetration (courtesy of Dr. R. Schmauz)

the urethra and are usually associated with stricture or perineal fistula (see Chapter 8). The tumour usually develops in the coronal sulcus but in most cases the growth was too large to be certain of its precise origin. KYALWAZI (1966) has described different growth patterns and these are illustrated in Figs. 3, 4 and 5. Histologically most tumours are well differentiated keratinizing squamous carcinomas and metastasis to inguinal nodes occurs late. Clinically the differential diagnosis of carcinoma from venereal diseases such as lymphogranuloma venereum or granuloma inguinale may sometimes present problems. Histologically, differentiation from giant condyloma or Buschke-Loewenstein lesion (DREYFUS and NEVILLE, 1955) may be problematic but in the majority of cases the diagnosis is all too easy. The growth may continue for many years and it gives rise to considerable morbidity. Mortality is low and is usually a result of sepsis or local haemorrhage rather than widespread dissemination. During the past decade only three patients with carcinoma of the penis have come to necropsy. All these showed widespread lymph node involvement and only one patient had metastatic deposits in the lung. These findings are essentially the same as those of DODGE and LINSELL (1936).

About 90% of Ugandans are not circumcised. Circumcision is practised by Moslem Africans (about 5% of the population) and a minority of small tribes, most

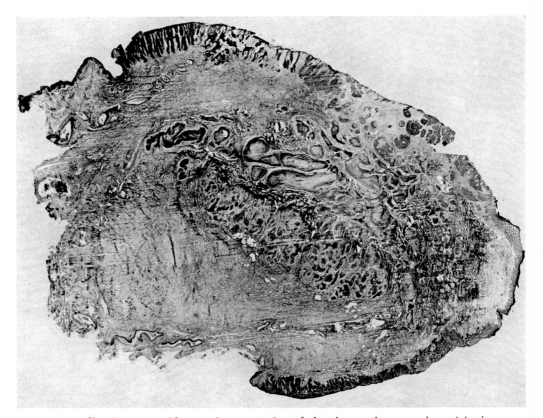

Fig. 4. Infiltrative type with extensive permeation of the glans and corpora but minimal disturbance of the external dimensions of the penis (courtesy of Dr. R. SCHMAUZ)

notably the Bakonjo in the west of the country and the Bagishu in the east (Dodge and Kaviti, 1965). Circumcision is carried out at different times of life and is often a bloody and rather inefficient operation. Nevertheless, circumcising tribes have a lower incidence than uncircumcised tribes (Table 7). The highest proportional rate is

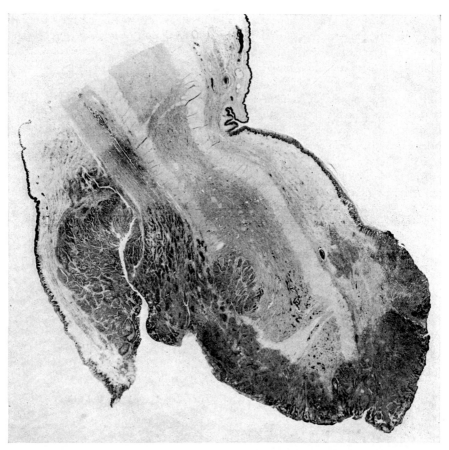

Fig. 5. Ulcerative desctructive growth pattern with extensive necrosis of tumour and destruction of penile tissue (courtesy of Dr. R. Schmauz)

found in the Bunyoro, in which tribe carcinoma of the penis accounts for 41.4% of cancer of males. A very high rate is found among their neighbours in Toro. There is a considerable variation in rate in tribes who do not circumcise. These findings are very similar to those of Dodge and Linsell (1963). It is uncertain why the Kiga and Lugbara should have rates much lower than their neighbours, but this is assumed to be a result of social habit and cleanliness. Schmauz and Jain (1971) have analyzed the epidemiology of carcinoma of the penis in detail and they found that Baganda people living close to Bunyoro had a higher incidence of penile cancer than Baganda living in other parts of Buganda. They also suggested that Ruandans living in high-

Table 7. Proportion of total cancer accounted for by carcinoma of the penis
and cervix in different tribes

Tribe	ca. penis (%)	ca. cervix (%)
Bunyoro	41.4	21.8
Toro	31.2	24.3
Teso	25.1	20.9
Ankole	12.6	16.3
Ganda	12.0	27.3
Ruanda/Rundi	10.7	17.5
Acholi	10.5	30.9
Soga	7.6	26.0
Kiga	4.2	14.8
Lango	3.5	23.1
Lugbara	3.0	10.1
Circumcising tribes [a]	2.4	10.5

[a] Bwamba, Bakonjo, Bagishu, Pokot and Sebei.

rate areas had a higher rate than those living in low-rate areas. This might suggest
that some factor, possibly infective (e. g. herpes simplex genitalis) is more common
in these areas. Unfortunately there is little information available as to the incidence
of penile carcinoma in Ruanda or Burundi though CLEMMESEN et al. (1962) believed
it to be frequent.

Precancerous lesions may be found if sought but patients seldom present at this
stage. Ulceration of the coronal skin with intraepithelial dysplasia is very common
among the Bunyoro and Toro. Investigation of the frequency and significance of
these lesions is currently being undertaken (SCHMAUZ, personal communication, 1971).

Both carcinoma of the cervix and carcinoma of the penis can be produced by
smegma. It might be expected, therefore, that these tribes with a high proportion of
penile cancer would also have a high rate of cervical tumours. The proportions of
penile and cervical cancer in different tribes are compared in Table 7. It will be seen
that there is a tendency for tribes with a low proportion of cervical tumours to have
a low proportion of penile cancer. The Lango and Soga do not conform to this trend
in that the proportion of penile cancer is fairly low but cervical neplasms appear to
be common. There is thus some limited support for the concept that there might be a
common aetiology for both these tumours and it is possible that both might be a
result of poor genital hygiene in the male.

The frequency of carcinoma of the penis in other African countries varies widely.
In Kenya it is less frequently encourtered than in Uganda (LINSELL and
MARTYN, 1962) and this is associated with the far more widespread practice of
circumcision among Kenyan tribes. The majority of cases on the files of the Kenya
Cancer Registry came from the Luo and Turkana tribes, who do not circumcise,
while the disease is extremely uncommon among the Kikuyu, the largest tribal group
in the country (DODGE and LINSELL, 1963; DODGE, 1965). The geographical distribution of tribal circumcision was plotted for the East African countries by DODGE and
KAVITI (1965). Circumcision is practised in areas near the coast, where Arab influence

is marked, or where Nilo-Hamitic populations, such as the Masai, have established themselves in otherwise largely Bantu areas. These areas comprise almost the whole of Kenya, a small area of eastern Uganda, and roughly the eastern half of Tanganyika (Tanzania) and the island of Zanzibar. Infant circumcision appears to be universal in Ethiopia (Huber, 1960) as well as in the Moslem countries of north and north-east Africa, and carcinoma of the penis is said not to occur in Ethiopians (Boldt, 1959). Chapman (1958) noted that carcinoma of the penis accounted for 7% of all male cancers among Africans in Durban, whereas in Johannesburg (Higginson and Oettlé, 1960), Cape Town (Grieve and Linder, 1970) and Bulawayo (Skinner, 1970) it was very much less common. In view of the findings in Uganda it would be interesting to know if these are a result of circumcision practice in the different African groups of southern Africa. In Lourenco Marques, Mozambique, carcinoma of the penis accounted for 0.8% of all tumours in African residents (Prates and Torres, 1965). Circumcision in this area is carried out in some Africans in childhood or at puberty, but not in others. Further, more detailed information as to the relation between circumcision practice, genital hygiene and cancer incidence in these areas would be of value.

In West Africa little information is avilable. Edington and Maclean (1965) recorded only 6 cases of carcinoma of the penis out of 1,920 malignant tumours. Burkitt, Nelson and Williams (1963) state that the disease "is virtually unknown in Nigeria where tribal circumcision is routine. In parts of Ghana, however, i. e. the Ashanti region, it is occasionally seen. Circumcision there is by no means universal." First-hand information from these and other African countries is needed.

Studies of the geographical pathology of cancer of the penis in Uganda reveal that factors other than the uncircumcised state are important in the pathogenesis of the disease and that these vary with geographical location. Careful comparisons of the incidence rates among uncircumcised populations in other areas with an overall high frequency of the disease may shed further light on the nature of these factors.

Chapter 8

Malignant Tumours of the Kidney, Bladder and Urethra

P. P. ANTHONY

With 14 Figures

Nephroblastoma appears to have a very similar incidence, appearance and clinical course in all countries in which it has been studied including Uganda. Patients in Uganda present late and tend to have less well differentiated tumours. Renal tubular carcinoma (hyper-nephroma) is much less common than in Caucasians, but the reasons for this are obscure. Tumours of the bladder are commonly seen particularly in Buganda. They are most frequently of squamous type but adenocarcinomas are also common. Both these tumour types are associated with urethral stricture. Transitional cell tumours are less common and do not appear to be associated with strictures. Schistosomiasis was not a factor in the development of these tumours. Urethral tumours are seen commonly, often in association with strictures.

Primary malignant tumours of the kidney, bladder and urethra accounted for a total of 262 cases in the five years 1964 to 1968. This figure includes histologically proven cases only. The distribution by site and histological type is shown in Table 1. A further 19 cases were diagnosed clinically without histological confirmation. These comprised 15 tumours of the bladder and 4 of the kidney.

The World Health Organization International Classification of Diseases (I.C.D.) (7th ed., 1957) divides tumours of the urinary tract into two categories: 1) malignant neoplasms of kidney (I.C.D. No. 180) and 2) malignant neoplasms of bladder and other urinary organs (I.C.D. No. 181). Figs. 1 and 2 show the total age- and sex-specific incidence rates for this series.

Table 2 shows a comparison of incidence rates in different countries. It is evident from these figures that considerable differences exist between various parts of the world. Uganda occupies low (I.C.D. 180) and middle (I.C.D. 181) positions in this table but this very rough division into two categories hides important differences in histological type that may relate to aetiology. Most cases of malignant tumour of the kidney in Uganda are childhood nephroblastomas whilst adenocarcinoma of the kidney is quite rare. Involvement of the kidney by Burkitt's lymphoma is common but will not be considered in this chapter. In the industrialized countries of the West transitional cell carcinoma of the bladder predominates whereas in Uganda squamous cell carcinoma is by far the commonest type. The ratio of urethral to bladder cancer is unduly high in Uganda, yet another contrasting finding. These important comparisons will be further analyzed under the individual headings below.

Table 1. Malignant tumours of the urinary tract: distribution of 262 cases by site and histological type

Kidney
Nephroblastoma	56
Adenocarcinoma	19
Carcinoma of the renal pelvis	4
Fibrosarcoma	1
Total	**80**

Bladder
Transitional cell carcinoma	19
Squamous cell carcinoma	75[a]
Adenocarcinoma	26
Anaplastic carcinoma	7
Other	11
Total	**138**

Urethra
Transitional cell carcinoma	1
Squamous cell carcinoma	38
Adenocarcinoma	3
Total	**42**

[a] Two cases diagnosed by cytology alone are excluded.

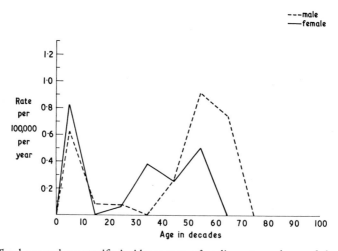

Fig. 1. Total age and sex specific incidence rates of malignant neoplasms of the kidney

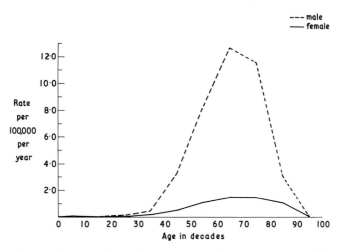

Fig. 2. Total age and sex specific incidence rates of malignant neoplasms of the bladder and urethra

Table 2. Incidence rates per 100,000 per year of malignant neoplasms of the kidney (ICD 180) and of the bladder and other urinary organs (ICD 181) from 16 selected countries (from DOLL, PAYNE and WATERHOUSE, 1966) and Uganda (present series, Kyadondo) based on a Standard African Population

	ICD 180 Males	Females	ICD 181 Males	Females
Mozambique	1.1	0.6	11.1	10.0
Nigeria	0.0	0.3	2.5	1.1
South Africa	0.6	0.4	—	—
Canada	3.5	2.0	6.5	1.6
Puerto Rico	0.8	0.7	4.2	2.0
U.S.A.	3.6	1.9	9.0	2.9
Israel	3.4	2.6	6.9	1.8
Denmark	3.1	2.1	5.8	1.8
England and Wales	2.3	1.1	6.5	1.7
Finland	2.3	2.0	3.3	0.8
Netherlands	2.6	1.2	3.9	1.1
Norway	3.0	1.8	2.5	1.0
Sweden	4.2	2.6	4.5	1.5
New Zealand	3.5	1.6	5.4	1.1
Singapore	0.9	0.6	1.2	0.3
Japan	0.5	0.7	—	—
Uganda	0.5	0.5	4.6	1.0

The Kidney

The total incidence rate figure for malignant neoplasm of the kidney conceals the important fact that the majority, 56 of 80 cases, are childhood nephroblastomas. The incidence of nephroblastoma is probably no greater than excepted (see Chapter 19), but precise figures are not available for the population at risk. The incidence of adult adenocarcinoma of the kidney is unduly low if one considers the proportional rate of this type of tumour: 0.25% in Uganda compared to around 1—2% in most parts of the world. Other types of renal cancer are uncommon and small numbers observed during the period of study do not allow further comment.

Nephroblastoma

Synonyms: Wilms' tumour, adenocarcinoma, "mixed tumour" of the kidney.

The incidence of this tumour is similar throughout the world, Uganda being no exception as far as can be ascertained. It accounts for some 20% of all childhood malignancy. Nephroblastoma may be found in the fetus, in premature infants and in the newborn. A significant number, perhaps as much as one-tenth, are present at birth though they may not become manifest until a few months of age. Rarely, they develop in adolescents or even in early adulthood. In most parts of the world, however, the peak age of children affected by this tumour is one to three years. Boys have been stated to be more commonly affected than girls but the reverse and an equal sex distribution have also been recorded. Age has an important influence on prognosis: the younger the patient on first presentation the better is the chance of ultimate survival following adequate treatment. Occasionally the tumour appears in both kidneys simultaneously. It is not known whether this is due to synchronous development of two separate primary tumours in each kidney or whether one is a metastasis from the other. The histological appearances are usually the same on both sides. There is a statistically significant association with certain congenital defects such as aniridia, "renal ears" and renal malformations (DORN and CUTLER, 1955).

Age and Sex

Table 3 shows the age and sex distribution of 56 cases of nephroblastoma. This shows a very similar distribution to other parts of the world, half the cases falling

Table 3. Age and sex distribution of 56 cases of nephroblastoma

Age in years	Boys	Girls	Total
0—1	3	6	9
—2	7	6	13
—3	6	9	15
—4	1	5	6
—5	3	2	5
—6	1	1	2
—7	—	1	1
—8	1	1	2
—9	—	1	1
—10 and over	1	—	1
Age and sex not known			1
Total	23	32	56

into the age group 1 to 3 years. The youngest patients was 3 months old on first presentation and the oldest 13 years. There was no significant difference between the sexes.

Tribal and Geographical Distribution

The number of cases occurring in each tribe and area was proportional to the size of the population at risk.

Macroscopic Features

Twenty-three tumours occurred in the right and 18 in the left kidney. Four were bilateral. Two arose from single "horseshoe" kidneys. In one the side was not known. Most tumours were described as large or very large and a history of a slowly enlarging abdomen over the preceding weeks or months was the commonest complaint.

The tumours presented as soft, bulky, sometimes fluctuant masses enclosed in a thin, ragged fibrous capsule which had, in some cases, already been broken through. Regional lymph nodes were often involved and the renal vein rarely. On sectioning, a variegated appearance was the rule, made up of soft, solid, brain-like areas divided by tough fibrous strands sometimes enclosing islands of cartilage or bone and cysts filled with clear fluid (Fig. 3).

Microscopic Features

These varied greatly but the two main components were closely aggregated round cells of embryonic character and loose masses of primitive mesenchyme, individual tumours being made up of a mixture of these. The commonest pattern seen was tubular epithelial structures in various stages of development, their cells mingling imperceptibly with the surrounding sarcomatous tissue (Fig. 4). Rosette formation occurred imparting a neuroblastomatous appearance to the tumour. The cells of more mature, better differentiated tubules were columnar, showed mucus secretion and were often arranged in layers. Strips of transitional epithelium were occasionally seen, rather like pelvicalyceal lining (Fig. 5). Glomerulus-like structures were rarely present. The mesenchymal component varied from well-differentiated fibroblastic tissue, with abundant, mature collagen to frankly sarcomatous proliferation of poorly differentiated spindle cells. Muscle, cartilage and bone were occasionally present. Degeneration and necrosis resulted in cyst formation and haemorrhage.

Most authorities consider that these tumours result from a neoplastic deviation of the normal process of development from nephrogenic blastema to nephrons of the adult kidney (WILLIS, 1967).

There have been attempts to subdivide nephroblastoma into histological types according to the predominant tissue component. In the classification of WHITE and BODIAN (BODIAN and RIGBY, 1964) the degree of resemblance to normal kidney resulted in seven types. This classification is shown in Table 4, which also compares the distribution of the various types in the United Kingdom and Uganda. Seventy-five percent of types A, B, C and D, which were made up of better differentiated tissues, occurred under the age of two in both series and had a much better survival

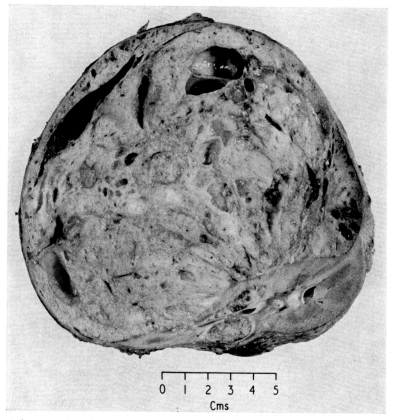

Fig. 3. A large partly solid and partly cystic nephroblastoma compressing the kidney to one
side (bottom right)

Table 4. Nephroblastoma: distribution by histological type in the United Kingdom
(WHITE and BODIAN, 1964) and in Uganda (present series)

Types	U.K.	Uganda
A. Reniform	1	0
B. Tubular	13	2
C. Papillary	4	0
D. Mesenchymal	6	2
E. Focal blastemal	10	20
F. Mixed mesenchymal blastemal	27	16
G. Massive blastemal	28	12
Total	89	52[a]

[a] These figures exclude cases in which insufficient
material was available for histological assessment.

than types E, F and G which were composed of undifferentiated tissues and tended
to occur later in life. Fig. 6 shows an example of an undifferentiated type-G tumour.

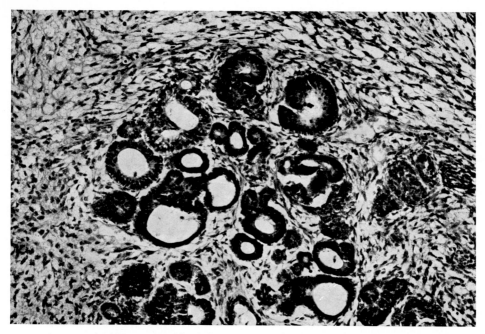

Fig. 4. Nephroblastoma: renal tubular structures of variable differentiation (HE × 40)

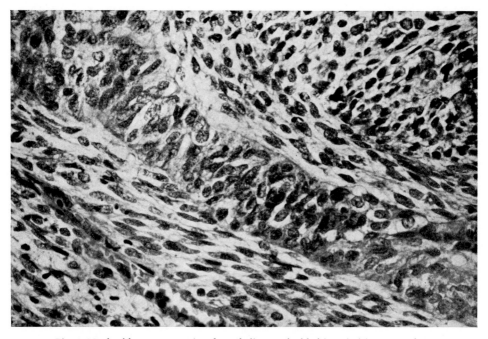

Fig. 5. Nephroblastoma: a strip of urothelium embedded in primitive mesenchyme
(HE × 100)

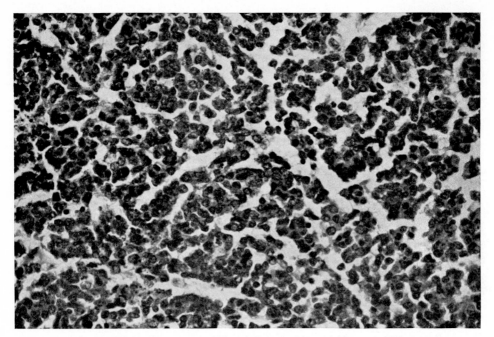

Fig. 6. Nephroblastoma: a mass of undifferentiated renal blastema (HE × 100)

The overall proportion of undifferentiated tumours is higher in Uganda (48 out of 52, or 92%) than in the United Kingdom (65 out of 89, or 73%). This may be an additional factor in the very poor survival of Ugandan children with this tumour. Prime importance, however, should be attached to early detection and adequate treatment.

Spread, Treatment and Prognosis

Nephroblastoma tends to remain circumscribed and spread through the pseudo-capsule of compressed fibrous tissue is a late occurrence. It was nevertheless already present in eight of 14 cases in which resection was carried out, which is an indication of late diagnosis. Metastases, in order of frequency, were seen in regional lymph nodes (5 cases), liver (4 cases), lungs (2 cases) and testis (1 case). The renal vein was involved in 3 cases. In the vast majority of cases (40 out of 56) no form of curative surgery was attempted and documentation is incomplete. There were only 2 cases in which the tumour was still confined to the kidney; both were operated on and one of them was known to be alive and well after 2 years. In recent years a more vigorous approach has been adopted towards treatment which, ideally, should include removal of all tumour tissue if feasible and subsequent radiotherapy or chemotherapy. This scheme may be excepted to result in very much improved survival figures, particularly in the better differentiated group of tumours of infants and very young children. White and Bodian (Bodian and Rigby, 1964) reported 2-year survival rates of 75% and 100% in their B and C types respectively.

Aetiology

The association with congenital abnormalities ("renal ears", aniridia, horseshoe kidney) indicates the presence of some carcinogenic influence in intra-uterine life, but the nature of this is unknown (PELLER, 1965).

Adenocarcinoma of the Kidney

Synonyms: hypernephroma, clear-cell carcinoma of the kidney, Grawitz tumour.

Adenocarcinoma of the kidney is rare in Uganda, and represents only 0.25% of all malignant tumours. This is in contrast to most recorded figures from Western Europe and North America which are usually in the 1—2% range but in keeping with the rest of Africa, similar low rates being known to obtain in all the sub-Saharan portion of the Continent (DAVEY, 1968). This low incidence is only partly accounted for by the low proportion of the middle-aged and elderly people in African populations (HIGGINSON and OETTLÉ, 1962).

In most areas of the world the majority of patients with this tumour present in the fifth and sixth decades. Rarely, adenocarcinoma of the kidney develops in children or in extreme old age. Males are affected twice as often as females. The growth may arise in either kidney and is occasionally bilateral. The majority originate from the renal cortex near the upper pole. This is also a common site for "adrenal rests" which is why renal adenocarcinoma was once supposed to originate from these islets of adrenal tissue entrapped under the capsule of the kidney ("hypernephroma").There is a superficial histological similary but electron microscopy has demonstrated its origin from renal tubular epithelium (OBERLING, RIVIERE and HAGUENAU, 1960).

Adenocarcinoma has excited considerable interest because of its association with certain systemic, haematological and biochemical phenomena. Patients with this tumour commonly present with pyrexia of unknown origin, anaemia and an elevated erythrocyte sedimentation rate. These features are apparently not due to necrosis or haemorrhage within the tumour or to the presence of metastases. In about 2% of cases polycythaemia is present, characterized by erythrocytosis without leukocytosis or thrombocythaemia and a normal arterial oxygen saturation content. High levels of erythropoetin have been found in the blood and in the tumour itself after removal. Hypercalcaemia may also occur in the absence of skeletal metastases. Finally, in about 7% of cases amyloid is present in both kidneys as well as elsewhere in the body. The commonest form of presentation, however, is the classical triad of haematuria, a mass and pain in the flank.

Age and Sex

Table 5 shows the age and sex distribution of adenocarcinoma of the kidney in Uganda, which shows no significant difference from other parts of the world. The youngest patient was 18 and the oldest 60 years of age. Most cases occurred in the 30 to 50 age group but this may be explained by the small proportion of people over 50 in the population at risk. Both sexes were affected equally.

Tribal and Geographical Distribution

Nine of these 19 cases occurred in Buganda. This is slightly more than would be expected but the low figures do not allow any comparisons of significance.

Table 5. Age and sex distribution of 19 cases of renal adenocarcinoma in Uganda

	Males	Females	Total
0—10	—	—	—
11—20	—	1	1
21—30	1	1	2
31—40	—	4	4
41—50	5	2	7
51—60	3	—	3
61—70	—	—	—
70 and over	—	—	—
Age unknown	1	1	2
Total	10	9	19

Macroscopic Features

In common with many other types of visceral cancer in Uganda, these tumours also presented when large or very large. The largest recorded example weighed 4 kg. Both kidneys were affected with equal frequency but none was bilateral. The usual naked-eye appearance as that of a rounded lobulated mass displacing the remainder of the kidney to one side and surrounded by a flimsy pseudo-capsule of thin connective tissue. The appearance of the cut surface was variable and depended to some extent on the histological type. Growths mainly composed of clear cells, at least in part, were of a typical golden-yellow colour. Others, made up chiefly of granular cells, presented a whitish, mottled appearance. Areas of fresh or old haemorrhage and necrosis were usually evident. Degeneration followed by liquefaction produced cysts in an otherwise solid tumour. Areas of fibrosis were common, either as thin strands dividing the tumour into lobules or as more extensive areas of scarring. A papillary growth pattern was sometimes evident to the unaided eye, giving rise to cystic spaces filled with yellow-brown cauliflower or frond-like projections sprouting from the wall. Large, dilated vascular spaces were nearly always present. The capsule and/or the renal vein showed naked-eye evidence of tumour infiltration in some cases.

Histological Features

Renal adenocarcinomas show a wide range of structural variation depending on arrangement, cell type and degree of differentiation. Fifteen of the 19 tumours in this series were predominantly solid and were composed of variable mixture of clear and granular cells. Clear plant-like cells are usually disposed in a solid, alveolar fashion, bounded by slender connective-tissue septa. The nuclei are regular, round and usually small, with dense, darkly staining chromatin. The clarity of the cytoplasm is due to the accumulation of lipid and glycogen, both of which are lost in routine histological processing, leaving a seemingly empty cell. The cytoplasm of tumour cells may also be finely, but densely granular. The next commonest appearance, in four tumours, was that of clear or granular cells arranged in tubular, papillary or cystic patterns. Finally, some tumours are made up of spindle and giant cells with marked variability in size and shape, bizarre, gigantic nuclei and numerous mitoses. Only one tumour in this series was of this anaplastic type.

Attempts to relate these diverse histological patterns to clinical behaviour have largely failed but there is evidence from several sources mainly the series of GRIFFITHS and THACKRAY (1949) that grade of differentiation has a statistical significance in prognosis. Grading is not based on cell type but on general criteria of malignancy. Tumours which show well marked tubule formation or are neatly organized into papillary and cystic formations qualify for Grade I so long as their cells are fairly uniform in size and staining with few mitoses. Survival in this is 10 or more years even though many patients eventually develop metastases. The cells of Grade III tumours, at the other extreme, are grossly pleomorphic and exhibit many mitoses. Most patients in this group are dead within three years. Grade II tumours are intermediate between Grades I and III in all respects. In this series there were five tumours in Grade I, 13 in Grade II and only one in Grade III. It would seem that renal adenocarcinomas are better differentiated in Ugandan Africans and should carry a better prognosis.

Spread, Treatment and Prognosis

Adenocarcinoma of the kidney expands as it grows, stretching the kidney and surrounding soft tissues around itself and a pseudocapsule is formed. Local spread results in breach of this capsule with invasion of perinephric fat and adjoining structures, particularly colon. There is a tendency for growth into the renal vein which may be continued up the inferior vena cava and may even reach the heart. At operation metastases to regional lymph nodes are present in about one-third of cases. More common and of greater importance is, however, dissemination via the blood stream to many distant organs. The extent of spread was known in 13 of 19 cases in this series; there was none in two, local in 6, lymphatic in 5 and blood-borne in 5, to liver, lung and bone. Treatment was by surgical resection. Prognosis is determined by grading, as referred to above, and even more, by extent of spread. The fate of those treated is not known.

Aetiological Factors

Little is known about the aetiology of adenocarcinoma of the kidney in man. Its incidence begins to rise in the fourth decade and this continues throughout life. Males are more commonly affected than females, which may indicate the effect of sex hormones on tumour initiation and growth. Such an effect has been demonstrated in some animal species. The protracted administration of oestrogens to male Syrian hamsters, for example, often induces multiple renal adenocarcinomas but fails in females unless preceded by castration. Studies of the effects of hormones on renal adenocarcinoma in man are, as yet, inconclusive (BLOOM, DUKES and MITCHLEY, 1963). More important, perhaps, is a trend for renal adenocarcinoma to increase with urbanization and this is most evident in males of social class 1 at the top end of the economic scale (CASE, 1964). Occupation, however, is without effect.

It is often difficult to distinguish a renal cortical adenoma from an adenocarcinoma. Lesions considered benign may be solid, papillary or cystic and be composed of clear or granular cells. They are most frequently found under the capsule and vary from a few millimeters to several centimeters in size. They are rarely encapsulated, but lack other evidence of malignancy, such as increased mitotic activity, necrosis or haemorrhage. Bell (1938) found that the majority of those under 3 cm in diameter are truly benign and will not recur or metastasize after removal. The distinction, however, is purely arbitrary in many cases. Many adenomas arise in contracted kidneys scarred by arteriosclerosis or chronic infection (Rees and Winstanley, 1958).

It is of interest to note that in 9 of 19 cases of renal adenocarcinoma in this series the tumour bearing kidney was grossly scarred by chronic pyelonephritis and in 3 multiple renal adenomata were present. One of these is shown in Fig. 7.

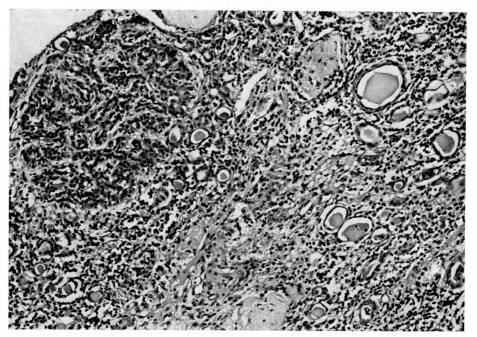

Fig. 7. One of several renal adenomata (top left) in an area of chronic pyelonephritis. A renal adenocarcinoma was also present in the same kidney (HE × 40)

Carcinoma of the Renal Pelvis

Four tumours were seen in this category, of which two were transitional cell carcinomas and two squamous cell carcinomas. One of the latter was associated with renal calculus. Calculus is only very rarely seen in Ugandan Africans.

Other Malignant Tumours of the Kidney

One case of fibrosarcoma was seen in a female patient aged 31.

The Bladder

The incidence of carcinoma of the bladder varies considerably throughout the world. Several large-scale investigations have determined the relative frequency of these tumours in different geographical areas, in different races, in both sexes, and have analyzed the patterns of general and specific populations, clinical findings and autopsy records (STEINER, 1954; DORN and CUTLER, 1955; CLEMMESEN, NIELSEN and LOCKWOOD, 1957; SEGI and KURIHARA, 1964, 1966; DUNHAM and BAILAR, 1968; DOLL, MUIR and WATERHOUSE, 1970). The situation is a complex one and is liable to fluctuations even in the same area or group of people. The findings of these and numerous other studies have been summarized by HUEPER (1969) and may be briefly stated as follows:

The evidence for geographical variability is impressive. In general, the highest mortality rates prevail in the most highly industrialized and urbanized countries though there are remarkable exceptions to this, Japan and Sweden for example. Hereditary, genetic or racial factors seem unimportant and even where differences exist between races living in the same area, such as whites and negroes in South Africa, these are most likely to arise from environmental factors (OETTLÉ, 1964). Males are more commonly affected than females in all countries except in Mozambique where bladder tumours occur slightly more frequently in females (PRATES, 1962). In most countries carcinoma of the bladder is a disease of middle age and beyond but this is not always so, even in industrialized countries such as Japan, Norway or Sweden and a slight shift into younger age groups definitely occurs in many parts of Africa. The incidence of bladder cancer appears to be rising in England and Wales (CASE, 1956), Denmark (CLEMMESEN, 1965), Japan (SEGI and KURIHARA, 1966) and other industrialized countries. Town dwellers are more prone to bladder cancer than rural inhabitants. This may be influenced by numerous occupational hazards that are known to exist, particularly in the dye, rubber and cable industries, most of which have been traced to the presence of 2-naphthylamine (CASE, 1966). The risk of exposure may also occur in other people through pollution of public waterways. Cigarette smoking may increase liability by a factor that has been variably estimated from two- to five-fold (KERR and BARKIN, 1970).

International comparisons suffer from inaccuracies common to many other tumours with, in addition, two further complications. One is a lack of agreement on what constitutes a transitional-cell papilloma as distinct from carcinoma, which confuses bladder cancer statistics in areas where this histological type is common. The various schemes of classification and grading have been discussed by JACOBS (1967). The other is that there are at least two histological types of carcinoma of the bladder that may be aetiologically different: transitional-cell carcinoma and squamous-cell carcinoma. The former accounts for about 90% of cases in Europe and North America (PUGH, 1959; MOSTOFI, 1968) whereas the latter is much commoner in Africa (OETTLÉ, 1955; DIMETTE, SPROAT and SAYEGH, 1956; DODGE, 1962). The third major type, adenocarcinoma, forms a small minority of cases. The importance of registering bladder cancer by histological type has recently been emphasized by TULINIUS (1970).

Much of the controversy in Africa regarding aetiology of bladder cancer has centred on the role of chronic schistosomal infestation. The strength of the evidence for and against varies in different parts of Africa (Case, 1962). The situation in Uganda will be discussed below.

Carcinoma of the Bladder in Uganda: General Data

Fig. 2 shows the total age- and sex-specific incidence rates of cancers of the urinary tract in Uganda and Table 2 the comparative age-corrected incidence rates in selected countries as defined by ICD. Number 181 may be usefully divided into two further categories: carcinomas of the bladder and carcinomas of the urethra. The latter will be considered separately, though it is recognized that an overlap may exist between these two tumour sites.

Age and Sex Distribution

Table 6 shows the age and sex distribution of 127 cases of carcinoma of the bladder. The youngest patient was 20 and the oldest 95 years of age but the majority, 89 of 127 cases, fall in the 40—70 age group with a mean of 54.8 years. The age distribution was similar in all histological types.

It is also evident from Table 6 that males predominate over females to quite an unusual extent, the ratio of male to female being 8.1:1. This ratio was also similar in all histological types.

Table 6. Age and sex distribution of 127 carcinomas of the bladder
of all types in Uganda

	Males	Females	Total
0—10			
11—20		1	1
21—30	3	2	5
31—40	5	2	7
41—50	28	6	34
51—60	33	3	36
61—70	18	1	19
70 and over	22	1	23
Not known	1	1	2
Total	110	17	127[a]

[a] Excludes 11 non-epithelial tumours.

Tribal and Geographical Distribution

Seventy or just about half of all patients were Baganda, and a further 18 cases were of other tribes but also residing in East and West Mengo districts. This concentration of cases in the most urbanized part of the country is unlikely to be due entirely to selection by availability of hospital facilities as these exist throughout the country. A possible source of bias is the existence of sophisticated urological skill and, in particular, diagnosis by cystoscopy, both of which tend to be concentrated in the main Kampala hospitals. Many cases, however, present with such gross disease, namely tumours fungating through cystotomy tracks and abdominal fistulas, that the correct diagnosis is perfectly obvious on simple clinical examination.

Transitional Cell Carcinoma

This histological type was the least common epithelial neoplasm with 19 cases out of a total of 127 in this series (14.9%). This is in contrast to experience in England (PUGH, 1959) and North America (MOSTOFI, 1968) but similar to experience in other parts of Africa (OETTLÉ, 1955; DIMETTE, SPROAT and SAYEGH, 1956; DODGE, 1962).

Site

Reliable information existed in only 10 of 19 cases. The growth was situated on the trigone in 6 cases, on the lateral and posterior walls in one each and was multiple in 2.

Macroscopic and Microscopic Features

Most tumours were described as large. Seven were frond-like, papillary growths, 10 solid, infiltrative and ulcerated; two were partly papillary and partly solid. All these tumours were made of transitional type of cells arranged either on a tree-like framework of slender connective tissue papillae or in broad, anastomosing masses. All were invasive.

Grading was carried out according to generally accepted criteria of degree of resemblance to normal tissue, nuclear pleomorphism and number of mitoses. Four tumours were of low, 6 of average and 9 of high grade.

Squamous metaplasia was present in 7 tumours. Its presence did not bear any relationship to grade.

Bladder mucosa away from the tumour was available for study in only 4 cases; 2 of these showed carcinoma in situ.

Two patients had urethral strictures on first presentation and gave histories of 2 and 4 years' difficulty in micturition. In one of these squamous metaplasia was present in the tumour.

Spread and Prognosis

Information on these points is incomplete. In only two cases was the tumour still confined to the submucosa. Muscle only was invaded in one. There was local spread to the soft tissues of the pelvis in 7 cases, 2 of which presented with vesicovaginal or rectal fistulae. There was no attempt made at regular follow-up of these patients during the period of study, and none of them came to autopsy.

Squamous Cell Carcinoma

This histological type was by far the commonest with 75 out of a total of 127 epithelial tumours of the bladder (59%). Squamous metaplasia occurs in transitional cell carcinomas but tumours made up purely of squamous cells are uncommon in England (PUGH, 1959) and North America (MOSTOFI, 1968), accounting for only

6—7⁰/₀ of cases. In most parts of Africa, on the other hand, squamous cell carcinoma is quite common: 55⁰/₀ in Egypt (DIMETTE, SPROAT and SAYEGH, 1956), 57⁰/₀ in South African negroes (OETTLÉ, 1955), 59⁰/₀ in Portuguese East Africa (GILLMAN and PRATES, 1962). In an earlier study DODGE (1964) recorded that 40⁰/₀ of bladder cancer in Uganda was of squamous cell type.

Site

In 13 cases the site of the tumour could not be established from the records available. In 28 it was stated to fill the whole of the bladder. In 21 cases the base was chiefly involved and in the remaining 12 the growth arose from the walls of the organ.

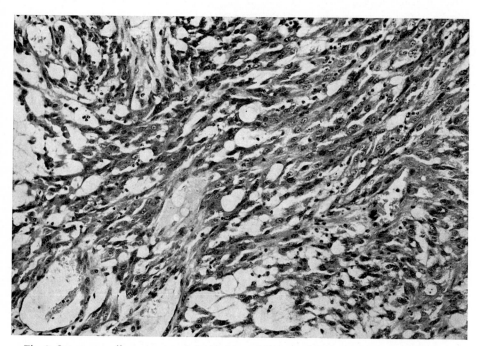

Fig. 8. Squamous cell carcinoma of the bladder with a pseudosarcomatous spindle cell pattern
(HE × 100)

Macroscopic and Microscopic Features

Squamous cell carcinomas formed shaggy, necrotic, infected masses, frequently ulcerated and sometimes covered by crusts made up of keratin, tissue debris and fibrin. Histologically they were made up purely of squamous cells. The degree of differentiation was assessed in three grades: low (17 cases), average (27 cases), and high (31 cases), denoting increasing anaplasia. Fig. 8 shows a highly undifferentiated squamous cells carcinoma with a pseudosarcomatous spindle-cell pattern.

Bladder mucosa away from the tumour, or not destroyed by it, was available in 38 cases. Squamous metaplasia was seen in 13 of these and carcinoma in situ in 7, in 3 cases both being present. PRATES and GILLMAN (1959) regarded squamous metaplasia as a complication rather than a precursor of cancer. CONNERY (1953), however, followed up 45 cases with metaplasia, and 15 of these patients eventually developed cancer. Further follow-up studies are clearly necessary.

Stricture of the urethra was present in 32 of 75 cases of squamous cell carcinoma of bladder with a history of difficulty in micturition for some years preceding. The usual site of the stricture was the posterior part of the penile urethra. It is of interest to consider the effect of urethral strictures on the presence of squamous metaplasia and carcinoma in situ. In all 10 cases of stricture in which non-tumorous bladder mucosa was available either squamous metaplasia or carcinoma in situ was present. By contrast, in 28 cases without stricture only 4 showed squamous metaplasia and 3 carcinoma in situ.

Spread and Prognosis

No information was available in 32 cases. In 6 the tumour was confined to the blader wall. In 27 the pelvis had been invaded, with lymph node metastases in 13. Widespread metastases were present in 4 when first seen. Four presented with anterior abdominal fistulae with tumour fungating through; in 2 vesicorectal and in one vesicovaginal communications were present. Prognosis is difficult to determine as regular follow-up was not possible. In the majority of cases survival is unlikely to have been prolonged because of the extensive nature of the disease. Fifteen patients came to autopsy, but the fate of the remainder was not known.

Adenocarcinoma

The proportion of cases of adenocarcinoma amongst patients with bladder cancer in England and North America is no more than 1—2% (PUGH, 1959; MOSTOFI, 1968). Some of these are accounted for by a definite predisposing condition such as exstrophy of the bladder. In Uganda 26 of 128 cases (20.3%) were of this type, the frequency being rather higher than that of transitional-cell carcinoma but considerably lower than squamous-cell carcinoma.

Site

In 12 cases the site was not recorded. The whole of the bladder was involved in four, the base in 8 and the fundus in 2.

Macroscopic and Microscopic Features

Adenocarcinomas of the bladder formed an interesting group with varied features. The majority, 18 cases, were solid, 4 were grossly mucoid and 4 papillary. FRIEDMAN and ASH (1959) pointed out that since the lining of the bladder derives partly from the primitive endoderm of the cloaca and partly from a portion of the Wolffian duct, tumours may manifest histogenetic potentialities common to the entire cloacal-urogenital complex. This may explain the tremendous variability of pattern in

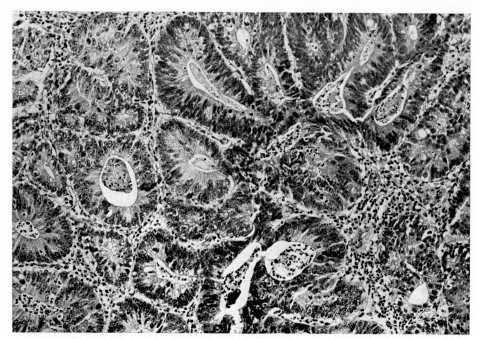

Fig. 9. Adenocarcinoma of the bladder: glandular spaces lined by columnar, intestinal type of epithelium (HE × 40)

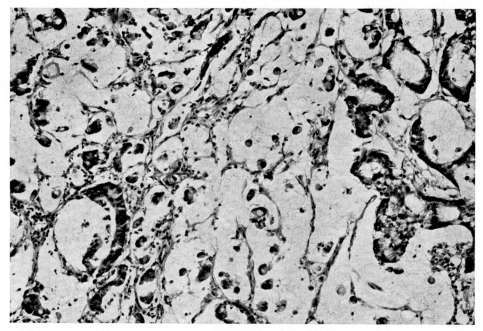

Fig. 10. Mucoid adenocarcinoma of the bladder: the tumour cells, some of "signet-ring" cell type, lie in pools of mucus. Strips of columnar cell epithelium are also present (HE × 40)

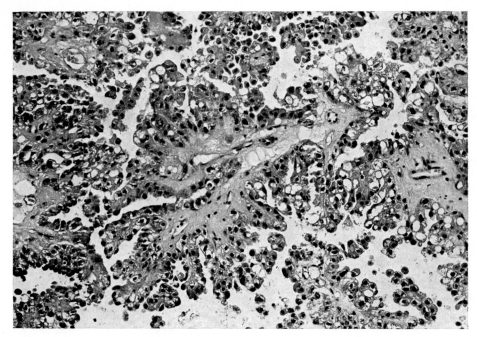

Fig. 11. Papillary adenocarcinoma of the bladder with a toothed, peg-like surface epithelial
lining resembling neoplastic mesothelium (HE × 40)

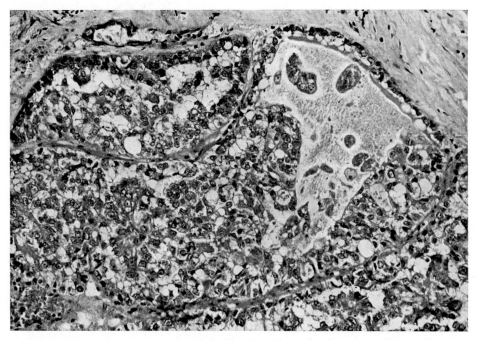

Fig. 12. Clear cell adenocarcinoma of the bladder with an alveolar pattern (HE × 40)

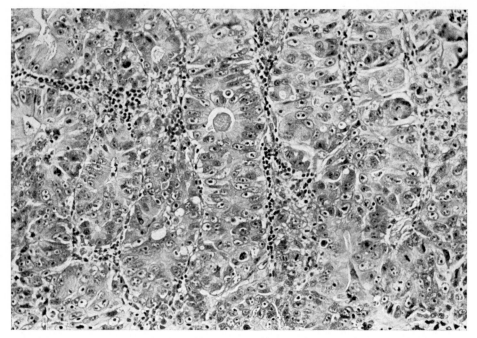

Fig. 13. Adenocarcinoma of the bladder resembling müllerian epithelium (HE × 100)

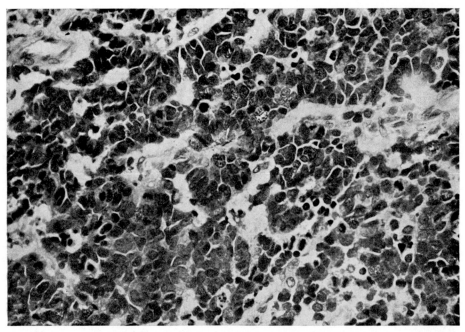

Fig. 14. Anaplastic carcinoma, with no recognisable pattern of differentiation in any part of the tumour (HE × 100)

adenocarcinomas, resembling urachal, intestinal, endometrial, nephrogenic and mesothelial tissues. Fig. 9 shows the commonest pattern which is clearly intestinal and is
almost indistinguishable from that of carcinoma of the colon (12 cases). Four further
cases were grossly mucoid and were made up almost entirely of signet-ring cells
(Fig. 10). In others (4 case) a papillary and cystic pattern was evident with a surface
lining of cuboidal cells sometimes of a peg-like or toothed appearance rather
resembling mesothelium (Fig. 11). One of these also showed the presence of clear
cells, forming alveolar structures, cysts and tuft-like projections somewhat reminiscent of ovarian "mesonephromas" (Fig. 12). One case showed a close resemblance to
müllerian epithelium (Fig. 13) and one was partly adenoid and partly squamoid
("adenoacanthoma"). This variability is well covered by the term of FRIEDMAN and
ASH (1959) who called them all "dysontogenic tumours."

Nine of these 26 adenocarcinomas were associated with a pre-existing stricture of
the posterior urethra. In 4 glandular metaplasia of the bladder mucosa was also
present. The relationship of this metaplastic change to adenocarcinoma is of interest.
MCINTOSH and WORLEY (1955) showed that in exstrophy of the bladder normal
transitional cell type of mucosa is present at birth which later undergoes glandular
metaplasia and eventually adenocarcinoma develops.

Spread and Prognosis

In 10 cases the extent of spread was not recorded. The pelvis was invaded in 9,
with lymph node metastases in 4. Four patients presented with fistulae, 2 on the
anterior abdominal wall and 2 in the rectum. Two patients had widespread metastases. Nine came to autopsy, the fate of the remainder was unknown.

Anaplastic Carcinoma

Seven cases could not be assigned to any of the above categories. All of them
were thought to be undifferentiated tumours of epithelial origin (Fig. 14). There were
no distinguishing features of interest.

Non-Epithelial Malignant Tumours of the Bladder

There were 4 embryonal sarcomas, 2 with rhabdomyosarcomatous differentiation
and one leiomyosarcoma, all of them in children. Three malignant lymphomas
and one fibrosarcoma were seen in adults. Two cases of phaeochromocytoma in the
bladder wall were seen.

Aetiological Factors in Bladder Cancer in Uganda

A number of seemingly disparate factors have been incriminated in the aetiology
of carcinoma of the bladder. Table 7 summarizes these according to the histological
type of malignancy. Some of these may be operative in Uganda, others are clearly not.

Table 7. Aetiological factors in carcinoma of the bladder listed by histological type

Transitional cell carcinoma
Carcinogenic chemicals encountered in industry:
      2 naphthylamine
      4 aminodiphenyl benzidine
Endogenous carcinogens:
      abnormal tryptophan metabolites
      excess β-glucuronidase
Cigarette smoking
Schistosomiasis
Non-specific chronic inflammation associated
  with stones and diverticula

Squamous cell carcinoma
Schistosomiasis
Urethral stricture
Leukoplakia
Abnormal tryptophan metabolites
Excess β-glucuronidase
Non-specific chronic inflammation associated
  with stones and diverticula

Adenocarcinoma
Exstrophy of the bladder
Cystitis glandularis
Non-specific inflammation associated with
  stones and diverticula

Schistosomiasis

There was not a single case of vesical schistosomiasis in 127 carcinomas of the bladder in this series.

Much has been written on the association, or lack of it, of squamous cell carcinoma of the bladder with chronic infestation by *Schistosoma haematobium*. Most of the evidence comes from Egypt, where 70 to 90% of the population has been stated to harbour the parasite (Ibrahim, 1948). Hashem (1961) found that carcinoma of the bladder comprised 12% of all cancer encountered in 4447 autopsies in the Pathology Department of the Cairo University Hospital and that 83.1% of bladder cancer occurred in bladders infested with schistosomiasis. This suggests a highly significant association but others have not always found it so. Gillman and Prates (1962) writing of Portuguese East Africa, an area in which schistosomiasis is endemic, argued in favour of a causal connection between infestation and bladder cancer. Edington (1956) reported strong evidence of such a connection from Ghana: schistosomal ova were found in 71% of autopsies on bladder cancer cases while the prevalence of schistosomiasis in the general population was only 1.4%. Higginson and Oettlé (1962) were more guarded in their assessment of the situation in South Africa and suggested the severity of the infestation ought to be taken into consideration as well as its mere presence. Payet (1962) went so far as to say that there was no proof that schistosomiasis was involved in the aetiology of bladder cancer in former French West African territories where infestation with *Schistosoma haema-*

tobium was endemic but there was no appreciable difference in the incidence of bladder cancer from areas where it was infrequent or absent.

Those who believe in a causal connection between *Schistoma haematobium* infestation and cancer in the bladder have pointed out that tumours occur in younger age groups, are usually of squamous cell type and do not involve the base of the bladder. Males predominate in Egypt but females are more commonly affected in Mozambique. A credible explanation of this phenomenon may be the fact that agriculture in Egypt is an essentially male occupation in contrast to Mozambique where for the most part women cultivate the fields (HIGGINSON and OETTLÉ, 1962).

In Uganda, though squamous cell carcinoma is the commonest type, evidence of vesical schistosomiasis is totally lacking. DODGE (1962) found a single instance out of 83 cases and in this series there was none out of 127 cases. These findings are in striking contrast to those in other parts of Africa and tend to invalidate the argument for a causative role of schistosomiasis in the undoubtedly high incidence of squamous cell carcinoma in most parts of the Continent. *Schistosoma haematobium* only occurs with any frequency in the Lango district of central Uganda (BRADLEY, 1968). This series includes 3 cases of bladder cancer from this area, all of which were of the transitional cell type. *Schistosoma mansoni* is more widespread and ova are not infrequently seen in rectal and liver biopsy material in the diagnostic histopathology service of the Pathology Department of Mulago Hospital, Kampala, which covers the whole of Uganda. In a review of 30,700 biopsies and 3,369 post mortems ANTHONY and McADAM (1972) found 122 instances of schistosomal infestation. In the vast majority (117) the liver and the gastrointestinal canal were affected. There were 2 cases of bladder infestation, both in biopsies sent from the Shirati district of Tanzania. One of these was associated with transitional cell carcinoma, the other with mucoid adenocarcinoma.

A shift in the incidence of bladder cancer towards younger age groups is absent in Uganda. Males predominate over females in a ratio of 8.6 to 1, yet, as in Mozambique, females tend to work in the fields and not males as in Egypt. The base of the bladder is not conspicuously spared.

The failure to incriminate vesical schistosomiasis in the aetiology of bladder cancer in Uganda must direct attention towards other possibilities and of these urethral stricture seems the most important.

Urethral Stricture

Table 8 shows that in 43 of 120 cases of histologically classifiable bladder cancer a pre-existing urethral stricture was present. In squamous cell carcinoma this figure rose to 32 of 75 or 42.6%. These strictures were situated in the posterior penile urethra. Their aetiology is unknown, though there is a strong belief among clinicians in Uganda that they are post-gonococcal. DODGE (1964) had come to similar conclusions in an earlier study, recording a 35% incidence of stricture in bladder cancer in Uganda. There often is several years' history of difficulty in micturition and patients may present with tumours fungating through cystotomy tracks in the anterior abdominal wall. DODGE (1964) recorded 8 such cases and there were 6 in this series.

It is a matter for speculation how strictures may enhance the development of cancer in the bladder. Assuming that most bladder cancer is induced by some constituent or other of the urine, the longer it is in contact with the mucosa the greater the effect. DODGE (1964) postulated that this was due to an abnormal pattern of tryptophan metabolism and increased β-glucuronidase activity in the urine. Dietary tryptophan is either incorporated into the body proteins or broken down to serotonin, 5-hydroxyindole-acetic acid (5-HIAA) or nicotinic acid. Several compounds are found along these metabolic pathways that are themselves or that are converted to carcinogenic ortho-aminophenols. Detailed investigations showed an increase of these in the urine of patients with bladder cancer (KERR, BARKIN and MENCZYK, 1964). Matoke, which is a preparation of steamed green bananas, forms the staple diet of Ugandan Africans. Serotonin is known to exist in high concentration in bananas and matoke-eaters excrete abnormally large amounts of 5-HIAA in the urine (CRAWFORD, 1962). The possibility of other tryptophan derivatives being present in bananas also exists. The ortho-aminophenols excreted are normally in the form of conjugates, mainly glucuronides. The presence of β-glucuronidase would

Table 8. Urethral stricture and main types of carcinoma of the bladder in Uganda

	Total	Urethral stricture present	%
Transitional cell carcinoma	19	2	10.5
Squamous cell carcinoma	75	32	42.6
Adenocarcinoma	26	9	34.6
	120 [a]	43	35.8

[a] Excludes anaplastic carcinomas that could not be classified further.

convert them to free and actively carcinogenic ortho-aminophenols (BOYLAND, 1963). It is therefore possible to postulate, with DODGE (1964), that elevation of this enzyme would convert an innocuous urine to one that was carcinogenic and this could be highly significant in those with urinary retention due to urethral strictures. It may be noted also that in vesical schistosomiasis elevated levels of both ortho-aminophenol derivatives and of β-glucoronidase have been found with or without the presence of a tumour (FRIPP, 1965). The current situation with regard to these recent biochemical developments has been reviewed by KERR and BARKIN (1970) and is rather more complex than had been suggested. It is possible, however, that both chronic urinary retention due to urethral strictures in Uganda and vesical schistosomiasis as seen, say, in Egypt could contribute to bladder cancer through stasis of altered urinary constituents. This still does not explain why squamous-cell carcinoma is so common in Africa unless one postulates that stasis also leads to chronic inflammation and squamous metaplasia in the bladder. There is some evidence in support of this from the findings presented above, namely that in all 10 cases of stricture in which non-tumorous bladder mucosa was available either squamous metaplasia or carcinoma in situ or both were present in contrast to 28 cases without stricture only four of which showed these changes.

Other Possible Causes and Predisposing Factors

Chemical carcinogens of industrial origin are unlikely to have any significant role in Uganda. Ninety-four percent of the population live off the land and the type of industrial activity that might produce a carcinogenic risk is all but non-existent even in the capital. The habit of smoking is increasing but it is unlikely to be an important cause of cancer in Uganda where squamous-cell carcinoma predominates. In Western populations with a high consumption of cigarettes transitional-cell carcinoma remains the commonest form of bladder malignancy. Bladder stones are rare anywhere in Africa and none were encountered in this series. Diverticula may predispose to carcinoma through, it is assumed, urinary stasis and chronic infection but again there were none in this study. Those born with exstrophy of the bladder are highly liable to subsequent development of glandular metaplasia and adenocarcinoma and this is occasionally seen in Uganda, but there were none in this material.

The Urethra

In the period covered by the study 42 histologically confirmed carcinomas of the urethra were seen. The bladder-urethra cancer ratio is 3:1 which is higher than the ratio of 5:1 recorded earlier by DODGE (1962) and considerably higher than the 40:1 in Europeans.

Table 9 shows that the age and sex distribution was similar to that of bladder cancer with the same heavy preponderance of males over females: 8.3 to 1. Thirty-four out of 42 patients were from the Baganda tribe.

Table 9. Age and sex distribution of 42 carcinomas of the urethra

	Males	Females	Total
0—10			
11—20			
21—30			
31—40	4		4
41—50	8	3	11
51—60	9	1	10
61—70	11	1	12
70 and over	1	1	2
Not known	3		3
Total	36	6	42

These tumours were situated in the posterior urethra in all but 3 cases where they presented as indurated, clinically palpable swellings. Six presented with extravasation of urine into the soft tissues of the perineum and scrotum and multiple discharging fistulas. The usual mode of spread of these tumours was into the urethral bulb first

(8 cases) then to the perineum (20 cases), base of penis (6 cases), scrotum (5 cases) and buttocks (1 case). Metastases were present in the inguinal lymph nodes in 6 cases. Only one case came to autopsy and was found to have widespread dissemination of tumour to many organs.

Thirty-eight of 42 cases were squamous cell carcinomas. They were graded into low (15), average (13) and high (10). Two of these were situated near the external meatus. Three were adenocarcinomas and one transitional cell carcinoma, the latter in the mid-shaft of the penis.

Twenty-one cases were associated with stricture of the posterior urethra, known to have been present for up to 10 years before the development of the tumour. All but one of these were squamous-cell carcinomas. In none of the 42 cases was there any evidence of urinary schistosomiasis.

The overall picture is similar to that described for carcinoma of the bladder and the same deliberations may be applied to aetiology.

Chapter 9

Melanoma

M. G. LEWIS

With 5 Figures

Benign naevi are probably as common in Ugandan Africans as in other peoples. They, are, however, only rarely excised. Malignant melanomas most frequently arise on the feet and as a rule are only found in parts of the body which are normally not pigmented. Thus melanomas of the trunk or choroid are very rare. About 11% of melanomas are found only in lymph nodes and evidence suggests that in such cases the primary tumour has regressed, probably as a result of immune rejection. The reasons why the pigmented portions of the skin should be so resistant to tumour growth are unknown.

Malignant melanoma was diagnosed in 195 cases, 191 of which were histologically confirmed. Biopsy specimens were taken of 34 benign melanocytic tumours during this period.

Melanomas accounted for 2.7% of malignant tumours overall, a figure very similar to that found in other countries. The black cancer has been familiar in Africa for many years; for example ALBERT COOK described a case in 1904 (DAVIES et al., 1964). Many references in the literature suggest that negroes are less likely to develop melanoma than whites (MATAS, 1896; PACK, 1948; RAVEN, 1966). In fact, the incidence in Uganda is 0.55 per 100,000 persons per year and in Kyadondo County it is 1.7 cases in females and 0.7 cases in males per 100,000 persons per annum (all figures corrected for an African standard population). These figures are very similar to returns of many cancer registries from different parts of the world in many different races (DOLL et al., 1970).

Four patients were under 25 at the time of diagnosis; age-specific incidence rates are shown in Table 1. The fall in ratio among old people is probably an artefact due to inability or unwillingness to come to hospital, but the age-specific incidence curve in all registries shows only a slow rise with age in contrast with the exponential rise with some tumours. This suggests that the carcinogenic stimulus for malignant melanoma is not an accumulative one.

There were 98 females and 97 males. The incidence among females in Kyadondo County is significantly higher than in males and proportional rates in many different tribes show a higher figure than in males (Table 2).

The geographical variation of malignant melanoma is quite marked (Table 2). The Bakiga and Lugbara both show high proportional rates while other tribes living

Table 1. Age-specific incidence rates of malignant melanoma for Uganda.
Cases per year per 100,000 persons

	Female	Male
15—24	0.03	—
25—34	0.4	0.4
35—44	1.3	0.9
45—54	1.8	2.0
55—64	2.8	2.8
65—74	1.7	1.6
75+	0.3	0.3

Table 2. Malignant melanoma in different tribes, expressed as a
proportion of total cancer

Tribe	Male	Female	Both
Bantu			
Kiga	7.7	4.8	6.1
Ankole	3.0	2.6	2.8
Toro	0.7	6.1	3.1
Bunyoro	1.4	1.3	1.4
Ganda	1.5	1.5	1.5
Soga	3.6	3.7	3.6
Ruanda/Rundi	2.8	3.2	3.0
Nilotic			
Acholi	1.0	2.8	1.9
Lango	2.5	3.5	3.0
Nilo-Hamitic			
Teso	3.0	1.8	2.4
Karamojong	5.1	—	3.7
Sudanic			
Lugbara	5.2	7.1	6.0
All tribes	2.4	2.9	2.7

in the west of the country show much lower rates. These rates will be influenced by
the quality of medical care available in different parts of the country and the use
that people make of them. However, there does not appear to be any correlation
between rates and accessibility to hospitals or to geographical factors (Lewis, 1968).
The incidence of melanoma in different tribes is difficult to obtain since questions as
to tribal background were not asked in the 1969 Census. If one assumes that the
proportion of the population accounted for by different tribes in 1966 was similar to
that in 1959 (Uganda Census, 1959) some idea of the relative incidence can be
obtained (Table 3). This suggests that the incidence in the Lugbara is almost four
times the incidence in the Bunyoro and shows the tribes in a very similar ranking
order to that obtained using proportional rates. Proportional rates in the different
ethnic groups show a tendency for Sudanic people to have a slightly higher rate than
Bantu, but differences are not significant (Table 4).

Table 3. To show the number of cases of melanoma and the relative frequency
in different tribes

Tribe	Cases	% of melanoma cases	% of population	Relative frequency
Lugbara	14	7.2	3.7	1.9
Kiga	22	11.3	7.1	1.5
Toro	8	4.1	3.2	1.3
Soga	17	8.7	7.8	1.1
Lango	12	6.2	5.6	1.1
Ganda	32	16.4	16.1	1.0
Gisu	10	5.1	5.1	1.0
Ankole	13	6.7	8.1	0.8
Acholi	7	3.6	4.4	0.8
Teso	11	5.6	8.1	0.7
Kumam	2	1.0	2.0	0.5
Bunyoro	3	1.5	2.9	0.5

Table 4. Malignant melanoma as a proportion of total cancer
in different racial groups

	Males		Females	
	Cases	Proportional rate	Cases	Proportional rate
Bantu	58	2.5%	56	2.2%
Nilotic	8	2.0%	16	3.8%
Nilo-Hamitic	10	3.0%	7	2.5%
Sudanic	7	3.5%	7	5.0%

The sites of origin of melanomas in Africans (Table 5) are very different from those in Caucasians. In Africans the majority of tumours arise on the foot, usually close to the lateral margin of the sole at the junction of pigmented and unpigmented skin. This distribution is found in all African countries and not only in Uganda (HEWER, 1935; EDINGTON, 1956; THYS, 1957). Melanomas occurring in American negroes also occur fairly frequently on the foot. Other areas in which melanomas occurred were the mouth, nose and conjunctiva. All these areas are normally not pigmented, but can often be seen to have areas of ectopic pigmentation (LEWIS, 1967a). In Africans it is extremely rare for malignant melanoma to arise in pigmented skin (LEWIS and JOHNSON, 1968) or in the uveal tract (see Chapter 13).

The different sites at which melanoma arises in Ugandan Africans have been reviewed (BROOMHALL and LEWIS, 1967; LEWIS, 1967a; LEWIS and MARTIN, 1967). At all these sites the presence of isolated areas of pigmentation are to be found surrounded by normally unpigmented skin. Examination of the feet of Africans reveals that many subjects have pigmented spots on the normally unpigmented skin of the sole. Many of these are pale, rather diffuse patches of pigment but some are discrete junctional naevi which appear much darker in colour and have a distinct edge. The distribution of such naevi on the feet correlates well both anatomically and geographically with the distribution of melanoma (LEWIS, 1968). It is postulated that these isolated areas of pigment-bearing cells are instrinsically unstable, whereas normally pigmented tissues are remarkably resistant to tumour growth, either primary or secondary. The nature of such tumour-resistance to pigmented skin is unknown, but obviously worthy of more detailed study. No case of melanoma was

Table 5. Site of origin of melanomas

Foot	131
Hand	7
Mouth	7
Site not stated	7
Nose	3
Forearm	3
Eye	3
Buttock	2
Lymph nodes	24
Other sites	8 [a]
	195

[a] 1 case each vulva, knee, back, chest wall, scalp, anus, lip.

found in an albino during this study. Such cases are described and it would be of interest to discover the anatomical distribution of melanomas in the unpigmented skin of albinos.

Macroscopically the primary tumour varied in size from pin-head to enormous fungating masses. The tumour was sometimes surrounded by a densely pigmented zone or melanotic blush (Fig. 1). In other cases there was a hypopigmented halo (Fig. 2). Lateral growth was extensive but often ceased abruptly when the tumour encountered normally pigmented skin. This produced a polypoid appearance (Fig. 3). The colour of the tumour varied from coal black to white and often showed variable degrees of pigmentation in different parts of the tumour. The differential diagnosis from Kaposi's sarcoma may be difficult in some cases (LEWIS and KIRYABWIRE, 1968 b).

The histological appearances of malignant melanoma are similar at all sites of origin. Tumours contained variable amounts of melanin and diagnosis may be difficult when only small amounts of melanin are manufactured. Tumours may be classified by the dominant cell pattern present. Spindle-cell type (Fig. 4), alveolar arrangements of round cells and pleiomorphic types are relatively easy to distinguish but mixed cell patterns are common. Junctional activity at the margin of tumours helps to distinguish primary tumours from secondary deposits and such areas must be excised if recurrence of tumour is to be avoided. The macroscopic appearance of this area of junctional activity is the melanotic blush found surrounding some tumours.

Others are surrounded by a hypopigmented zone. Satellite nodules are fairly commonly seen on the sole of the foot but only very rarely spread to the dorsum.

Metastatic spread to involve local lymph nodes occurs commonly and early, particularly when the primary site is in the mouth. However, satellite nodules of tumours occurring along the course of lymphatics are very rarely seen. Twenty-one patients, 11°/o of all cases, were seen in whom there were large inguinal nodes which

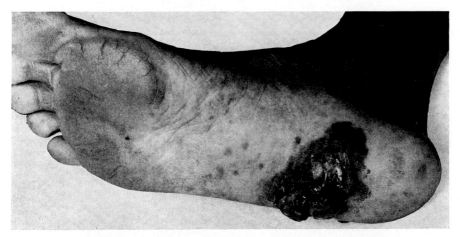

Fig. 1. Malingnant melanoma on the sole of the foot with surrounding "melanotic blush"

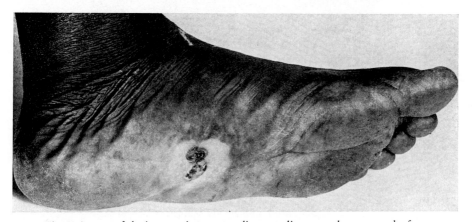

Fig. 2. A zone of depigmentation surrounding a malignant melanoma on the foot

often resulted in a fungating tumours mass (Fig. 5) with the primary on the foot. Similar cases have been described from other countries (PACK and MILLER, 1961; SMITH and STEHLIN, 1965) A few of the more observant of these patients gave a history of having had a small black spot on the foot which had disappeared spontaneously. This suggested that some factor most likely to be an immunological response had "cured" the primary tumour but that metastases had persisted (LEWIS

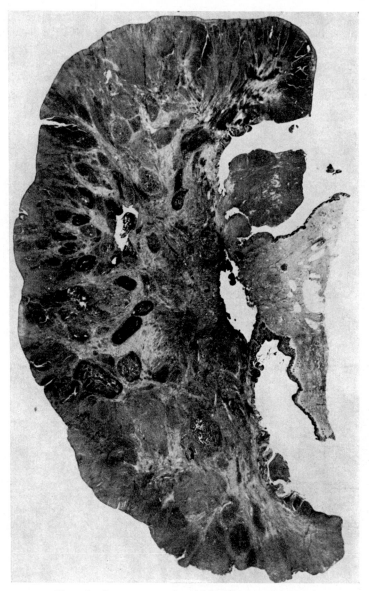

Fig. 3. Section across a polypoidal malignant melanoma

and Kiryabwire, 1968 a). Following this line of reasoning, antibodies to tumour tissue were discovered (Lewis, 1967 b) and their presence was found to correlate with the behaviour of the tumour which remained localized for long periods. As dissemination proceeded antibodies disappeared from the patient's serum (Lewis et al., 1969). Antibodies could be reformed by such patients following injection of the patient's own irradiated tumour cells but this procedure was without clinical effect (Ikonopisov et al., 1970).

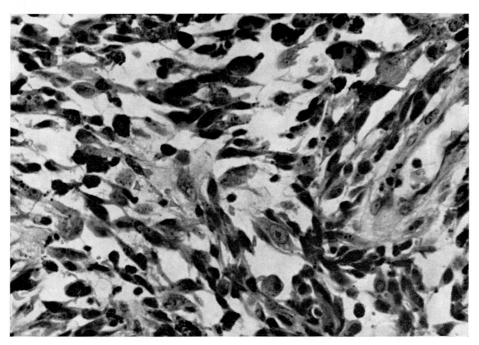

Fig. 4. Histological appearance of a spindle cell type of malignant melanoma

Naevi seem to be as common in Africans as in Europeans (LEWIS and JOHNSON, 1968). But because of the pigmentation of the surrounding skin these are much less obvious, though easily discernable if actively sought. Perhaps for this reason they are seldom excised. We received specimens from 31 naevi from Africans, 24 from Europeans and four from Asian subjects. The majority of tumours in Africans were excised from the region of the face (Table 6). Most of the cases were compound or junctional naevi and showed no extraordinary features. Four cases of blue naevi were seen, two on the scalp and two on the forearm. The spindle-cell arrangement of these lesions sometimes caused confusion with connective-tissue tumours.

Table 6. Site of benign naevi excised from African subjects

Head and Neck		21
(conjunctiva	5	
eyelid	5	
other sites	11)	
Forearm		3
Abdominal wall		1
Vulva		1
Leg		2
Multiple		2
Unstated		1
		31

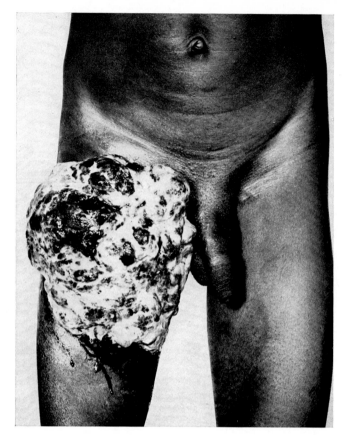

Fig. 5. A large fungating malignant melanoma arising from the lymph nodes of the groin in an African

Aetiology

The proportion of cases of malignant melanoma which are derived from pre-existing naevi is a matter of controversy. Estimates vary from almost 100% (ALLEN and SPITZ, 1953), through rather less than 50% (AFFLECK, 1936; WEBSTER et al., 1944; ACKERMAN, 1948 b, and LENNOX, 1960), to as low as 25% (BECKER, 1948). In fact, the proportion probably varies considerably in different parts of the body. Naevi on the feet are probably particularly likely to become malignant (BUTTER-WORTH and KLAUDER, 1934; HESELSON, 1961). In Ugandan Africans the close correlation between naevi and malignant melanomas on the foot makes it almost certain that most such tumours arise in preexisting junctional naevi (LEWIS, 1968).

It has been suggested that trauma to the feet might possibly induce malignant melanoma. Such trauma could be mechanical (STEVENSON, 1925; HEWER, 1935; SEQUEIRA and VINT, 1934; ELMES and BALDWIN, 1947; ENOS and HOLMES, 1951), or physicochemical due to wood smoke or cautery (CHESTERMAN, 1931), or heat (DAVIES et al., 1968). It may be that such stimuli act upon naevi and increase the liability to malignant change. However, DAVIES (1959) noted no reduction in incidence among shoe-wearing urban Africans compared with rural dwellers although squamous carcinoma of the lower leg had been markedly reduced.

HANDLEY (1931) considered that the liability to malignant transformation was an inherent property of the naevus and was not likely to be influenced by external stimuli.

The highest incidence of malignant melanoma in the world is found in Queensland (DAVIS et al., 1966), particularly among people of Celtic descent. These workers suggest that exposure to ultraviolet light increases the incidence of melanomata and that such tumours need not arise in areas which are directly exposed to sunshine. This factor is most unlikely to influence the rate of melanoma in an African population. The incidence is also low in India (SIRSAT, 1952, 1956; REDDY et al., 1954); in Japan (YOSHIDA, 1955) and in China (STEINER, 1954). In Ceylon and Java the incidence appears to be higher (STEINER, 1954). There is some difference of opinion on the relative frequency of melanoma in American negroes and Caucasians. Some authorities state that the incidence in Caucasians is higher (MUELLING and BURDETTE, 1950; MORRIS and HORN, 1951; ALLEN and SPITZ, 1953) while others suggest it is equal (MACDONALD, 1959). In New Zealand the incidence among Europeans is much higher than among Maoris (ROSE, 1970). In summary, there is no clear-cut relationship between depth of pigmentation and incidence of melanoma. High rates are found among Celtic people and low rates in Chinese and Japanese with intermediate levels in Negroes.

Chapter 10

Tumours of the Skin

ULLA IVERSEN and OLAV HILMAR IVERSEN

With 11 Figures

Cancer of the skin in Ugandan Africans is found almost exclusively in association with some previous damage. The most frequent predisposing lesion is a tropical phagedenic ulcer usually located on the lower leg. Tumours also occurred following burns or bites. Tumours were found more commonly among people from the west of the country. The cause of this regional variation is unknown. Tumours were predominantly well differentiated squamous carcinomas. Basal-cell tumours were only rarely seen. Tumours induced by solar damage were seen in albinos and on the conjunctiva but rarely on normally pigmented skin.

A wide range of tumours of skin accessories was seen but these showed no great differences from tumours in Caucasian subjects.

This chapter is concerned with epithelial tumours arising in the skin, except for melanomas, which are discussed in Chapter 9. Skin cancer from border regions between mucous membranes and skin is generally not included, thus cancers of the lip, anus, penis and vulva are discussed elsewhere. Eyelids, however, are included here. Connective-tissue tumours of the dermis are considered with other soft-tissue tumours (Chapter 15).

Table 1 shows the number of diagnoses made each year. There is a slight increase each year more or less in proportion to the total number of biopsies taken (Chapter 1). Altogether 696 malignant epithelial tumours were diagnosed, that is 9.5% of cancer

Table 1. Number of histologically verified skin tumours 1964—1968

Year	Squamous-cell carcinoma				Other epithelial tumours	Total
	Men	Women	Sex not recorded	Total		
1964	65	49	2	116	11	127
1965	74	54	0	128	18	146
1966	66	57	2	125	23	148
1967	88	59	1	148	18	166
1968	76	68	2	146	16	162
Total	369	287	7	663	86	749

overall. Histological examination confirmed squamous-cell carcinoma in 663 of these cases. A further 3 patients were presumed to have squamous-cell carcinomas on clinical grounds but no biopsy was taken. There were 13 basocellular carcinomas; and 73 tumours of skin appendages were seen, 20 of which were thought to be malignant.

The incidence of skin cancer (melanomas not included) in Uganda is 1.45 cases per 100,000 persons among women and 1.86 in men, corrected for an African standard population. The age at diagnosis varied from 8 to 90 years. There were only 26 patients under the age of 25 years, and most patients were aged between 25 and 65 years. Age-specific incidence rates showed a curve rising to the age of 60—70 and falling in older people.

There were 301 females and 388 males, and 7 patients in whom the sex was not stated.

Squamous-Cell Carcinomas

Incidence

Squamous-cell carcinoma of the skin was diagnosed in 663 cases during this five-year (1964—1968) period. The age-specific incidence rates in each sex, based upon the biopsy material, are shown in Table 2. Virtually every case of carcinoma of the skin diagnosed as such was biopsied. Table 2 includes 92 cases of unknown age and 7 cases of unknown sex who were all assigned to age and sex according to the distribution of cases of known age and sex.

Table 2. Age- and sex-specific incidence rates of cutaneous squamous-cell carcinomas (all figures annual incidence per 100,000)

Age group	Men	Women
0— 9	—	—
10—19	0.11	0.14
20—29	1.32	0.99
30—39	3.31	2.98
40—49	6.53	4.35
50—59	6.91	5.30
60—69	6.50	6.76
70+	2.46	1.60
All ages	1.70	1.33

The overall annual incidence rate of histologically confirmed squamous cell carcinomas of the skin in Uganda per 100,000 population was 1.70 for men and 1.33 for women. The incidence rate increases up to the age of 50 to 59 for men, where it reaches 6.91 new annual cases per 100,000 population. In the age group 60+ the incidence falls again. There is generally a slightly lower incidence among females than among males, except for the age group 60 to 69, where the incidence rate for women is slightly higher, and reaches the maximum for women, 6.76.

In the whole material there were very few cases before the age of 25, only 13 men and 13 women altogether.

Localization

Table 3 shows the anatomical localization of the 663 squamous-cell tumours. The lower limb is much the most frequent site, followed by head and neck and trunk with almost the same numbers, and then the upper limb.

In 553 cases tumours were found arising on the lower limb. The vast majority (79.8%) arose on the skin, closely overlying the tibia or the fibula. A few cases (13%) occurred on the foot and in the region of the ankle. Other parts of the leg were rarely involved. No significant difference was found in the distribution between males and females.

Table 3. Showing the anatomical localization of histologically confirmed squamous-cell carcinomas

Sex	Head and neck	Trunk	Upper limb	Lower limb	Site not recorded	Total
Men	12	23	12	311	11	369
Women	16	7	5	238	21	287
Sex not recorded	1	1	1	4	0	7
Total	29	31	18	553	32	663
Percentage	4.4	4.7	2.7	83.4	4.8	100.0

Twenty-nine cases presented with tumours on the head or neck. Eleven of these were on the scalp, 4 on the eyelid, and 5 on the cheek. Nose, ear, chin and forehead were very rarely involved. Tumours on the trunk were relatively unusual. Thirty-one cases are recorded and 16 of these occurred on the scrotum or inguinal region. Carcinoma of the penis is very commonly seen in Uganda, but all such cases arise in the coronal region and differential diagnosis is easy (see Chapter 7). More problematic are tumours which arise in perineal fistulas following gonococcal strictures. It is difficult to be sure whether such cases arise in the urethra, the skin or the fistula itself. Thirty-eight such cases were seen during the period of this survey and all have been classified as tumours of the urethra (see Chapter 8).

Squamous carcinomas elsewhere on the trunk occurred on the buttocks, lumbar region and chest wall. Only one case was found arising from the skin of the breast.

Of the 18 squamous cell carcinomas occurring on the upper limb, 4 were found on the fingers, one on the palm, 4 on the back of the hand, 6 at the elbow, 2 on the upper arm, and one on the shoulder.

Preceding Lesions

Table 4 shows the preceding lesions as reported by the patients. Of the 663 patients 477 reported that the new growth started as an ulcer that proceeded directly to tumour. There was no record of a previous lesion observed at the site of the subsequent tumour in 111 cases. In 43 cases previous scarring had been noted. Traumatic lesions such as bites, healed tropical ulcers, other infections, and burns due to lightning or wood fires were mentioned in equal numbers as the cause of scarring. No

Table 4. Showing the preceding lesions in patients with squamous-cell carcinomas of the skin

Age	No information	No previous lesions	Ulcer that proceeded directly to tumour	Previous scarring due to						Total
				Unknown lesion	Burns or lightning	Tropical ulcer, infection, leprosy	Bites of animals, snakes	Trauma operation	Albinos	
0— 9	1	0	0	0	0	0	0	0	0	1
10—19	1	3	4	1	0	0	0	0	1	10
20—29	2	8	42	1	0	1	0	2	1	57
30—39	4	15	105	5	1	1	0	2	1	133
40—49	8	21	111	4	3	2	0	2	0	151
50—59	4	17	79	4	3	4	1	1	0	113
60—69	4	23	47	1	0	1	0	1	1	78
70+	0	5	17	0	0	0	0	0	0	22
Age not recorded	4	19	72	1	2	0	0	0	0	98
Total	28	111	477	17	9	9	1	7	4	663

Table 5. Showing the proportion of cases with preceding lesions of various types at each anatomical site

Site	No information	No previous lesion	Ulcer that proceeded directly to tumour	Previous scarring due to						Total
				Unknown lesion	Burns or lightning	Tropical ulcer, infection, leprosy	Bites of animals, snakes	Trauma operation	Albinos	
Head and neck	0	62.1	20.7	0	3.4	0	0	0	13.8	100
Trunk	0	64.5	32.3	0	0	0	0	3.2	0	100
Upper limb	5.6	16.7	61.0	0	16.7	0	0	0	0	100
Lower limb	3.8	12.5	77.0	3.1	0.9	1.4	0.2	1.1	0	100
Site not recorded	18.8	6.3	71.8	0	0	3.1	0	0	0	100
All regions %	4.4	16.7	71.6	2.6	1.4	1.4	0.2	1.1	0.6	100

significant difference was found in the age distribution of patients with different preceding lesions.

Table 5 shows the proportion of previous lesions at the site of development of squamous cell tumours in different parts of the body. In all 71.6% of the tumours started as ulcers proceeding directly to tumour without an intervening period in which the ulcers healed. Most of the tumours on the head, neck and trunk started without obvious preceding lesion, whereas most of the tumours on the limbs started in a phagedenic ulcer that proceeded directly to a tumour. Remarkably few tumours (6⁰/₀) occurred in well healed scars, except in the case of scars after burns on the upper limb. No previous lesion was noted in about 17⁰/₀ of the cases overall.

Duration of Symptoms

Table 6 shows the duration of symptoms of the 663 squamous cell tumours. In more than one-third of these cases no time was recorded. A few patients in every age group reported a history of less than 5 months. In these cases it is impossible to differentiate between the duration of the tumours themselves and the duration of the preceding disease. There is a remarkable number of tumours with a long duration of symptoms, and this was seen even among patients under the age of 30. No difference was apparent in the duration of symptoms in the different age groups.

Table 6. Duration of symptoms of 663 squamous-cell carcinomas by age groups

Age group	Duration in months						No time recorded	Total
	< 5	6—11	12—23	24—59	60—119	120+		
0— 9	0	0	1	0	0	0	0	1
10—19	0	0	1	1	1	0	7	10
20—29	2	4	5	8	1	16	21	57
30—39	7	7	14	26	11	30	38	133
40—49	10	4	16	21	14	30	56	151
50—59	4	4	15	21	4	20	45	113
60—69	5	5	12	8	8	8	32	78
70+	2	1	2	2	4	4	7	22
Age not recorded	10	3	7	13	10	11	44	98
Total	40	28	73	100	53	119	250	663

In Table 7 is shown the duration of symptoms in months of tumours in different parts of the body. Many of the tumours of the limbs had a very long duration, whereas tumours on the head, neck and trunk generally had a short duration.

Table 7. Duration of symptoms of 663 squamous-cell carcinomas in different anatomical sites (percentages)

Site	Duration of symptoms in months						No time recorded	Total
	< 5	6—11	12—23	24—59	60—119	120+		
Head and neck	17.2	0	20.7	6.9	6.9	0	48.3	100
Trunk	29.0	16.1	9.7	9.7	3.2	6.6	25.7	100
Upper limb	16.7	0	11.1	16.7	5.6	11.1	38.8	100
Lower limb	3.8	4.2	11.3	16.4	9.0	20.0	35.3	100
Site not recorded	6.3	0	6.3	3.2	0	15.4	68.8	100
All sites	6.0	4.2	11.0	15.1	8.0	18.0	37.7	100

Ethnic and Geographical Distribution

The crude annual incidence rate is highest in Western region with 1.9 cases per year per 100,000 population. The figures for other regions were Eastern 1.7, Northern 1.3 and Central (Buganda) 1.2. The higher incidence rate in the Western than in the Central region is surprising since hospital facilities are best and the biopsy rate highest in the Central region. Table 8 shows skin cancer as a proportion of cancer overall in the major tribes of Uganda. The proportional rates are markedly high among the Bakiga and incidence rates are also high in this region. High rates are also seen among the pastoral Karamojong and the immigrant Ruanda people.

Table 8. Skin cancer as a proportion of cancer overall
in the major tribes of Uganda

Tribe	Males	Females	Both sexes
Kiga	21.4	31.7	27.5
Lugbara	12.6	18.2	15.0
Karamojong	17.9	6.7	14.8
Ruandan	13.8	15.6	14.6
Lango	10.5	14.1	12.7
Nkole	10.4	13.3	11.6
Soga	13.2	7.3	10.4
Teso	11.1	6.2	8.7
Toro	10.6	4.3	7.8
Acholi	6.3	6.1	6.2
Baganda	4.4	2.2	3.3
All tribes	9.9	9.0	9.5

Histology

All cases have been histologically reviewed and classified in different types and grades of differentiation. A tumour was assigned to a type or a grade of differentiation if the dominant part of the tumour showed the criteria mentioned below. The squamous-cell tumours have been classified as follows:

1. Carcinoma *in situ*. There is only one case with this histological picture.

2. Squamous-cell carcinoma, *well differentiated*. These are tumours consisting mainly of well differentiated squamous epithelium with keratinization, and horny pearls (Fig. 1). The differential diagnosis from pseudocarcinomatous hyperplasia is extremely difficult in many cases. This was a problem throughout and one which we were unable to solve satisfactorily. Most tumours showed an absence of the granular layer and produced parakeratotic material whereas in many reactive states there is often a prominent granular layer. Islands of epithelium were often an artefact, and in many cases the diagnosis of malignancy was only made on a combination of histological, clinical and X-ray evidence.

3. Squamous-cell carcinoma, *moderately differentiated*. These are tumours consisting mainly of squamous-cell epithelium with moderate signs of keratinization, and with few or not fully developed horny pearls (Fig. 2).

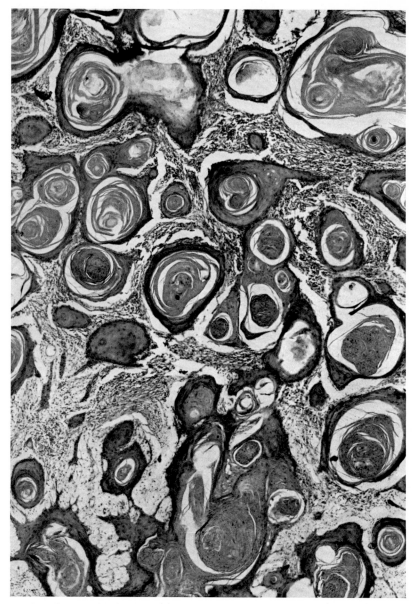

Fig. 1. Microphotograph of a well differentiated squamous cell carcinoma with abundant keratinization and formation of horny pearls

4. Squamous-cell carcinoma, *undifferentiated*. These are tumours consisting mainly of squamous-cell epithelium, with no or very scanty single-cell keratinization, and no horny pearls (Fig. 3).

5. Squamous-cell carcinoma, *spindle-cell variety*. These are squamous-cell carcinomas with almost exclusively spindle-formed cells, and with no or very little keratinization (Fig. 4).

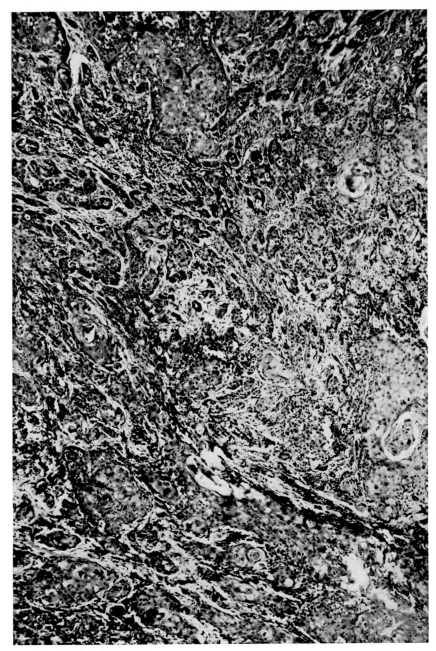

Fig. 2. Microphotograph of moderately differentiated infiltrating squamous cell carcinoma with single cell keratinization and formation of a few small horny pearls

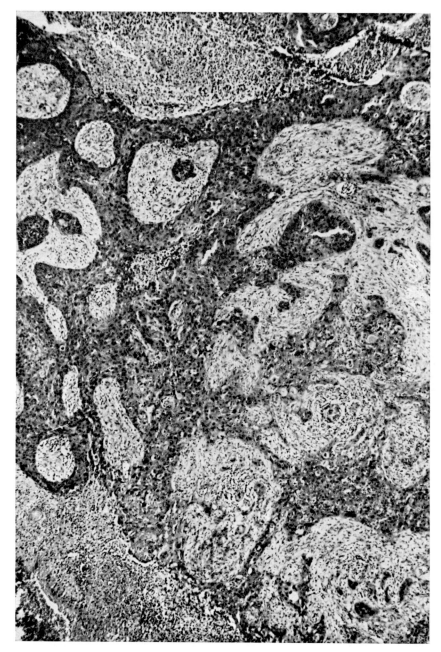

Fig. 3. Microphotograph of an undifferentiated squamous-cell carcinoma almost without single-cell keratinization and with no horny pearls

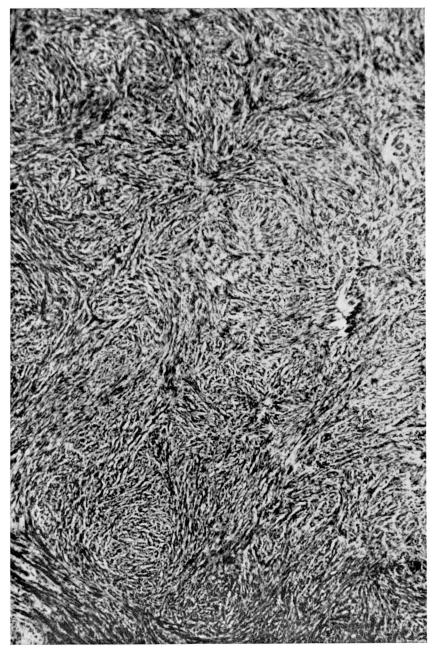

Fig. 4. Microphotograph of a squamous-cell carcinoma of the spindle-cell variety

Table 9. Showing the age distribution of histological types of squamous-cell carcinoma

	Mixed types			Well differen-tiated			Moderately differen-tiated			Undiffer-entiated			Spindle variety			All types			Total
	M	F	?	M	F	?	M	F	?	M	F	?	M	F	?	M	F	?	
0— 9	—	—	—	—	—	—	—	1	—	—	—	—	—	—	—	—	1	—	1
10—19	—	—	—	2	2	—	1	2	—	1	—	—	—	1	—	4	5	—	9
20—29	3	1	—	19	18	1	4	6	—	1	3	—	1	—	—	28	28	1	57
30—39	3	1	—	54	41	1	12	15	1	5	—	—	—	—	—	74	57	2	133
40—49	—	2	—	71	34	—	20	16	—	2	4	—	2	—	—	95	56	—	151
50—59	3	1	—	53	30	—	11	11	—	2	1	—	1	—	—	70	43	—	113
60—69	3	—	—	30	16	1	4	16	1	5	2	—	—	—	—	42	34	2	78
70+	1	1	—	9	5	—	5	1	—	—	—	—	—	—	—	15	7	—	22
Age not recorded	—	—	—	24	40	2	12	16	—	2	2	—	—	—	—	38	58	2	98
Total	13	6	—	262	186	5	69	84	2	18	12	—	4	1	—	366	289	7	662 [a]
Both sexes	19			453			155			30			5						

[a] plus one case of *carcinoma in situ* in a 10 year old boy.

6. Squamous-cell carcinoma, *mixed types*. These are squamous-cell carcinomas in which two or more of the histological types mentioned above are distinctly present in almost equal amount.

The proportion of these histological types at different ages is shown in Table 9. There were 453 well differentiated tumours, 155 moderately differentiated, 30 undifferentiated, 5 of the spindle-cell variety, one carcinoma *in situ* (which occurred in

Table 10. Showing the proportion of patients with short and long duration of symptoms compared with the histological type of tumour

Histological type	% < 24 months	% > 24 months
Mixed	33.3	66.7
Well differentiated	32.1	67.9
Moderately differentiated	39.0	61.0
Undifferentiated	47.7	52.3
Spindle cell variety	25.0	75.0
Total	34.4	65.6

a 10-year-old boy), and 19 cases of mixed type. The age distribution in all histological types was similar to that of the total material. There is, however, some difference between the sexes in that in some age groups there were more moderately differentiated tumours among females than among males, especially in the age group

60—69, even though there are more men than women (M/F = 6/5) in the population at risk.

Table 10 shows the duration of symptoms in months in relation to the different histological types of tumour. The values have been divided into those with a duration of less than 24 months and those with a duration of more than 24 months. There are more undifferentiated than well differentiated tumours in the group of short duration, and conversely more well differentiated than undifferentiated tumours which were of long duration. If grade of differentiation is considered to be a sign of growth rate, the mixed types have a growth rate similar to the well differentiated types, whereas the spindle-cell variety is characterized by a still slower growth rate in spite of its apparent dedifferentiation. The proportion of histological patterns is very similar in different parts of the body. There is perhaps a slight tendency for the trunk to have a relatively greater proportion of undifferentiated tumours, and for the lower limb to have more well differentiated tumours, but the differences are small.

Table 11. Showing the proportion of tumours of each histological type in relation to the different preceding lesions (percentages)

Histological type	No information	No previous lesion	Ulcer that proceeded directly to tumour	Previous scarring	Albinos	Total
Mixed type	—	26.3	57.8	15.9	—	100
Well differentiated	2.9	14.6	74.6	7.5	0.4	100
Moderately differentiated	8.3	17.4	71.6	2.0	0.7	100
Undifferentiated	6.6	29.0	51.6	9.6	3.2	100
Spindle cell variety	—	60.0	40.0	—	—	100
Total	4.2	16.6	72.0	6.6	0.6	100

Table 11 shows the proportion of each histological type in relation to previous lesions. There is a tendency for the well differentiated and moderately differentiated tumours to start as ulcers proceeding directly to tumours. A greater proportion of spindle-cell tumours than of other types of tumour had no discernible predisposing lesion.

Clinical Staging

The majority of tumours occurred on the leg and in this site grew slowly for a very long period. Macroscopically they were often fungating (Fig. 5) or ulcerating (Fig. 6). Metastases were only rarely seen. Only 3.4% of well differentiated tumours showed deposits in the regional nodes and for poorly differentiated tumours this figure rose to 13.8%. The majority of cases arose on the shin and direct extension to involve the underlying bone was seen in 11.1% of cases (Figs. 7, 8 and 9). Well and poorly differentiated tumours showed an equal tendency for bone involvement to occur. Haematogenous spread was not seen in this series.

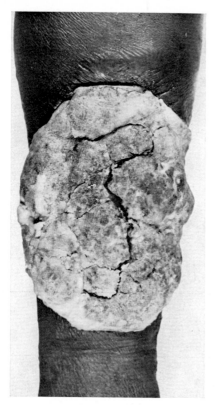
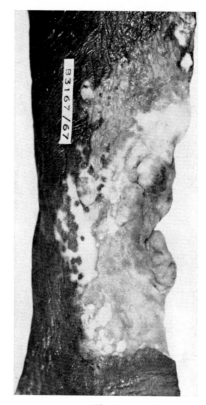

Fig. 5　　　　　　　　　　　　　　　　　　　　　Fig. 6

Fig. 5. Fungating variety of a squamous-cell tumour on the shin, arising from a tropical ulcer

Fig. 6. Ulcerating form of a squamous-cell carcinoma on the shin arising from a tropical ulcer.
Note the depigmented areas around the ulcer

Basal-Cell Carcinomas

Only 13 cases of basal cell carcinoma were noted in the five-year period surveyed, and three of these occurred in albino Africans (Table 12).

About half these tumours occurred on the head and neck and only one on the trunk (Table 13). Basal-cell carcinomas were also found in the anal region but these cases are not considered here. Three patients gave a history of development of an ulcer preceding the tumour, but in the other 10 patients no prior lesion had been noted. The ages of the patients at diagnosis are shown in Table 12.

Tumours of Skin Accessories

A total of 73 cases of tumours of skin accessories were diagnosed. In this particular group of tumours it is often difficult to delineate precisely the distinction between benign and malignant behaviour. Twenty of these appeared to be malignant and 53 were benign. Under the heading of benign skin-accessory tumours are included

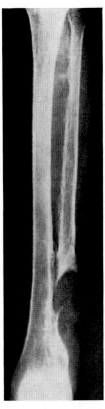

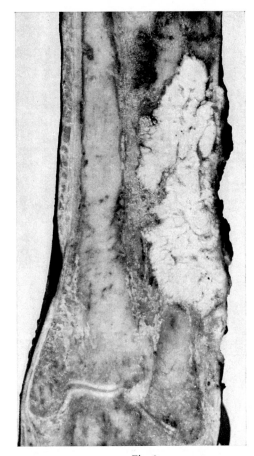

Fig. 7   Fig. 8

Fig. 7. X-ray of a squamous-cell carcinoma on the lateral side of the right lower leg, showing erosion of fibula

Fig. 8. Frontal section through the lower part of the leg in the same patient as illustrated in Fig. 7

7 calcifying epitheliomata (Malherbe tumour), 8 pleiomorphic adenomata, 4 examples of syringocystoadenoma papilliferum, 3 turban tumours and sundry examples of trichoepithelioma, clear-cell hidradenoma, sebaceous adenoma, sweat-gland adenomata of both eccrine and apocrine type. Thirteen of the 20 skin-accessory malignant tumours were diagnosed as undifferentiated, four were thought to be sebaceous-gland carcinomas, and three were considered to have arisen in sweat glands.

The age distribution is shown in Table 12 and the site of origin in Table 13. The majority of these tumours (45%) occurred on the head, a particularly common site being the nose. Most occurred in patients under the age of 50 years. The sex incidence in benign adenomata was equal, but there was a male excess of 12/8 cases among the malignant tumours.

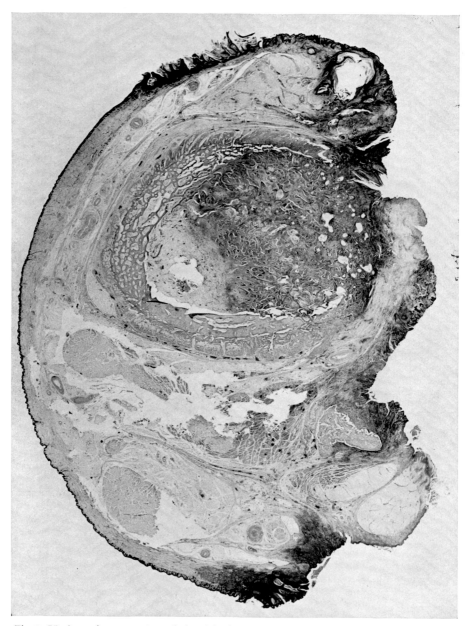

Fig. 9. Horizontal cross-section of the right leg in a patient with an anterior squamous-cell carcinoma of the shin. The large ulceration with invasion of the tibia is clearly seen

Table 12. Skin-appendage tumours by age and sex

Age group	Adenomas of sweat gland, sebaceous gland, hair bulb and unclassified		Sweat-gland carcinomas		Sebaceous-gland carcinomas		Undifferentiated skin-appendage carcinomas		Basal-cell epithelioma		All types	
	Male	Female	Male	Female	Male	Female	Male	Female	Male	Female	Male	Female
0—9	1	1	—	—	1	—	—	—	—	—	1	1
10—19	4	1	—	—	1	—	—	—	—	—	5	1
20—29	1	4	1	—	—	1	—	1	3	—	2	5
30—39	9	6	—	—	—	—	1	1	1	1	13	9
40—49	3	7	2	—	—	—	3	—	1	1	5	8
50—59	4	3	—	—	1	—	1	2	—	1	10	6
60—69	3	2	—	—	—	—	—	1	—	1	5	4
70+	—	—	—	—	—	—	1	—	—	—	—	1
Age not known	1	3	—	—	—	—	1	2	1	2	3	7
Total	26	27	3	—	3	1	6	7	6	7	44	42

Albinos

The anatomical distribution and histological appearance of skin tumours in albinos is very different from that in normally pigmented individuals. These tumours have therefore been dealt with separately (see Tables 4, 5 and 11).

The majority of tumours occur on the face (Fig. 10) and ears and in some cases on the shoulders and the backs of the hands.

Histologically the tumours were 4 squamous carcinomas, 3 basal cell tumours and one trichoepithelioma. Squamous carcinoma usually showed an undifferentiated

Table 13. Showing the site of origin of skin-appendage tumours

Localization	Adenomas of sweat gland, sebaceous gland, hair bulb and unclassified	Sweat-gland carcinomas	Sebaceous-gland carcinomas	Undiff. skin-appendage carcinomas	Basal-cell epithe-liomas	All types
Head and neck	24	1	3	5	6	39
Trunk	17	1	1	4	1	24
Upper limb	4	—	—	—	3	7
Lower limb	7	1	—	4	3	15
Unknown	1	—	—	—	—	1
Total	53	3	4	13	13	86

appearance in marked contrast with "ulcer cancer" where the vast majority were well differentiated tumours. Basal-cell tumours are quite frequently seen and often multicentric. Albino subjects accounted for 23% of all basal cell carcinomas, from which it is calculated that albinos are at least 1000 times more likely to develop such

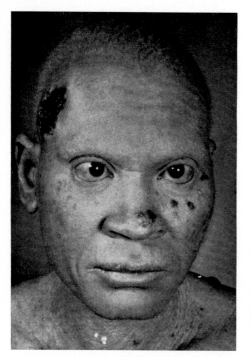

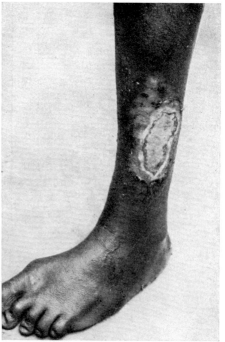

Fig. 10

Fig. 11

Fig. 10. Male African albino with multiple basal-cell carcinomas

Fig. 11. A typical tropical ulcer in a young male African

tumours than normally pigmented patients. Tumours in albinos quite frequently show evidence of "in-situ" change at the edges of the tumour whereas this was seen only once in 659 cases in pigmented individuals.

Discussion

This chapter concerns a review of all cases of skin cancer received at the Department of Pathology, Makerere Medical School during the years 1964 to 1968 inclusive. The slides were reviewed microscopically and classified according to histology. The material thus comprises virtually all histologically verified skin cancers in the country. The cases registered represent only a minimum incidence since cases are obviously missed, particularly in rural areas. The proportion of undiagnosed cases is probably lower than with any other type of tumour since the history is long and painful and most patients probably come to hospital eventually.

The typical skin cancer of Uganda is a well differentiated squamous-cell carcinoma occurring on the shin of a man about 60 years old, living in the Western region and belonging to a Ruanda-Rundi or Bakiga tribe. Such a tumour usually develops in a so-called tropical ulcer (Fig. 11), which does not heal completely but may show considerable variation in size at different times. The ulcer has been present for more than 24 months before malignancy develops. Involvement of bone is a late event, metastasis to lymph nodes is unusual, and haematogenous spread is rare.

Table 14. Annual incidence rates of squamous-cell carcinomas of the skin in different countries (all figures corrected for an African standard population per 100,000 people per year)

	Males	Females
Africans in Uganda (this study)	1.7	1.3
Bantus in Johannesburg (OETTLÉ, 1963)	1.7	3.0
U.S. negroes (OETTLÉ, 1963)	2.6	3.4
Four northern U.S. cities, whites (HAENZEL, 1963)	8.9	5.3
Four southern U.S. cities, whites (HAENZEL, 1963)	32.3	14.3
Cape Province, whites (GRIEVE and LINDER, 1970)	79.5	44.4
Cape Province, coloured (GRIEVE and LINDER, 1970)	2.3	2.0
Cape Province, Bantu (GRIEVE and LINDER, 1970)	0.5	1.0

The overall incidence of skin tumours is found to be very much lower in negro peoples than among Caucasians. Thus the incidence in Cape Province, South Africa, among whites is about 50 times that in Bantu (Table 14). As a general rule, the highest incidence figures are found among Anglo-Saxon peoples and the lowest in Chinese and Japanese. The annual incidence rate in Ugandan men is about the same as for male American negroes and Johannesburg Bantu. Among women in Uganda, the skin cancer rate is somewhat lower than that among female American negroes. The incidence rate in Uganda is very low compared with that of a white population in the southern part of the U.S.A. or Cape Province, South Africa.

The age-specific distribution in Uganda shows a similar curve to that seen in other parts of the world, except that over the age of 60 years in men and 70 years in women the annual incidence appears to fall whereas it continues to increase in Europe and U.S.A. It is possible that there is a genuine reduction in incidence but there is almost certainly some reduction in hospital attendance among old people either as a result of difficulty or unwillingness.

In lightly pigmented people sunshine plays the greatest role as skin carcinogenic factor, and the exposed areas on head, neck and hands usually show the highest frequency of skin cancers. In pigmented Ugandans only 4.4% of the skin cancers occurred on head and neck. In our material from Uganda, the lower limb is the dominant site. OETTLÉ (1963) found 59% of squamous-cell carcinomas on the lower limb, while in our material 83% of the squamous-cell carcinomas were localized on the lower limb, both in men and women. Most of these cancers were found on the shin, and remarkably few on the foot. This distribution of lesions has been noted on many occasions in Africa (DAVIES et al., 1968; CAMAIN et al., 1972), and is a result of the overwhelming importance of tropical phagedenic ulcer as the antecedent lesion of carcinoma. In Anglo-Saxons the commonest sites for the development of tumours of the skin are on the exposed parts of the upper extremities, the head and neck. In white Australians, for example, 93% of all malignant skin tumours occur in these sites (TEN SELDAM, 1963). In Uganda the European population also suffers from this sun-induced tumour, whereas the Asian and Negro residents are largely immune (TEMPLETON and VIEGAS, 1971). In albino Africans the distribution of tumours is similar to that in Europeans and is discussed below.

It is difficult to be certain why tropical ulcer should be so liable to develop malignancy. It has been estimated that about 9% of chronic ulcers will eventually develop tumours (JANSSENS et al., 1958) and about 2% were found to be malignant in an outpatient survey in Uganda (SHEPHERD, 1966). This is a considerably higher figure than pertains for varicose ulceration in Caucasians. It is possible that the micro-organisms responsible manufacture carcinogenic materials or that treatment with various herbs exerts this effect. SHEPHERD (1966) was impressed by the frequency in which the skin around an ulcer appeared to be the site of tumour development and he thought that it might be that the scar itself was predisposed to malignancy. It may also be that sunshine incident upon the unpigmented border of proliferating epithelium contributes to the development of cancer, or possibly contact with soot from the open fireplaces increases the liability to malignant change. The popular opinion that scarring plays a very important part in skin carcinogenesis is not supported by our material. The rather long duration from the first symptom until frank malignancy may point to relatively weak or slow-acting carcinogenic factors.

SHEPHERD (1966) showed that there was a higher frequency of skin cancer among the Ruanda-Rundi tribes than among the Baganda tribe of Uganda. Of 108 epitheliomas investigated more than three times more than expected were found in patients belonging to this immigrant group. Our investigation confirms the excess among patients from these tribes. The difference is unlikely to be due to genetic factors. People belonging to these tribes are often refugees living in poor conditions and are probably less likely to have tropical ulcers treated early than indigenous people.

Our material shows an excess of cases in Western region. In most tumours the incidence among the Baganda appears to be much higher than in any other tribe so that this excess of skin cancers in Western District is probably very considerable. In addition to the tribal factor this excess may point to additional local exogenic carcinogenic factors, particularly common among the Bakiga.

Squamous-cell carcinomas in Uganda are usually very highly differentiated tumours with many horny pearls. Five cases of squamous-cell carcinomas with a spindle-cell pattern were noted, 4 in men and one in a woman. The age distribution was similar to other types. Rather contrary to expectation they seem to grow relatively slowly and none showed bone involvement, nor were there any signs of metastases. They usually had a long duration of preceding symptoms, possibly indicating a slow growth rate. The spindle-cell variant of squamous-cell carcinoma has been recognized for many years in the oral region and the upper respiratory tract, but is rare in the skin (LICHTIGER et al., 1970). The lesions may easily be mistaken for sarcomas, but in our five cases the transition from squamous epithelial cells to spindle cells was quite obvious in small areas of the biopsy material.

Basal-cell carcinomas are extremely rare but were seen from time to time. These did not show actinic changes in the surrounding collagen and are assumed to have arisen from skin-accessory glands. Other types of skin-accessory tumours were seen and examples of a wide range of tumour types were noted.

In addition to solar-induced tumours other actinic and senile conditions were rare. These include senile keratoses, naevus sebaceous, inverted papilloma, and so forth. This is in part a function of the population structure of Uganda with its excess of younger age groups but even among older people these conditions are rare. Keratoacanthoma was never seen in a negro patient during this five-year survey, though three examples were seen in Asian patients and one in a European. DAVIES et al. (1968) recorded a few examples in Ugandan Africans but the condition appears to be exceedingly rare in all areas of Africa (OETTLÉ, 1963). This apparent immunity is as yet unexplained.

The number of albinos in an African population varies markedly in different parts of Africa. In South African Bantu the incidence has been calculated at 1 in 5000 overall with considerable variations from place to place (OETTLÉ, 1963). The site of tumour involvement in African albinos is very similar to that seen in Europeans in the tropics. The distribution fits in well with the suggestion that exposure to ultraviolet light (sunshine) is responsible for tumour production. Histologically the dermal collagen usually shows extensive elastotic degeneration. This change is seen in tumours in Caucasian subjects but is not present in the tumours arising from scars or ulcers.

In most respects the African skin seems to be particularly well adapted to the environment. Melanoma is only seen in depigmented areas and solar-induced tumours either of squamous or basal cell pattern are seen mainly in albinos or on the conjunctiva. Tumours of skin accessories may be slightly more frequent in negroes than in Caucasians but it is very difficult to be certain of this. If tropical ulcer were always cured in the early stages of development (as is easily possible with antibiotics) malignant tumours of the skin would become rarities. This places a considerable onus on the medical profession of Uganda, who have at their disposal the ability to prevent approximately 100 cases of malignant tumours each year.

Chapter 11

Tumours of the Brain

A. C. Templeton

Tumours of the central nervous system are infrequently diagnosed. Controversy exists as to whether this is due to inadequate facilities or to a genuinely low incidence. Diagnosis is undoubtedly deficient but it seems likely that there is a true deficiency in the number of cases occurring.

During the period under review 26 malignant tumours and 50 benign tumours were diagnosed. Of these, 79% were seen in Mulago Hospital, Kampala, and only a few were referred from up-country hospitals. During most of this period no specialist neurosurgical facilities were available in Uganda. It is likely therefore that a considerable proportion of intracranial tumours seen in Uganda were not registered or diagnosed. For example, when a specialist neurosurgeon arrived in Uganda he was able to record 17 pituitary tumours seen within 18 months (Bailey and Thomas, 1971). The probable extent of under-diagnosis has been surveyed by Bailey (1971). Pituitary tumours and acoustic neuromas are considered in rather greater detail in chapters 13 and 15 respectively.

Table 1. Primary tumours of the central nervous system

Glioma	17
Medulloblastoma	1
Pinealoma	1
Haemangioblastoma	1
Hortega-cell tumour (microglioma)	1
Meningeal melanoma	2
Neurinoma (1 spinal, 3 on 8th nerve)	4
Meningioma	12
Pituitary adenoma	5
Craniopharyngioma	4
Secondary tumours (symptomatic)	2
Lymphoma/Leukaemia	18

Astrocytoma

There were 16 cases of astrocytoma, including glioblastoma multiforme. The age range was from 4½ to 54 with a mean of 31 years. Three cases occurred in children aged 4½, 10 and 11 years. There were 10 males and 6 females. The tumours were distributed as follows: frontal lobe 3, parietal and central area 3, occipital and temporal 2, midbrain 2, hindbrain and cerebellum 6. All 3 tumours of childhood were found in the cerebellum. One tumour was of the very well differentiated type (Grade 1), five were Grade 2 and ten grade 3 or 4; many of the latter would be classified as glioblastoma multiforme. Adult patients had significantly less well differentiated tumours than children.

Medulloblastoma

There were 3 cases of medulloblastoma. One, in a 13-year-old male, was a typical midline cerebellar tumour. One, in a 4-year-old female, was also a midline cerebellar tumour; in this tumour some of the tumour cells resembled oligodendroglia but the basic cytology was compatible with a medulloblastoma. The other tumour occurred in the roof of the fourth ventricle in a 29-year-old man.

Cerebellar Haemangioblastoma

A typical cystic cerebellar haemangioblastoma was seen in a 28-year-old adult male. The tumour formed a very small nodule in a large cerebellar cyst.

Pinealoma

One case of typical germinoma (atypical teratoma) of the pineal gland has been seen in a 22-year-old man. The patient had marked increase in his appetite and was grossly obese but there were no other signs of endocrine disturbance.

Microglioma

One primary lymphoreticular tumour was diagnosed. This occurred in the frontal lobe in a 25-year-old male. The cytology was pleomorphic with many multinucleate cells.

Malignant Melanoma

A case of diffuse meningeal melanomatosis was seen in a 7-year-old boy with signs of hydrocephalus (LEWIS, 1969).

Meningioma

There were two cases of malignant meningioma with invasion and destruction of the skull. Seven benign meningiomas were diagnosed; in 6 cases the diagnosis was made at post mortem, and the tumour had apparently not given rise to symptoms.

Intraspinal Tumours

One malignant glioma of the cord was seen in an 8-year-old male. This was a neuroectodermal tumour of primitive cell type. The diagnosis of ependymoblastoma was considered but insufficient tissue was available for proper assessment.

Three meningiomas of the spinal canal were diagnosed.

Discussion

It has been suggested that cerebral tumours are rare in Africans (Muwazi and Trowell, 1944; Gelfand, 1957), though Smith et al. (1934) reported three "gliosarcomas" in an analysis of 500 umours in Nigerians. In 1948 Davies analysed 2,162 tumours in cases over 10 years of age who came to post mortem in Uganda between 1931 and 1947; he found seven brain tumours in adult males, 4 of which were astrocytomas. In a clinical study Billinghurst (1966) found 57 cases of cerebral tumour in a total number of 122,159 admissions between 1953 and 1965.

When allowance is made for the problems of hospitalization and diagnosis, particularly in neurological disorders, it is evident that cerebral tumours are not uncommon in Ugandan Africans. It is even possible that their incidence is similar to that seen elsewhere. With the development of facilities, an increasing number of cases are being reported in sub-Saharan Africa in Kenya (Ojiambo, 1966), in Nigeria (Odeku and Janota, 1967) and in Senegal (Collomb et al., 1963).

Secondary Deposits

During the period of this survey only two patients developed symptoms of an intracranial space-occupying lesion as a result of metastatic deposits. In one case the primary site was unknown and in the other it was a bronchial tumour. Secondary tumours in the brain are not common in Uganda and this is probably because of the relative rarity of carcinoma of the bronchus. During a recent survey of intracranial lesions 16 secondary tumours of the brain were found among 5,541 necropsy records (Poltera and Templeton, 1972). The primary sites from which these were derived is shown in Table 2.

Table 2. Secondary deposits found in the brain
in 5,541 necropsy examinations

Malignant melanoma	4
Lung (1 alveolar)	4
Choriocarcinoma	2
Breast	2
Stomach	
Retinoblastoma	1 case each
Sphinoidal sinus	
Nasopharynx	

Extension of lymphoma or leukaemia to involve the nerve roots or meninges represents the commonest tumour of the intracranial cavity found in Uganda. The major stumbling block in the therapy of Burkitt's tumour is that there is no really satisfactory method of treating such involvement (Ziegler et al., 1970).

Chapter 12

Tumours of the Eye and Adnexa

A. C. TEMPLETON

With 5 Figures

Tumours of the eye and adnexa were seen frequently. Carcinoma of the conjunctiva, retinoblastoma and Burkitt's lymphoma involving the orbit account for the majority of cases. Conjunctival squamous carcinoma develops in preexisting piguecula and frequently penetrates the globe causing collapse of the eye. Retinoblastoma occurs with approximately equal frequency in many parts of the world. Unfortunately Ugandan children are often brought to a hospital late in the course of the disease when successful treatment is impossible.

Other tumours of the eye, including melanoma, are rare in Ugandan Africans.

The tumours of the eye and adnexa occurring in Uganda in the years 1961—1966 have been reviewed earlier (TEMPLETON, 1967 a), and this present series is very similar in basic pattern (Table 1). In European practice tumours of the ocular apparatus are dominated by intraocular melanoma and basal cell carcinoma of the eyelid. In Uganda both these conditions are rare, and the majority of tumours discussed under this heading comprise Burkitt's lymphoma, retinoblastoma and carcinoma of the conjunctiva.

Involvement of the orbit is frequently seen in Burkitt's lymphoma. In a large proportion of cases this occurs in conjunction with a maxillary tumour. It is then difficult to say exactly where the tumour arose. In 29 of the cases listed here there appeared to be orbital involvement without a large maxillary mass. Involvement of the globe itself was not seen in this series of cases but has been seen in specimens submitted for opinion from other countries. Destruction of the globe following exposure keratitis is distressingly common. Iritis has been noted in association with Burkitt's tumour but its cause is unknown. In relapse following therapy cranial-nerve involvement is common and external ophthalmoplegia or individual pareses occur (ZIEGLER et al., 1970). The nerve trunks may be infiltrated with tumour cells and this occurs more commonly in the third, fourth and sixth nerves than in the optic nerve. The differential diagnosis of Burkitt's tumour from the other causes of orbital swelling seen in Ugandan children is discussed more fully elsewhere (TEMPLETON, 1971).

Retinoblastoma

There were 57 cases in the period under survey. The cases seen in each succeeding year were 11, 11, 9, 14 and 12 respectively. This level has been remarkably steady for the past decade in spite of a rising registration rate of other tumours. This suggests that the majority of such tumours are being registered.

Table 1. Tumours and tumour-like conditions involving the eye and adnexae

Orbit		118
Burkitt's lymphoma	59	
Sinuses and nasopharyngeal (including 2 nasopharyngeal carcinoma, 1 aesthesioneuroblastoma)	16	
Soft tissue sarcomata	4	
Pseudotumour	9	
Chloroma (myeloblastic sarcoma)	10	
Encephalocele	6	
Fibrous dysplasia	6	
Others [a]	8	
Lacrymal gland		13
Intraocular		58
Retinoblastoma	57	
Melanoma	1	
Conjunctiva		102
Squamous carcinoma (+ in situ)	53 (+36)	
Dermoid cyst	4	
Naevus cell tumour	6	
Malignant melanoma	2	
Kaposi's sarcoma	1	
Eyelid		23
Squamous carcinoma	4	
External angular dermoid	4	
Neurofibroma	4	
Kaposi's sarcoma	3	
Accessory gland tumours	2	
Basal cell carcinoma	2	
Naevus cell tumour	4	
Total		314

[a] Others: 2 haemangiomas, 1 case each multiple myeloma, osteosarcoma, retinal anlage tumour, metastatic neuroblastoma, malignant tumour ? nature, secondary tumour ? from stomach.

Retinoblastoma represents a large proportion of tumours of the eye and this fact led early observers to conclude that the incidence in Africans was high (ELMES and BALDWIN, 1947). This marked increase in frequency is a result of the population structure in African countries in which about one-fifth of the population are under the age of five years. The incidence per child at risk is in fact similar to that recorded in other countries. During the period of this survey the rate of cases was 1 in 27,000 surviving to the age of one year. A series from the U.S.A. calculated the rate at 1 in 23,000 (FALLS and NEEL, 1951). No evidence has been found of the rising incidence reported in other countries in recent years.

There were 32 males and 25 females. The age ranged from 5 months to 6 years (mean 2.9 years). The mean age is somewhat higher than in many countries but this is probably a result of delay in arrival at hospital rather than a difference in behaviour of tumours.

There was no predominance of any tribal or ethnic group, nor any evidence of geographical variation. The previously noted excess among the Ankole people (TEMPLETON, 1967 a) has not persisted into the period of this survey.

Presentation

Patients presented at hospital late in the course of the disease. In 38 out of 57 patients there was extensive involvement of the orbital tissues. A further 16 patients had invasion of the optic nerve and in only three cases was the tumour confined to the globe. This is a result of poor parental appreciation of the significance of early signs such as a yellow reflex which had often been noted at least one year prior to arrival in hospital. In addition to parental ignorance the structure of primary medical care in Uganda makes it difficult to get specialist attention unless there is an easily appreciable lesion. Radiotherapy is unavailable in Uganda and surgery is unlikely to be curative. Treatment has been undertaken using various cytotoxic agents such as cyclophosphamide and vincristine sulphate. Initial response has sometimes been dramatic but is seldom sustained. The prognosis is therefore dismal in the extreme.

The histological pattern was very similar to that seen in other countries. Rosette formation was seen much less frequently and in no case was a true rosette seen in tumour tissue outside the globe. Whether the presence of rosettes determined the extent of spread or whether the extent of spread determined the ability to form rosettes is arguable. Rosettes were only found in the globe where it was reasonable to suppose that intraocular pressure had been maintained. Thus if the sclera was breached or the anterior chamber invaded rosettes were not found. In addition rosettes seemed to be more numerous in the region of the choroid than in other parts of the tumour. It is suggested that some factor in the region of the choroid may contribute to the formation of rosettes and that the stage of spread determines whether they are present.

Squamous Cell Carcinoma of the Conjunctiva

Fifty-three cases of invasive squamous carcinoma were seen and a further 36 lesions with moderate or marked dysplasia of the epithelium were examined.

This tumour appears to be common in many parts of Africa. High rates are reported from Sudan (DAOUD et al., 1968), Senegal (QUÉRÉ, CAMAIN and LAMBERT, 1964), Ethiopia (JUDGE, personal communication, 1969), Malawi (TICHO and BEN SIRA, 1970). Other countries which report high incidence rates include Afghanistan (SOBIN, 1969) and Iran (HAGHIGHI et al., 1971). All these countries have in common a high sunshine rate and often a dusty atmosphere, and many lie at high altitudes. These facts suggest that ultraviolet light and perhaps minor trauma from dust are involved in the pathogenesis. Cattle are well known to suffer from a similar disease known as cancer eye (RUSSELL et al., 1956) and it has been found that the incidence in different parts of the U.S.A. is roughly parallel to the number of hours of sunshine in each area. In Uganda, indigenous Zebu and Ankole long-horn cattle do not suffer from cancer eye but a number of cases have been seen in exotic breeds such as Herefords which have been introduced to improve the quality of local strains. This dif-

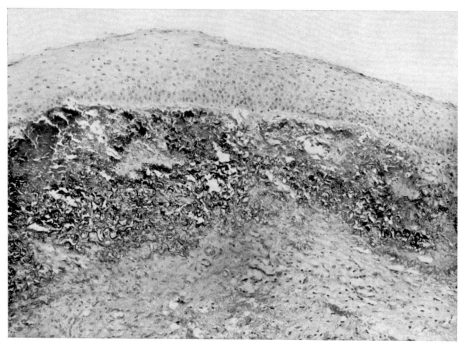

Fig. 1. Pinguecula showing thickening of the epithelium above an area of elastotic degeneration

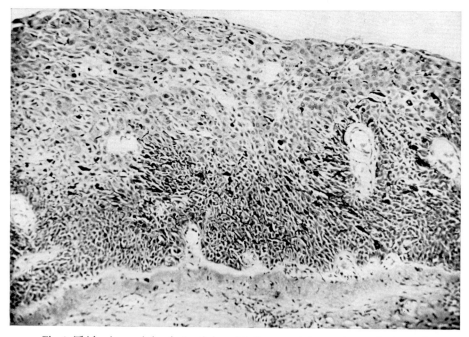

Fig. 2. Thickening and dysplasia of the epithelium overlying a pinguecula. Note the melanocytic proliferation which often occurs at this phase

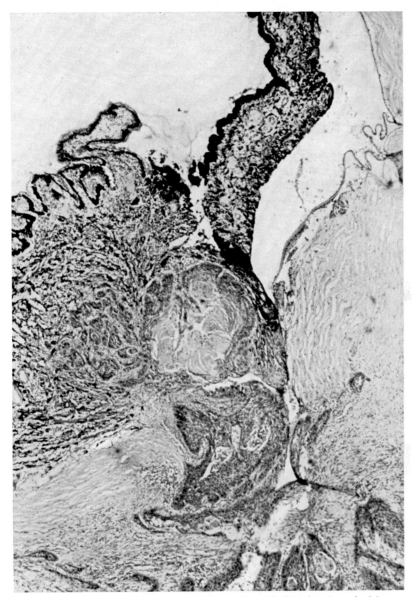

Fig. 3. Infiltration of squamous carcinoma through the sclera into the iris

ferential sensitivity is almost certainly a result of variations of pigment distribution in the two strains.

Tumours almost invariably occurred close to the limbus, usually on the nasal aspect but more rarely laterally. The most common pattern of development was from an area of dysplastic proliferation overlying elastotic degeneration of the collagen. The preceding lesion was a pinguecula in most cases and the lesion progressed through phases of dysplasia, intraepithelial carcinoma, usually with a heaped-up rather papillary structure, to invasive tumour. Superficial lateral spread of the tumour over the surface of the cornea and conjunctiva was often seen, but deep invasion with perforation of the globe occurred frequently. Metastases to cervical nodes occurred when deep penetration had taken place but was not seen when the lesion was superficial.

Squamous carcinoma and its predisposing lesions were therefore classified into three groups:

1. Pingueculae with no dysplasia or only keratinization (Fig. 1);
2. Pinguecula with dysplasia of the overlying epithelium (Fig. 2);
3. Invasive carcinoma (Fig. 3).

These stages can be distinguished clinically with a reasonable degree of accuracy. The first group presents a raised, smooth, glistening nodule. The second shows a roughened surface, is often raised, and most frequently pigmented (Fig. 4). The third is larger than 3 mm and often appears either even more raised and ulcerated. These correlations are very similar to those reported from Malawi (TICHO and BEN SIRA, 1970).

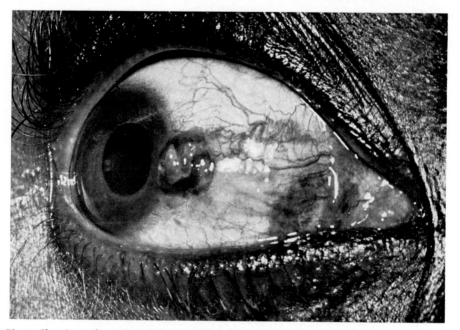

Fig. 4. Showing a heaped-up lesion overlying the media limbus; a leash of vessels leads to the dysplastic area

Biopsies of pingueculae and all dysplastic epithelial proliferation were studied, a total of 96 cases. This represented only a tiny fraction of the true incidence of these lesions, the vast majority of which are never seen in hospital and only a small proportion of which are examined microscopically. The relative proportions of each group are therefore considerably distorted but they serve for comparison.

Patients with pinguecula were slightly younger in mean age than those with cancer (Table 2). The lesions appeared faintly yellowish with a smooth shiny surface.

Histologically the collagen showed extensive elastotic degeneration with a few in-flammatory cells, mainly lymphocytes, at the periphery. The epithelium was usually slightly thickened and often showed keratinization.

Table 2. Distribution of patients by age and sex

	Cases	Males %	Age range	(mean) years
Pinguecula	23	60	13—70	(31.9)
Dysplastic lesions	34	64	15—70	(35.5)
Carcinoma	49	75	13—70	(41.2)

The dysplastic lesion showed collagenous degeneration with rather greater in-flammatory infiltrate in the stroma. The cells found included many mast cells and a few plasma cells were usually present. The lesion usually appeared quite dark in colour often with a grey crust and was frequently misdiagnosed as a naevus cell tumour. The colour was a result of melanocytic proliferation in the epidermis. The dendritic processes of the proliferating cells were very easily seen as long fronds between the squamous cells (Fig. 2). The melanocytic hyperplasia increased in in-tensity in proportion to the degree of dysplasia until the stage of carcinoma in situ was reached, when it was less marked. When invasive change took place the pigment cells were much less obvious but pigment was usually visible in macrophages in the stroma. It would appear therefore that the stimuli inducing dysplasia of the epi-thelium induced a proliferation of melanocytes but once the epithelium became suf-ficiently disorganised the pigment cells no longer survived.

The epithelial dysplasia was seldom extensive and usually only covered 2 mm. Elastosis of the underlying collagen was always present if the specimen was sufficient to contain stroma. A Bowenoid pattern of diffuse change in the area was very unusual and the Borst Jadahsohn lesion was found in the majority of cases. This latter pattern showed spherical patches of dysplastic cells apparently arising from a small area, possibly even a single cell, with more normal areas of epithelium between them.

The epithelium was often thrown into folds at this stage, but only rarely became overtly papillary in structure. The basement membrane remained intact but in a few cases the intensity of the underlying inflammation made it difficult to be certain.

The age of patients with invasive tumours varied widely. The mean age was slightly higher than that of patients with dysplasia (Table 2) but with such a wide range this did not reach significant levels. The mean age was considerably lower than in patients with tumours of the lid (56.7 years), and though numbers are too small to be certain the age-specific incidence rate did not rise sharply with age. All the histo-logical and epidemiological features suggest that this tumour is a result of exposure to sunlight. Most such tumours show an exponential increase in incidence with age, and the failure to rise in similar fashion suggests that there is some additional factor at work; perhaps some mechanical or dietary factor makes the eye susceptible to development of malignancy early in life.

Differential diagnosis in the early case from pterygia and pingueculae is relatively straightforward (vide supra). The heaped-up, rather crusted nature of the lesion helps to separate it from the uncomplicated lesion. If melanocytic hyperplasia is extreme then differentiation from naevi may be difficult unless a reliable history of recent development is obtained. Subconjunctival nematode infections may give rise to raised nodules but these are usually multiple and often in an unexposed area of the conjunctiva. In later stages of development the diagnosis is unfortunately only too easy but in very extensive cases it may be difficult to be certain whether the tumour arose on the lid or the conjunctiva.

Invasive tumours were often very superficial and did not penetrate beyond the superficial parts of the sclera. Sometimes apparently extensives lesions were found to be attached only at a single point, rather like a water-lily leaf, and were easily removed by local surgery. Recurrence of the tumour if removed at this stage was unusual, even without the aid of radiotherapy. Tumours showed a wide range of histological grading from well differentiated keratinizing tumours to poorly differentiated somewhat basaloid lesions. This latter appearance was found in a greater proportion of the few cases arising lateral to the cornea than of those medial to it. In a number of cases the globe of the eye was penetrated and usually ruptured. In such cases lymph-node involvement was found quite commonly and one patient is known to have died with widespread metastases from a moderately differentiated tumour. Penetration of the globe probably occurred in the region of the canal of Schlem. In two cases tumour was found penetrating the sclera to involve the ciliary body. In other countries penetration and perforation of the eye is very unusual following carcinoma of the conjunctiva (REESE, 1963). This is probably a result of earlier treatment but it might be that the sclera of the eye in Africans is for some reason more penetrable than in Caucasians. It has been suggested that childhood malnutrition might affect the collagen structure and thereby render invasion easier (DAVIES et al., 1968). Frank keratomalacia due to vitamin A deficiency is rare in Uganda today, though there is evidence that it used to be more widespread. Bitôt's spots are found frequently in Burundi (YASSUR, personal communication, 1970) but are rarely seen in Uganda. The cornea shows extensive abnormality during the period of kwashiorkor (EMIRU, 1970), but there is no certain evidence of permanent damage. The histological evidence of solar damage is limited to the superficial areas immediately under the epidermis and it seems very unlikely that scleral damage is produced by this mechanism.

Tumours of the Eyelid

In contrast to the frequency of conjunctival carcinoma, tumours of the lids are rare. Thus only four squamous cell and two basal carcinomas were seen. Five of these patients were female and there was only one male patient aged 45 who had a squamous cell tumour at the outer canthus of the eye which may possibly have arisen from the conjunctival reflection. All the other tumours arose on the upper lid. The five female patients were all aged between 50 and 70 years. Of the three patients with squamous carcinoma two came from the north of the country and the third had lived most of her life in central Tanzania, whereas both patients with basal carcinoma were Baganda. Tumours of the skin in Ugandans usually arise in previously scarred tissue and normal skin is remarkably resistent to cancer (see Chapter 10). It is not known whether any of these patients had scars on the eyelid but all patients with squamous carcinoma of the lid came from areas where trachoma is found, in contrast to conjunctival cancer which was found most commonly in Buganda. Basal-cell carcinomas are rare in Ugandans, and tend to be found in regions of the body which suggest origin from glands rather than surface epithelium, such as the eyelid and axilla. These are probably not a result of solar damage except in albinos.

Two tumours seem to have arisen from accessory glands. A 54-year-old male Muganda presented with a pea-sized mass just below the lacrymal punctum which was not ulcerating the surface. Histological examination showed a basaloid squamous-cell carcinoma intermingled with clear cells which contained mucus. This "muco-epidermoid" tumour was thought to have arisen from the lacrymal sac or duct. The second patient, an 18-year-old male, had a pleiomorphic adenoma arising on the inner aspect of the medial end of the right upper lid. This tumour was presumed to have arisen from a meibomian gland or possibly from ectopic lacrymal tissue.

Melanocytic Tumours

Intraocular melanomas are extremely rare in Africans. During the past decade only two cases have been seen in Uganda. Only one was seen in the period of this survey, compared with 57 retinoblastomas. This deficiency appears to be genetically determined and is found throughout Africa, and in American negroes to a lesser extent. In Uganda the sites at which melanomata develop are those which are normally depigmented (LEWIS and MARTIN, 1967). Thus in the eye melanomata of the conjunctiva are much more commonly seen than tumours of the ciliary body or choroid.

Six naevi of the conjunctiva were seen. In an earlier report from Uganda, DAVIES et al. (1968) noted that junctional naevi in children sometimes behaved in a malignant fashion when the histological appearances and the age of the patient suggested a benign course. We have seen no such lesion in recent years. Two cases of malignant melanoma of the conjunctiva were seen, both of which occurred in adults and both showed all the histological hallmarks of malignancy.

Soft Tissue Sarcomas

Sarcomas of the face and jaws are seen quite frequently in children in Uganda and and are sometimes difficult to differentiate from Burkitt's tumour (ZIEGLER et al., 1971). Only four soft-tissue tumours involving the orbit were seen in the years of this study. This total is rather smaller than either before 1964 or since 1969. Two of these tumours were diagnosed as rhabdomyosarcomas; one occurred in the orbit of a 36-year-old female and showed cross-striations in strap cells, whereas the other, which developed in a 9-year-old girl, showed an embryonal appearance. The other two sarcomas seen both occurred in children; one was diagnosed as fibrosarcoma and the other as a malignant neurilemmoma (TEMPLETON, 1971).

Chloroma (Granulocytic Sarcoma)

Ten cases were seen in which patients presented with proptosis and eventually proved to have myeloblastic leukaemia. This represents an incidence many times greater than is found in other countries, where chloromatous deposits are rare (DAVIES and OWOR, 1965). There were 4 females and 6 males, the age range being from 1 to 40 years with a mean of 12.1 years. Eight of the 10 patients were diagnosed at Mulago Hospital and this suggests that the condition must be even more frequent in Uganda than is suggested by this report. Five of these patients presented with bilateral proptosis and 5 had unilateral involvement. In these 10 cases deposits of chloromatous tissue were found in the orbit and the eye itself was normal. Cases have been seen in which there was extensive intraocular involvement (TEMPLETON, 1967 a).

The clinical differential diagnosis from other tumours of the orbit is difficult and it is now standard practice to have a marrow examination performed in all cases of orbital tumours, particularly in childhood. Histological recognition may be difficult in anaplastic forms but if the condition is kept in mind eosinophilic myelocytes will often be found if sought. Staining for α naphthol ASD esterase (LEDER, 1964) confirms the myeloblastic derivation and greatly assists differentiation from histiocytic lymphoma.

Pseudo Tumour

Histologically these lesions showed all the features well described elsewhere (REESE, 1963). In the tropics, however, additional causes of orbital inflammation have

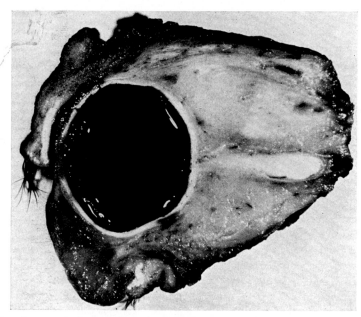

Fig. 5. Pseudotumour of the orbit. The orbital space is filled by granulation tissue with elongation of the optic nerve

to be considered. Worm infections of the orbital tissues are seen from time to time and fungi such as histoplasmosis duboisii are known to affect young children (TEMPLETON, 1971). Specific infections such as these have been excluded from consideration here but may be difficult to differentiate from tumours.

Nine cases of idiopathic inflammatory pseudotumour were histologically diagnosed. There were 6 males and 3 females. The age ranged from 8 to 60 years (mean 26.5 years). Five patients came from northern district but the reason for this excess is unknown. Bilateral involvement occurred in two cases. The history was usually of a few weeks' or months' duration, and the patient presented with painless proptosis. Two patients were under the age of 10 and were thought to have Burkitt's lymphoma but did not respond to cyclophosphamide. Solitary retro-orbital tumours may be very difficult to biopsy satisfactorily but this is mandatory if errors are to be avoided (Fig. 5). In addition to this the differential diagnosis from embryonal sarcoma or Burkitt's tumour is not easy on small pieces of tissue. The natural history of pseudotumour is regression over a period of some months, whereas the other tumours will continue to grow over a period of observation.

Anterior Encephalocele

This developmental defect seems to be at least as common as sacral meningomyeloceles in Uganda. The majority of cases occurred in the north of the country. The reason for this geographical variation is unknown.

Fibrous Dysplasia

Six cases were recorded in which the patient presented with proptosis caused by dysplasia of neighbouring bones. The condition is probably not unduly common but it is a slow-growing, immensely disfiguring process which brings the patient to hospital eventually, and these 6 cases derive from a population of 10 million people. The majority of patients were children and there were 3 males and 3 females. This condition is further discussed in the section on tumours of the bones and jaw.

Kaposi's Sarcoma

Four cases were seen. Three patients had lesions of the lid and the fourth a nodule on the limbus. All these patients were adults and one was female. Only one patient is known to have had cutaneous lesions elsewhere on the limbs but clinical details of the other 3 patients were sparse.

Ocular involvement in Kaposi's sarcoma is well recognized (Quéré et al., 1963). It usually occurs in association with lesions elsewhere in the body but may be solitary. In Tanzania ocular lesions were found to be quite frequent in children (Slavin et al., 1970) but in Uganda no such case was found. The development of nodules on the limbs and on the limbus of the eye suggest that previous trauma, either mechanical or radiant, might be associated with the localization of lesions. Trachoma is common in central Tanzania and less frequent in Uganda and it may be that such an infection could precipitate the development of ocular lesions in a predisposed patient.

Tumours of the Lacrymal Gland

Thirteen tumors were seen in the five-year period. Nine were pleomorphic adenomata and in one case adenocarcinoma had developed in a preexisting pleomorphic adenoma. There were 3 cases of adenocarcinoma. The age range of patients with pleomorphic adenoma was 30 to 58 years (mean 43.5) and there were 5 males and 4 females. Carcinomas were found at a younger age, mean 28 years, and 3 of the 4 patients were female.

Tumours of the lacrymal and salivary tissues are histologically similar and many diseases affect both types of gland. The distribution of lesions between the various glands is very different in different countries (Chapter 2). In Uganda the total number of tumours occurring outside the parotid is greater than those of the parotid itself, whereas among Caucasians parotid lesions outnumber the remainder by 3 to 1. It is difficult to be certain whether this altered ratio is due to decrease in the incidence of parotid tumours or increase in the tumours of other sites.

The distribution of tumour types was similar to that found in other countries (Böck and Feyrter, 1966), but that in the latter series 24% of tumours were adenoid cystic carcinomas. We have seen such lesions of the lacrymal gland but none occurred in the period of this review.

Chapter 13

Tumours of Endocrine Glands

A. C. Templeton

Tumours of the thyroid show a preponderance of follicular types but in other respects are similar to pattern described in other countries. Adrenal cortical tumours are rare. Phaeochromocytomas occur outside the adrenal more frequently than in the adrenal medulla. Autoimmune phenomena in the endocrine glands are extremely rare in Ugandan Africans.

In this chapter are included tumours of the pituitary, thymus, thyroid, parathyroid, islets of langerhans and the adrenal. Tumours of the chemoreceptor system are discussed in Chapter 15. Tumours of the endocrine portion of the ovary and testes are included under the heading of genital tumours of the respective sex. The total number of cases diagnosed is shown in Table 1.

Table 1. Showing the number of tumours of endocrine glands
which were diagnosed histologically

Pituitary		9
Craniopharyngioma	4	
Adenoma	5	
Thyroid		157
Adenoma	58	
Carcinoma	82	
Burkitt's lymphoma	17	
Parathyroid		—
Adrenal		22
Cortical carcinoma	2	
Medulla — Phaeochromocytoma [a]	3	
Ganglion neuroma	2	
Neuroblastoma	15	
Islets of Langerhans		2
Thymus		4
Total		194

[a] 5 Phaeochromocytomas developed in extra-adrenal locations.

Pituitary Tumours

Only 9 cases were diagnosed. There were 4 craniopharyngiomas and 5 adenomas. This incidence is certainly artificially low because of poor diagnostic facilities. After the period of this survey, Bailey and Thomas (1971) documented 17 cases of pituitary tumours in Uganda in the space of 18 months. It is likely that this latter figure represents a certain amount of "harvesting" of long-term cases which would previously have gone without treatment, but it indicates that there are a considerable number of cases in the country. ODEKU and JANOTA (1967) reported 4 pituitary adenomas and 3 craniopharyngiomas seen in a period of 4 years at Ibadan (Nigeria) out of a total of 44 intracranial neoplasms.

Three of the 4 craniopharyngiomata occurred in children aged 9, 11 and 18 years. The fourth case was a male of 56 years who had a tumour mass eroding the base of the skull and destroying the pituitary with involvement of the left petrous temporal. It is difficult to exclude the possibility that this tumour arose in the sphenoidal sinus but histologically it showed the typical central reticulate appearance of a cranio-pharyngioma. Pituitary adenomas occurred exclusively in adult life. Two of the patients with adenomata had symptoms and signs of acromegaly and were found to have eosinophilic adenomata. The three with chromophobe adenomas presented with the typical signs of homonymous hemianopia.

Secondary involvement of the pituitary by other neoplasms was only rarely seen. JANOTA (1966) in Nigeria found involvement of the pituitary in 21 of 23 patients with Burkitt's lymphoma who came to post mortem. Only 2 of 50 recent necropsies on children with Burkitt's tumour in Uganda have revealed such involvement. This marked difference is probably a result of more efficient intrathecal therapy which has recently become available rather than differences in the behaviour of the disease.

Tumours of the Thyroid

a) Benign Neoplasms (Adenoma of the Thyroid)

Fifty-eight cases were diagnosed, 52 in females and 6 in males. The mean age of patients in both sexes was 37 years.

The differentiation of true neoplasms from reactive states is often difficult. All the adenomas diagnosed in this series showed compression of thyroid tissue by a completely encapsulated growth that was homogeneous and different from the surrounding tissue (LAHEY et al., 1940). The criteria for diagnosis are not uniform from country to country, from one pathologist to another, or even the same pathologist at different times. The relative incidence in different communities is therefore virtually impossible to discuss. Histologically the majority of the adenomata recorded here were composed of micro-acini or the so-called fetal type of adenoma. Larger acini were sometimes seen within such nodules. A trabeculated structure was seen much more rarely.

The proportion of cases showing the so-called Hurthle cell change were small. Cells showing this appearance are rare in all glands in Ugandans. Thus oxyphilic cells are very rarely seen in salivary glands and no case of adenolymphoma (WARTHIN's tumour) has been seen in a Ugandan African. In spite of the fact that there are few old people in the population at risk this difference is probably real and is unexplained.

Adenomata are not associated with carcinoma in the vast majority of cases. In this series two anaplastic tumours showed remnants of material which could have been of a preexisting adenoma but no evidence of residual adenoma was found in other tumour types.

b) Carcinoma

Eighty-two cases were diagnosed, that is 1.1% of malignant tumours overall. This proportion is similar to that reported from most other parts of the world and other parts of Africa (JACKSON and REEVE, 1961). The incidence rates (corrected for an African population) in Kyadondo County were 1.6 cases per year per 100,000 people among females and 0.8 in males. These figures are very similar to those found in Europe, Africa and Asia but rather lower than those recorded from many American registries (DOLL et al., 1970).

The incidence in any country depends to some extent upon the diagnostic criteria used. The diagnosis of well differentiated follicular carcinoma is notoriously difficult. Papillary tumours are only marginally more easy to differentiate from reactive states. This problem is accentuated when large multilobular goitres are operated upon since degenerating nodules often contain papillary areas which can closely mimic the appearance of tumour. On the other hand, the more intense the sampling for micro-scopic examination, the more tumours will be diagnosed. The larger the goitre the greater the volume of tissue which remains unexamined. In this series from Uganda the degree of under-reporting is probably high. Large goitres are common and patients often unwilling to be operated upon. Specimens are examined carefully macroscopically but the number of blocks examined microscopically is smaller than in many university laboratories since only a small portion of tissue is sent from up-country hospitals. The diagnostic criteria employed were strict, and definite evidence of invasion or metastasis was required. In many metastatic tumours no evidence of invasion was found.

Material from 408 multi-nodular goitres was received in the Department of Pathology during the period under review. The incidence of multi-nodular goitre in Uganda is probably high, particularly in the region of Mount Elgon in Eastern Region. In a study in Kampala, CONNOR and FOLLIS (1966) found changes of thyroid hyperplasia suggesting relative iodine lack in all autopsy cases. They confirmed this impression by finding low iodine-excretion rates in school children in the same area (FOLLIS and CONNOR, 1966). However, increase in size of the thyroid gland is not commonly seen at post mortem. In a survey of thyroid weights in 400 adults at post mortem, less than 5% had thyroids heavier than 40 g and none was heavier than 100 g. These two pieces of information tend to contradict one another and indicate the need for carrying out large-scale systematic surveys in different parts of the country. The neighbouring areas of Sudan (WOODMAN, 1952), Congo (BAUDART, 1939) and Ruanda (MARNEFFE, 1958) have all been noted to have a high incidence of nodular goitre. POPOV (1967) in a survey in Ethiopia, noted that the incidence of goitre rose the further one went from towns or main roads. It is likely, therefore, that statistics based upon hospital practice will underestimate the extent of the problem.

The inter-relationships of cancer, adenoma and goitre are disputed. The early impression that cancer incidence rose parallel to the incidence of goitre has been challenged (SAXEN and SAXEN, 1954). One factor to be taken into account is that goitre increases the amount of thyroid material examined histologically, which in-creases the potential for finding occult tumours which may be clinically unimportant, and also increases the possibility of misdiagnosis. The proportion of multi-nodular goitres found to contain an unexpected cancer in this series was extremely small,

14 cases out of 400 goitres (3.5%). ZIMMERMAN and WAGNER (1960) record that the incidence of cancer in multi-nodular goitres has risen from 2% to about 10% over a period of 30 years. This rise is likely to be considerably influenced by diagnostic criteria and the diligence of search. In the same period the incidence of goitre decreased four-fold. There was no sustained increase in thyroid cancer in areas of Uganda where goitres seem to be common. The Bakiga people showed a slight excess of thyroid cancer but the tribes living around the area of Mount Elgon did not. The highest incidence rates quoted in "Cancer Incidence in Five Continents" (DOLL et al., 1970) come from volcanic areas. The incidence in Hawaii among all races is higher than all other registries quoted. High levels are also found in New Zealand Maoris and in Colombia. All of these areas also have a high incidence of goitre. It is possible that only certain types of thyroid cancer are associated with endemic goitre. WAHNER et al. (1966) in Colombia found that papillary carcinomas occurred much more frequently in non-goitrous glands than follicular or anaplastic tumours. There is no information on the state of the remaining thyroid in a considerable number of our cases, which makes it impossible to confirm this observation in Uganda. There did not appear to be any marked variation of the types of tumour seen in different geographical areas, except that 4 of the teenage patients came from Kigezi district which is located on high volcanic plateau (mean altitude 6000 ft.) in the southwest of the country. The Bakiga tribe accounted for 11% of cases of carcinoma of the thyroid compared with 4.9% of cancer overall.

The histological classification used here is a simple one into papillary, follicular, medullary and anaplastic types. Tumours showing papillary areas were diagnosed as papillary whether admixed with follicular areas or not. The diagnoses made and the distribution by sex are shown in Table 2.

Table 2. Showing the histological types of thyroid cancer diagnosed

	Males	Females	Total
Follicular	15	31	46
Papillary	7	14	21
Medullary	2	—	2
Anaplastic	3	7	10
Untyped	—	2	2
All cases	27	54	81

In many countries papillary tumours now account for the majority of thyroid cancers seen (WINSHIP, 1958). This is probably an effect of more efficient diagnosis and the undoubted change of criteria used in the classification of these slowly growing neoplasms while more anaplastic growths were always easily recognized. In Uganda and in Colombia (CUELLO et al., 1969) follicular carcinomas are much the most common type of tumour. These were mostly well differentiated and the follicles were surrounded by plump cuboidal cells, some with clear cytoplasm. Invasion of blood vessels was found in most cases but in some even the metastases appeared to be benign. The concept of benign metastasising goitre is now largely discredited but certain of these tumours are very sensitive to the effect of TSH. Proliferation of thyroid tissue in the lungs may occur following drug-induced hyperplasia of the thyroid without neoplastic growth (DALTON et al., 1948). DONIACH (1960) has suggested that there might even be two types of metastasis, one due to mechanical injection of the thyroid tissue into a vessel and the other a result of vascular destruction. Two medullary carcinomas were diagnosed, both of which contained stainable amyloid. Both patients were male and were aged 30 and 70 years respectively. Undifferentiated tumours were diagnosed in 10 cases. These were composed of giant cells in 4 cases and solid sheets of round cells in the remainder. Involvement of the thyroid in Burkitt's tumour is seen from time to time. This was seldom of great clinical importance since the size of such tumours was not large and was almost invariably associated with tumour masses in other areas, for example, the jaw or ovaries. No example of thyroid involvement by other types of lymphoma was seen. No case of Hashimoto's disease has been seen in Uganda and the number of lymphocytes present in the small number of cases of thyrotoxicosis which were seen was much less than in other parts of the world.

The age distribution of cases is shown in Table 3. Tumours at most sites in the body seem to occur at a considerably younger age in Ugandan Africans than in other people. With thyroid tumours this is not the case; no thyroid cancers were seen in childhood and only 22% occurred in patients under the age of 30. Correction for the

Table 3. The age distribution of different histological types of tumour

	10—19	20—29	30—39	40—49	50—59	60+	Unknown	Total
Follicular	4	8	9	4	9	8	6	48
Papillary	2	3	6	4	3	—	4	22
Others	1	—	3	1	5	2	—	12
Total	7	11	18	9	17	10	10	82

population at risk shows a rising incidence to the age of 65 and the incidence falls rapidly thereafter. The mean age of patients with papillary tumours (36 years) is younger than those with a follicular pattern (42.2 years), and other tumour types occurred in rather older people (47.5 years). This lowering of the mean age of patients with papillary tumours seemed to be a result of fewer old people rather than an excess of young patients (Table 3), since the majority (13 out of 18) of patients under the age of 30 had follicular tumours. No patient with papillary tumour was older than 60 years. Correction for the population at risk shows that the incidence of papillary tumours is highest in the fourth decade and steadily falls thereafter. By contrast, the incidence of follicular carcinoma rises in each succeeding decade, except in the very old. There were too few anaplastic tumours for meaningful calculations. In other parts of the world the vast majority of patients with thyroid tumours under the age of 30 showed a papillary pattern. The apparent absence of papillary tumours in the younger age group may be a result of tolerance of swellings of the neck for long periods, or possibly to a real deficiency of this type of tumour.

All diseases of the thyroid gland seem to be more common in females. The sex ratio shows a smaller excess of females in the case of cancer than with other thyroid masses, which explains the more sinister implications of a thyroid nodule in a male. In Uganda the male to female ratio in the cases of surgically treated nodular goitre was 1 male to 8 females and only 6 of the 58 patients with adenomas of the thyroid were male (1 male to 9 females). The ratio with carcinoma of the thyroid, however, was only a 2 to 1 excess of females (27 cases in males to 55 in females). This ratio was maintained in all histological types except medullary carcinoma where both tumours occurred in men. In a small survey of 25 cases seen at Mulago Hospital SHEPHERD and MANTHY (1963) found certain differences in the pattern of tumours occurring in males and females. In this series the age and histological distribution was essentially similar in both sexes.

The pattern of spread in the different tumour types is shown in Table 4. Cervical lymph nodes were noted to be enlarged in only a few cases, this is partly a result of inadequate clinical information. Papillary tumours showed nodal involvement more frequently than other histological types. Lung involvement was noted in 8 cases, and

Table 4. Metastases found in cases of thyroid cancer in each histological group

Histological type	Total cases	Cervical nodes	Extensive local infiltration	Distant metastasis
Follicular	47	9	7	17
Papillary	21	7	6	2
Others	14	2	12	3
Total	82	18	25	22

bone metastases were frequently found, particularly in follicular carcinoma. In a survey of 52 cases of secondary tumours in bone without a clinically detectable primary tumour (TEMPLETON, HUTT and DODGE, 1972) 12 cases were found to be from the thyroid. All of these cases had a follicular pattern. Extensive local invasion was found in all the anaplastic tumours, but distant and nodal metastases were less frequently seen in this type of tumour which often caused the patient's death without any distant spread. These patterns are very similar to those seen in other countries apart from the apparently low incidence of cervical node involvement.

The average duration of symptoms in patients with papillary tumours was 3.5 years prior to diagnosis. Follicular neoplasms had produced symptoms for an average of 2.8 years. Two patients with anaplastic tumours had had goitres for 10 and 15 years respectively, but in other patients symptoms were of less than 3 years' duration, with a mean of 1.2 years.

Parathyroid

No parathyroid tumours were seen during the period of this survey. Since the end of 1968 two examples of parathyroid adenoma producing extensive bone lesions have been diagnosed.

Adrenal
Cortex

Two patients with adrenal cortical carcinoma were found. Both were male. Bilateral tumours which had apparently been symptomless were discovered in a 90-year-old Busoga male at post mortem. The second patient aged 40 years had had abdominal pain for three months when the tumour was diagnosed at laparotomy, when it was found that neighbouring lymph nodes were involved.

No adrenal adenomata more than 1 cm in diameter were found at post mortem. (Approximately 3000 necropsy examinations on adults were carried out in this period.) This compares with an incidence of about 1.5% in Europeans (SYMINGTON, 1969). Small extra-capsular extensions were noted relatively frequently and many of the hypertensive patients investigated had nodularity of the adrenal cortex, but in no case did this give rise to nodules of more than 0.5 cm in diameter.

Other tumours most commonly involving the adrenal were Burkitt's lymphoma, hepatocellular carcinoma and Kaposi's sarcoma. Carcinoma of the bronchus is rare but adrenal metastases were found in a high proportion of necropsy examinations performed in this disease.

Medulla

Only 3 of the 8 phaeochromocytomas diagnosed developed within the adrenal medulla. Tumours of the adrenal medulla and the chemoreceptor system are discussed more fully in Chapter 15.

Islets of Langerhans

Two islet cell tumours were diagnosed. Neither appeared to be functional and neither showed specific staining on histological examination. Both came to light because they were growing in the head of the pancreas and had produced symptoms of pyloric stenosis. The differential diagnosis from carcinoid tumours of the duodenum in this situation was problematic but neither of these cases showed staining with diazo technique.

Cases of Zollinger-Ellison syndrome have been described in South African Bantu (BANK et al., 1965) but no functional islet cell tumour has been found in Uganda to date.

Thymoma

Four cases of thymoma were diagnosed. There were 3 epithelial tumours, 2 in females aged 18 and 34 years and one in a male of 50 years. Two of these cases were undifferentiated and the third showed a granulomatous appearance. The last was a lymphoid neoplasm occurring in a 25-year-old male.

One of these patients had hypertension with a positive Rogitine test. X-ray showed showed a mediastinal mass and he was thought to have a phaeochromocytoma. An anterior mediastinal mass was excised which proved to be an anaplastic epithelial thymoma, but the patient died 7 hours after operation. It is uncertain whether the thymoma was responsible for the hypertension and post-mortem examination was not performed.

None of these patients had evidence of myasthenia. In fact myasthenia gravis has not yet been confirmed in any Ugandan patient.

Chapter 14

Tumours of Bone and Jaw

O. G. DODGE

The most common malignant tumour of bone was osteosarcoma, which showed similar features to that found in other countries. Other tumours of bone were seen and showed no marked variation from experience elsewhere. Ewing's tumour, however, appears to be much less frequent in Africans than in Caucasians. Fibrous dysplasia, particularly of the facial bones, appeared to be more common but this may possible be a result of a harvesting effect.

Two hundred and eleven tumours of the skeleton (including tumours of the jaw but excluding Burkitt's lymphoma) were registered (Table 1). It should be noted that the series includes carcinomas metastatic to bone where the bone lesion was biopsied, and lymphomas of non-Burkitt type arising in, or metastatic to, bone. Ameloblastomas

Table 1. Tumours of bone and joints, 1964—1968

1. Primary malignant tumours of bone and joint		93
Osteogenic sarcoma	47	
Parosteal sarcoma	1	
Chondrosarcoma	13	
Giant-cell tumour	6	
Chordoma	4	
"Round-cell tumour"	15	
Synovial sarcoma	7	
2. Metastatic carcinoma		57
3. Malignant lymphoma (non-Burkitt)		26
4. Odontogenic tumours		35
Ameloblastoma	32	
Others	3	
		211
5. Primary benign tumours of bone and joint (not included in Cancer Registry)		134
Osteoma and osteochondroma	34	
Chondroma	10	
Chondromyxoid fibroma	4	
Myxoma of Jaw	3	
Ossifying fibroma	60	
Tendon sheath tumours	18	
Others	5	

are also registered although they are not, strictly speaking, malignant neoplasms. Synovial sarcomas are included in this chapter as well as in Chapter 15 on connective tissue tumours. Myelomas are included in Chapter 16.

The various types of bone tumour differ so widely in their age and site distribu-

Table 2. Relative frequency of some bone tumours in a North American (DAHLIN, 1957) and the Uganda series (Osteogenic sarcoma — 100)

	U.S.A. No. of cases	Uganda No. of cases
Osteogenic sarcoma	469 ... 100	47 ... 100
Chondrosarcoma	199 ... 42.5	13 ... 28
Giant-cell tumour	120 ... 26	6 ... 13
Osteochondroma	272 ... 58	34 ... 72
Chondroma	99 ... 21	10 ... 21

tion that there is little point in calculating frequency ratios or incidence rates for a group that includes such biologically disparate entities. There is no exactly comparable survey with which to compare relative frequencies, but DAHLIN's (1957) survey of nine years' experience of bone tumours at the Mayo Clinic offers in some respects an American parallel. His series includes, conveniently enough, almost exactly ten times the number of osteogenic sarcomas as the Uganda series. The numbers of some of the

Table 3. Lesions involving the jaws, 1964—1968
(Figures marked * are included in the totals given in Table 1)

Burkitt's lymphoma	143
Odontogenic tumours	35 *
Ossifying fibroma	48 *
Myxoma	3 *
Giant-cell lesions	10
Fibrous epulis	54
Dentigerous cysts	14
Rhabdomyosarcoma	6
Fibrosarcoma	1
Metastatic neuroblastoma	2 *
Non-Burkitt lymphoma	4
Total	320

other tumours can then be expressed as a proportion of the number of osteosarcomas (Table 2). Relative to osteogenic sarcoma there is a mild dearth of chondrosarcomas and quite a marked shortage of giant cell tumours in Ugandans. Benign tumours are, however, well represented in the Uganda series. The more striking features of the Ugandan list (Table 1) are, however, the high frequency of ameloblastomas and lesions of the ossifying fibroma group relative to primary bone tumours. All the former and most of the latter occurred in the jawbones, confirming the frequency of neoplastic disease in the jaw reported on in our earlier study (DODGE, 1965). This is shown clearly in Table 3, in which all the tumours and tumour-like lesions involving the jaws are summarized. Some of these are discussed in more detail below and others are dealt with in other chapters.

1. Osteogenic Sarcoma

The age and sex distribution of the 47 cases of osteogenic sarcoma are shown in Table 4. There are more patients in the youngest age groups, and fewer in the older

Table 4. Osteogenic sarcoma — age and sex distribution

	Male	Female	Total	% age	Dahlin (1957) % age
0— 4	—	—	— ⎫	11	6
5— 9	1	4	5 ⎭		
10—14	5	6	11 ⎫	50	53
15—19	6	5	11 ⎭		
20—24	3	3	6 ⎫	18	18
25—29	1	1	2 ⎭		
30—34	1	3	4 ⎫	11	9
35—39	1	—	1 ⎭		
40+	2	2	4	9	14
Total age known	20	24	44		
"Child"	1	—	1		
"Adult"	2	—	2		
Total	23	24	47		

Table 5. Osteogenic sarcoma — site distribution

Knee region:	Lower femur	13	
	Upper tibia	10	
	Upper fibula	1	
	"Knee" (bone not specified)	7	31
Ankle region:	Lower tibia	2	
	Lower fibula	1	3
"Femur", area not specified:		2	
"Leg", site not specified		2	4
	Total lower limb		38
Upper limb:	Humerus	3	
	Ulna	1	
	Total upper limb		4
Other sites:	Maxilla	1	
	Spine	1	
	Ribs	2	
	Ilium	1	5
	Total		47

ones, than in DAHLIN's (1957) series, but this can be accounted for by the very different age structure of the two populations. The oldest patient in the Ugandan series was 70 years old; none of the cases had any evidence of Paget's disease of bone. So far, not a single example of Paget's disease has been seen in Uganda Africans. The site distribution (Table 5) shows a marked concentration of cases in the lower limb (80%), mostly around the knee joint. This is not very different from Dahlin's series, in which some 65% of the osteogenic sarcomas arose from bones of the lower limb. It is likely that a crippling lesion in a weight-bearing bone will bring an African patient to hospital more surely than a lesion in, say, the ilium. In the table the sites are arranged by anatomical region where possible, rather than by individual bones, since the knee, and other joints, with the adjacent bone ends form functional units. The individual bone involved was known in 38 cases: femur 15, tibia 12, humerus 3, fibula 2, and others 6.

Tribal Distribution

Nine of these 47 tumours occurred in Baganda people (19%) and the rest were distributed among 17 different tribes. This represents the proportion of Ganda within the country fairly accurately, and it may be that in the case of this tumour the various tribes are equally well represented in the pathological material. The Baganda accounted for 29.5% of malignant tumours overall and it is possible that they have a lower incidence of osteogenic sarcoma than the other tribes. So far there is no other evidence to support this, but the relative paucity of Ganda seen in our earlier study of bone tumours in Ugandan Africans (DODGE, 1964) has been confirmed in this larger series.

Histological Features

The majority presented little diagnostic difficulty, showing small or extensive areas of tumour osteoid or bone production in a sarcomatous tumour. Four cases showed a mainly chondroblastic pattern, and one of these, in the tibia of a 16-year-old girl, had originally been reported as a chondrosarcoma. One tumour was mainly fibroblastic, and 6 were highly anaplastic, with only scanty osteoid production. One of these tumours, in the femur of an 11-year-old boy, was originally labelled as an undifferentiated tumour, but tumour osteoid was eventually seen on re-examination of the sections.

Aetiological Factors

Human osteogenic sarcoma most commonly arises in the area of bone adjacent to the epiphyseal lines of the distal femur and proximal tibia, shortly after the period of most rapid bone growth in adolescence (HEMS, 1970). In man, these two areas account for 55—70% of total increase in bone length (CAFFEY, 1961). Children developing osteogenic sarcoma seem on average to be taller than appropriate controls (FRAUMENI, 1967); large breeds of dogs develop more bone tumours than small breeds (TJALMA, 1966); and, as in man, it is the weight-bearing bones that are most commonly affected. Rapid growth and mechanical stress appear, therefore, to be important factors in the localization and age distribution of bone sarcoma.

In the Uganda series, the zones of rapid bone growth around the knee joint are, as in other series, the main site of osteogenic sarcoma. We have no information on the rates of bone growth and the times of epiphyseal closure in Ugandan children. The number of cases occurring is far too small to attempt any study relating stature to the risk of developing bone sarcoma.

Four tumours occurred in patients over 40 years; none showed any radiological evidence of Paget's disease of bone, and in spite of being specifically sought at necropsy, the disease has never been confirmed in a Uganda African.

The only agent in the external environment known to induce human bone sarcomas is ionizing radiation (GLASS and FRAUMENI, 1970). There are no radioactive sources (other than the natural background radiation) in Uganda and no possibility of any of the Ugandan patients having received any therapeutic or accidental radiation.

Parosteal Sarcoma

Only one tumour was placed in this category, from a 32-year-old male with a tumour arising from the "lower leg" (presumably tibia). This was a mainly periosteally-situated fibroblastic and osteogenic tumour.

2. Chondrosarcoma

Thirteen cases were registered. The age and sex distribution are shown in Table 6. More than half the cases occurred in the second decade. Although the numbers in the Ugandan series are small this is probably significantly earlier than in Dahlin's American series, where the highest incidence is in the sixth decade. Dahlin points out that the second decade of life, in which the peak incidence of osteogenic sarcoma occurs, is practically immune to chondrosarcoma in his series.

Table 6. Chondrosarcoma — age and sex distribution

	Male	Female	% in each decade	U.S.A. % in each decade (DAHLIN, 1957)
0— 9	—	—	0	0.5
10—19	4	2	54	0.5
20—29	—	1	9	11.5
30—39	1	1	18	20.5
40+	2	—	18	67
Unknown	2	—		
Total	9	4		

Four cases occurred in the bones of the lower limb (one in the femur, one in the fibula and 2 at the ankle), 4 in the innominate bone, and 5 at various other sites.

The relatively high proportions of cases arising in the leg bones, and of patients in the second decade, raise the doubt as to whether some of these tumours were not in fact chondroblastic osteogenic sarcomas. The histological diagnoses are all based on biopsy material and no amputation specimens were available at the time of review, so this possibility cannot be altogether excluded. As far as could be determined, all the tumours (with one exception, see below) showed differentiation towards cartilage in all areas, without areas of undifferentiated sarcoma or of differentiation towards fibrous or osteoid tissue, and all showed the rounded expansile edges characteristic of chondrosarcoma. Two cases provided some difficulty in diagnosis. In one, a girl of 10 years was said to have fractured the ankle some time previously, and had developed a mass at this site. Biopsy revealed what the surgeon believed to be a tumour, and histology revealed a uniform appearance typical of chondrosarcoma. The possibility of chondroid proliferation at the site of a malunited fracture seemed excluded by the absence of any other histological evidence of fracture repair. The other doubtful case was that of a woman of 32 who was said to have a very large abdominal mass (no further detail available); biopsy showed a malignant neoplasm which has been classified as a possible example of a mesenchymal chondrosarcoma. Only 2 of the 13 patients with chondrosarcomas were from the Ganda tribe; three were Lango from northern Uganda and others were from 7 different tribes.

3. Giant-Cell Tumours of Bone

Only 6 unequivocal examples of this tumour were recorded. All occurred in bones of the lower limb (one at the lower end of the femur, 3 in the upper tibia, one in the upper fibula, one in the talus). The youngest patient was a boy of 10, the oldest a woman of 35 years. The tumour in the 10-year-old boy showed a frankly malignant picture. In this case there was a history of being knocked down by a bicycle, followed three weeks later by severe pain in the knee. The tumour occupied the upper third of the fibula, and was infiltrating soft tissue. The other 5 tumours fall into the more benign categories (grades 1—2) of giant-cell tumour.

The common giant-cell lesions occurring in the jaw (mostly labelled "giant-cell epulis" or "reparative giant-cell granuloma") were not included in the cancer registry. One other case, originally diagnosed as a giant-cell tumour, has been excluded. The differential diagnosis from "brown tumour" of hyperparathyroidism and, in one case, from chronic osteomyelitis resulting from middle ear disease was sometimes difficult.

4. Chordoma

Four examples were seen. In three a reasonably confident diagnosis of chordoma was possible—these were tumours of the sacrococcygeal (1 case) and buttock areas (2 cases) in patients aged 2, 13 and 30 years. The histological features (mucinous and myxoid tumours with vacuolated "physaliferous" cells) were diagnostic. The fourth case, a retroperitoneal tumour in a man of 40, was a less clear-cut example, but this seemed the most probable histological diagnosis.

No case of intracranial or cervical chordoma was seen.

5. Round-Cell Tumours of Bone

This term has been used to describe a group of 15 bone tumours, all of them composed of small round cells, and none of them showing obvious differentiation. The diagnostic difficulties in this type of tumour are all too familiar to pathologists. The tumours which may fall into this group include metastatic neuroblastoma, metastatic

carcinoma, Ewing's sarcoma, and reticulum-cell sarcoma of bone. A differential histological diagnosis should not, ideally, be attempted without knowledge of the clinical
picture, the X-ray appearances, the pattern of catecholamine excretion, etc. As such a
favourable situation does not obtain in this series, it was felt wisest simply to group
the cases together, admitting that they probably represented a heterogeneous group of
primary and, possibly, secondary tumours of bone.

However, in view of the epidemiological features of Ewing's sarcoma revealed by
GLASS and FRAUMENI (1970), it was decided to attempt to separate the possible cases
of Ewing's sarcoma from the group. Table 7 gives details of the whole group, and
indicates those which on histological grounds might be classed as possible cases of
Ewing's sarcoma. In view of the apparent rarity of neuroblastoma in Ugandan
children (DAVIES, 1968) the two cases that are *histologically* suggestive of metastatic
neuroblastoma are also indicated.

Table 7. Round-cell tumours of bone

Age	Sex	Site	
1	M	Jaw	Possible neuroblastoma
9	F	Jaw	Undifferentiated round-cell tumour
11	F	Humerus	Possible Ewing's sarcoma
12	F	Knee	Possible Ewing's sarcoma
17	F	Femur	Possible neuroblastoma
18	M	Tibia	Possible Ewing's sarcoma
20	M	Skull	Undifferentiated round-cell tumour
23	M	Knee	Undifferentiated round-cell tumour
24	M	Tibia	Possible Ewing's sarcoma
25	F	Scapula	
25	M	Forearm	
45	F	Tibia	Undifferentiated round-cell tumour
50	M	Tibia	
60	F	Jaw	
Adult	M	Knee	

The status of Ewing's sarcoma as a disease entity is probably accepted by most
pathologists today, in spite of Willis's strongly-argued contention that Ewing's
tumour is a syndrome caused by several different kinds of tumours rather than a
pathological entity (WILLIS, 1967). Most writers on bone pathology have regarded it
as a relatively rare condition. In Dahlin's 1957 series, it accounted for 141 out of
1639 primary malignant tumours of bone (compared with 490 osteogenic sarcomas).
The analysis of death certificates of children dying of cancer in the U.S.A. carried out
by GLASS and FRAUMENI (1970) showed 482 cases of Ewing's sarcoma and 819 osteogenic sarcomas in a total of 1532 deaths from primary malignant bone tumours. Out
of these 482 cases only 12 (2.5%) were recorded in non-white children, whereas 127
(15%) of the osteogenic sarcomas were in non-whites.

The most frequent misdiagnosis of Ewing's sarcoma in children would lie in plac-
ing cases of metastatic neuroblastoma in this category, but as neuroblastoma is at least
as common in U.S. non-whites as in U.S. whites, it seems clear that Glass and
Fraumeni's data reveal that (1) Ewing's sarcoma is the second most frequent primary

bone tumour in U.S. white children, and (2) it is very much less frequent among U.S. non-whites. This discrepancy remains unexplained; the tumour has been reported as relatively common in India (BORGES et al., 1967) and Japan (IRIBE, 1969). Our previous study of bone tumours in Uganda (DODGE, 1964) revealed no example of a Ewing's sarcoma; the 4 possible cases in this series must be regarded with some caution. One case of Ewing's tumour has been recorded from Senegal (TESTU et al., 1963). Electron microscopic evidence (KADIN and BENSCH, 1971) suggests that Ewing's tumour might be derived from primitive myeloid cells. Myelosarcoma (chloroma) associated with acute leukaemia is frequently seen in Ugandan children (DAVIES and OWOR, 1965). It is intriguing that there might be a reciprocal relationship between these two entities.

6. Synovial Sarcoma

Seven tumours were placed in this group; all showed a spindle-cell sarcomatous pattern in which were embedded clefts, slits or pseudoglandular spaces lined by cuboid or columnar pseudo-epithelium.

The patients' ages ranged from 8 to 70 years. The patients all came from different tribes; 4 were female, 3 male. All the tumours were in the lower limb. The site and age distribution, and the histological features, seem to resemble those described in American or European series. Details of the patients are shown in Table 8.

Table 8. Synovial sarcomas

Age	Sex	Site
8	F	Hip joint
26	M	Hamstring muscles
30	F	"Knee"
40	F	Metatarsal
49	M	Achilles tendon
70	M	Second toe
Adult	F	"Thigh"

7. Metastatic Carcinoma and Malignant Lymphoma Involving Bone

In the period studied, 57 cases of malignant neoplasms metastatic to bone were recorded, making metastatic tumour the commonest type of bone tumour encountered. This total includes only those patients in whom the primary site was unknown at the time of the biopsy of the bone lesion. In the same period, 26 examples of malignant lymphoma (other than Burkitt's lymphoma) involving bone were recorded. It is not feasible to determine what number (if any) of these were primary in bone. (The lymphomas are discussed in Chapter 16).

The origin and distribution of bone metastases in Ugandan Africans has been the subject of a separate communication (TEMPLETON, HUTT and DODGE, 1972). The results of the survey are presented in Table 9. The relative infrequency of breast and

Table 9. Metastatic carcinoma and lymphoma in bone (primary site unknown before biopsy)

Site of Metastasis

	Skull	Vertebrae and sacrum	Sternum and ribs	Ilium	Mandible	Scapula and clavicle	Humerus	Femur	Tibia	Total
Primary diagnosed (30)										
Thyroid	3	—	1	1	—	—	2	2	1	10
Liver	2	2	1	—	—	2	—	—	1	8
Prostate	1	1	2	1	—	1	—	—	—	6
Neuroblastoma	—	—	—	—	2	—	—	—	1	3
Other	1	—	1	—	—	—	—	1	—	3
Primary not diagnosed (27)										
Adenocarcinoma	4	3	3	1	—	—	1	1	—	13
Squamous carcinoma	—	1	2	—	—	—	—	1	—	4
Anaplastic carcinoma	1	2	2	1	—	1	—	3	—	10
Malignant (26)										
Lymphoma [a]	3	3	2	1	4	—	1	10 [b]	2	26

[a] Excluding Burkitt's lymphoma.
[b] Includes 2 chloromas.

bronchial cancer in Ugandan Africans allows thyroid carcinoma to take first place on the Ugandan list. Hepatocellular carcinoma is frequently encountered in Ugandan Africans (see Chapter 3) and its appearance as a major source of bone metastasis is not surprising, though worth emphasizing as as clinical fact of some importance.

As in European and American studies, it is the bones of the axial skeleton which are among the most frequent sites of metastases from carcinoma. Among the non-Burkitt lymphomas involving the skeleton, the femur is the most frequently affected site, followed by the mandible. The jaw as a site of tumour localization in Ugandan Africans is discussed below.

8. Odontogenic Tumours

In the 1964—1968 period 35 odontogenic tumours were recorded by the Kampala Cancer Registry, of which 32 were ameloblastomas. The frequency with which ameloblastomas occur in African populations has been noted previously (see below), and in view of their clinical and epidemiological importance it was appropriate that these lesions should be included in the Cancer Registry, although these are not, strictly speaking, malignant neoplasms.

Ameloblastoma

The age and sex distribution are shown in Table 10. The largest number of tumours occur in the fourth decade. The youngest patient in the series was aged 4, the oldest aged 60.

Table 10. Ameloblastoma — age and sex distribution

Age	0—	5—	10—	15—	20—	25—	30—	35—	40—	45—	50—	55—	60—	Un-known	Total
Male	—	—	2	1	2	3	1	1	1	1	3	—	1	—	16
Female	1	—	—	2	—	—	5	2	2	1	1	1	—	1	16
Total	1	0	2	3	2	3	6	3	3	2	4	1	1	1	32

Twenty-five arose in the mandible, 2 arose in the maxilla, and in 5 cases it was unclear whether the origin was in upper or lower jaw. (No so-called adamantinomas of long bones were seen).

These features are similar to those described in European and American series. The histories varied from 2 months to several years. Many patients claimed that the lesion appeared following tooth extraction but it is likely that a loosened tooth was the first manifestation of the tumour. The tumours grow by expansion, with erosion of the cortical bone; in many cases the tumours had broken through the bone and periosteum and presented as rapidly-growing fungating infected tumours in the oral cavity. No evidence of metastasis was found in any case.

The histological appearances showed the same range of patterns as occurs in other series. No attempt was made to group the tumours into follicular and plexiform types, since both patterns could often be seen in the same section. One tumour showed

Table 11. Ameloblastoma — number of Ganda and non-Ganda cases per year, 1947—1970

	1947—1961	1962	1963	1964	1965	1966	1967	1968	1969	1970	Total
Ganda	15	1	3	2	1	2	2	—	3	2	31
Non-Ganda	9	5	1	5	4	2	3	10	4	7	50
Unknown	—	—	—	—	1	—	—	—	—	—	1
Total	24	6	4	7	6	4	5	10	7	9	82

conspicuous epidermoid differentiation within the tumour islands (so-called acantho-ameloblastoma), and 4 tumours were classed as granular-cell ameloblastomas. These showed the characteristic histiocyte-like cells laden with PAS-positive cytoplasmic granules within the tumour islands. The cases did not seem to differ from the other ameloblastomas in age, sex or tumour localization.

The tribal distribution shows interesting features compared with that found in the earlier series reported (DODGE, 1965). In that series, drawn from the years 1947—

1961, 24 ameloblastomas were recorded, of which 15 were from the Ganda tribe. In the current series, only 7 out of 32 tumours occurred in Ganda tribespeople. Twenty-four tumours occurred in members of 15 different other tribes, and 1 in a man of unknown tribe. Further, in the current series, only 3 patients lived in Kyadondo County, surrounding Kampala, and the rest were referred from medical centres in nearly every district of Uganda. This suggests that "harvesting" may have been occurring. The ameloblastoma is a conspicuous lesion, and a slow-growing one; patients may carry the tumour for many years before blocking of the oral cavity occurs, leading to death from starvation or from respiratory infection. It may be, therefore, that many of the tumours present in the nineteen-fifties among the Ganda tribe were seen at the local hospital at this period, and found their way into the Kampala Cancer Registry. We are now seeing larger numbers of cases from the hitherto unharvested regions beyond Kyadondo and the Buganda region (Table 11).

Ameloblastomas in African Populations

It has been realized for some years that ameloblastomas apparently occur rather frequently among Africans. In Uganda the common occurrence of jaw tumours was documented by SINGH and COOK (1956), DAVIES and DAVIES (1960) and DODGE (1965). The subject of ameloblastomas in East Africans was fully reviewed by SLAVIN and CAMERON (1969). Their study includes cases from Tanzania and Uganda, the latter drawn from the Kampala Cancer Registry records for 1962—1965 inclusive; there is therefore some overlap between their series and the present one, since 13 of the present series were included in Slavin and Cameron's study. The reader is referred to their paper for a detailed study of the histological features and histogenesis of these tumours. They pointed out that the impression of an unduly high frequency might be due to the "harvesting" of cases as adequate surgical services became available, and that the incidence might be expected to drop once the backlog of existing cases had been treated. ANAND, DAVEY and COHEN (1967) noted the apparent frequency of ameloblastoma in Nigerians and also thought that "harvesting" might well account for the large number of cases encountered. A further large series of ameloblastomas from Ibadan has been reported by AKINOSI and WILLIAMS (1969). Other African series have been reported from Ghana (KOVI and LAING, 1966), Senegal (REYNAUD, BEL and LY, 1961) and the Congo (THYS, 1957). From the West Indies, LAWRENCE (1966) reported that 16 of 38 primary bone tumours in the Jamaica Cancer Registry, were ameloblastomas.

It remains to be proved whether the apparent frequency of ameloblastoma (and other jaw tumours) in these different countries is simply a statistical artefact occurring during the early years of the epidemiological exploration of tumour incidence in these "underdeveloped" countries, or whether there is possibly a genuinely higher incidence of the tumour in people of African stock. The early delineation of Burkitt's lymphoma as a jaw lesion, and later realization of the multicentric nature of the tumour, offer an instructive parallel (see Chapter 16). Nothing is known of the aetiology of ameloblastoma other than its histogenesis from persistent islands of odontogenic epithelium; the writer is not aware of any comparative studies of the development of the teeth and jaws in African and non-African populations.

Other Odontogenic Tumours

This group consisted of one case of *Pindborg tumour* (calcifying epithelial odonto-genic tumour) in the maxilla of a 60-year-old woman who said that the lump had been present for 40 years; one case of *intra-alveolar clear-cell epidermoid carcinoma* of the mandible in a 40-year-old woman, with the clinical features of an amelo-blastoma; and one unclassifiable case which has been labelled as a *tumour of para-dental residues*.

9. Benign Tumours and Tumour-Like Lesions of Bone

These are not included in the Kampala Cancer Registry figures, but a note on this group may be appropriate here. During 1964—1968, 134 benign bone tumours or tumour-like lesions were seen in the Pathology Department of Makerere University College. The types of lesion are shown in Table 1. As with ameloblastoma, it is prob-able that the obvious presence of a mass, combined with the slow non-lethal evolution of the lesion, brings these patients to the local hospitals in misleadingly large num-bers, and as many of these tumours are amenable to surgical excision, they figure in the files of the pathology department with some frequency. *Osteoma* and *osteo-chondroma* (cartilage-capped exostosis) seem to occur in the same situations as in Europeans. In the group of *chondromas* 5 arose in bones of the hand and 2 in bones of the foot; these were clearly benign tumours. Two tumours of the knee area were diagnosed as chondromas on biopsy only, and it is not possible to exclude chondro-sarcoma in these. The *ossifying fibromas* form an interesting group, dominated by the jaw lesions. The patients' ages ranged from 8—50 years, with the 10—14 year group containing the most cases. The lesions showed the usual range of histological appear-ances, from the diffuse largely fibrous tumours indistinguishable from fibrous dys-plasia, to densely calcified tumour-like masses. The spherical calcified bodies ("cemen-ticles") were seen only in two lesions, both from the frontal bone.

Ossifying fibroma of the jaws has previously been reported from Uganda (DODGE, 1965), Senegal (REYNAUD and LY, 1961), the Congo (HENNEBERT and SEGHERS, 1964; SCOVILLE, 1964), and Ibadan, Nigeria (ANAND, DAVEY and COHEN, 1967). No attempt has been made in the present survey to distinguish between ossifying fibroma, fibrous dysplasia, fibro-osteoma, or other benign fibrous tumours of one.

As with ameloblastomas, the apparent frequency of this group of jaw lesions may be a statistical artefact. The other benign tumours seen seemed to resemble their counterparts in Europeans. The five "other tumours" mentioned in Table 1 include a benign chondroblastoma, an angioma, two osteoid osteomas, and one case of synovial osteochondromatosis.

Chapter 15

Soft Tissue Tumours

A. C. TEMPLETON

With 13 Figures

Tumours of soft tissues accounted for almost one third of the whole series. The outstand-
ing tumour of this group was Kaposi's sarcoma, which accounted for almost one twelfth of
malignancies of males. This tumour presents in one of three forms. Subcutaneous nodules are
found in many adult patients, while children with the disease usually present with generalized
lymph-node involvement and with few or no cutaneous tumours. Rarely adults present with
generalized cutaneous nodal and visceral lesions. Other connective-tissue tumours are probably
more common than in other countries but it is difficult to be certain if this is an effect of the
population distribution. The relative frequency and possible inter-relationships of tumour
types are discussed.

Soft-tissue tumours for the purpose of this chapter have been defined on the same
schema as that used in the manual on Histological Typing of Soft-Tissue Tumours
(ENZINGER, 1969), that is, all tumours of fibrous, adipose, muscular, vascular, synovial, mesothelial, peripheral, nervous, ganglionic and pluripotential mesenchymal
tissue, as well as certain tumours of debatable origin and other entities, probably of a
reactive nature which are easily confused with tumours. This group of cases accounts
for a very large proportion of tumours in this series. The heading embraced 2815,
tumours 670 of which were malignant. The diagnoses made are shown in Table 1.

Incidence

Tumours of soft tissues are very common indeed. There is no doubt that the
frequency is considerably underestimated by this review, particularly that of benign
tumours. Most such cases never reach hospital, those that do are usually not operated
upon, and of those tumours that are excised only a small proportion are submitted
for histological examination. Malignant tumours of superficial tissues are preferentially
selected over benign tumours of deeper regions.

The group as a whole, both benign and malignant, accounts for almost 30% of all
tumours registered. 9.1% of malignant tumours are derived from soft tissues, that is,
12.2% of all malignant tumours in males and 5.6% of malignant tumours in females.
This proportion is grossly in excess of any figures from other parts of the world. Proportional rates calculated from the registry returns published in Volume 2 of Cancer
Incidence in Five Continents (DOLL, MUIR and WATERHOUSE, 1970) show that soft-
tissue tumours are relatively most frequent in Africa. All three African registries

Table 1. Soft-tissue tumours

1. *Fibrous tissue*		329
A. Fibromas	60	
B. Fibromatoses	207	
C. Dermatofibrosarcoma protuberans	35	
D. Fibrosarcoma	27	
2. *Adipose tissue*		278
A. Lipoma	263	
B. Liposarcoma	15	
3. *Muscle*		1052
A. Smooth Leiomyoma	947	
Leiomyosarcoma	61	
B. Striated Rhabdomyosarcoma	44	
4. *Blood vessels*		408
A. Benign	396	
B. Malignant	12	
5. *Lymphatic vessels*		73
A. Benign	73	
6. *Synovial tissue* (Malignant)		7
7. *Mesothelial tissue* (Malignant)		3
8. *Peripheral nerves*		181
A. Benign	146	
B. Malignant	35	
9. *Sympathetic ganglia and paraganglionic tissue*		33
A. Benign	12	
B. Malignant	21	
10. *Pluri-potential mesenchyme* (Benign)		4
11. *Chordoma*		4
12. *Tumours of disputed histogenesis*		366
A. Benign		
1. Granular cell myoblastoma	16	
2. Nasal Glioma	8	
3. Myxoma	3	
4. Melanotic Progonoma	1	
5. Fibrous Hamartoma of Infancy	2	
B. Malignant		
1. Alveolar soft-part sarcoma	6	
2. Kaposi's sarcoma	329	
3. Clear-cell sarcoma of Aponeuroses	1	
13. *Related questionably neoplastic entities*		59
Juvenile xanthogranuloma	1	
Giant-cell tumour of tendon sheath	25	
Ganglion	33	
14. *Unclassified malignant tumours*		43
Total		2840

quoted (Ibadan, Bulawayo and Natal) show a proportion of soft-tissue tumours between 2.2 and 3.2% of cancer overall. Almost without exception cancer registries dealing with Caucasian populations have a proportion considerably less than 1%. The negro population of the western hemisphere shows an intermediate figure, 1.25% in Jamaica and 1.4% in Alameda County, California. The proportional rate in this Ugandan series was approximately three times the next most frequent area in the

world. Almost exactly half the malignant tumours were Kaposi's sarcoma but even
when these tumours are excluded the proportional rate of soft-tissue tumours is 4.2%
and 4.9% in males and females respectively, which is markedly higher than from
any other part of the world.

Proportional rate surveys are, of course, biased by the population at risk. In
Africa undue prominence is thereby given to tumours of young people. However,
incidence figures corrected for the population at risk (Table 2) show that the incidence

Table 2. Incidence of soft-tissue sarcomas in different communities. (All figures are corrected
for an African standard population of 100,000. All figures except Uganda are taken from
DOLL et al., 1970)

	Males	Females
Uganda (Kyadondo County)	4.7	3.5
Natal (African)	4.1	1.4
Colombia (Cali)	3.3	1.5
Uganda (whole country)	2.6	1.0
California (negro)	2.5	2.2
California (white)	1.9	1.8
Jamaica (Kingston)	1.2	1.5
India (Bombay)	0.6	0.6
Japan (Miyagi)	0.2	0.2

in Kyadondo County is higher than in other countries. The excess in males is largely
a function of the extreme frequency of Kaposi's sarcoma, but among women Kaposi's
sarcoma accounted for only 13% of cases of soft-tissue sarcomas. There has been
considerable dispute as to whether Africans are more likely to develop connective
tissue tumours than other races. In the case of Kaposi's sarcoma there is an undoubted
excess but this is not found among Africans in America. With other soft-tissue
tumours, DAVIES et al. (1965) in Uganda, and HIGGINSON and OETTLÉ (1960) in
South Africa found no excess and concluded that the proportional increase noted
previously in Africa (DES LIGNERIS, 1927; SHAPIRO et al., 1955) was a result of social
and population factors. In Alameda County negroes show a higher incidence than
whites (LINDON et al., 1970) but in West Indian negroes the rate is lower (BRAS and
WATLER, 1970). International comparisons of soft-tissue tumours are difficult to make
because registration practice is not uniform and diagnostic criteria of malignancy
vary. In addition the inclusion of many tumour types under a single heading makes
comparison of individual tumours impossible. Thus the differences in incidence in
Bantu people between Uganda, Natal (SCHONLAND and BRADSHAW, 1970) and
Cape Town (GRIEVE and LINDER, 1970) are almost certainly purely a result of differences in the incidence of Kaposi's sarcoma.

The sex distribution of tumours showed a marked male predominance but this
was entirely due to the strange distribution of Kaposi's sarcoma. Males with Kaposi's
sarcoma outnumbered females by 14 to 1, whereas in other types the sex ratio was
exactly equal. There were 316 males and 23 females with Kaposi's sarcoma, and 165
patients of each sex with other types of soft-tissue sarcomas.

The age distribution of soft-tissue tumours was similar to that found in other countries. There was a significant number of patients in every decade. There were 35 patients under the age of 5 years and 28 over the age of 70 years. Age-specific incidence rates showed a slow linear rise with age to the age of 65 and a slow fall thereafter in males; in females the fall in rates occurred much earlier and was more rapid (Fig. 1). The increase with age of Kaposi's sarcoma is an arithmetical progres-

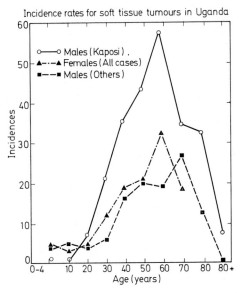

Fig. 1. A graph showing the age-specific incidence rates of soft-tissue tumours in Uganda

Table 3. Showing proportional rates of Kaposi's sarcoma and other connective-tissue tumours in different parts of the country

	Kaposi	Other soft-tissue sarcomas	All soft tissues
Lugbara	9.0	4.3	13.3
Toro	7.4	3.5	10.9
Ankole	7.1	4.7	11.9
Kiga	6.1	6.9	13.0
Soga	5.1	3.2	8.3
Gishu	4.5	6.9	11.4
Lango	4.5	5.5	10.0
Ruanda/Rundi	4.2	5.3	9.5
Nyoro	4.1	4.6	8.7
Ganda	3.6	3.5	7.1
Acholi	2.7	3.5	6.2
Teso	2.2	6.3	8.5
All tribes	4.5	4.5	9.1

sion, whereas in many carcinomas there is an exponential increase. This arithmetical increase is also found in some lymphomas and this similarity has been used to suggest that lymphomas and Kaposi's sarcoma are closely related (OETTLÉ, 1962). Kaposi's sarcoma may be similar to lymphomas but the age-related risk does not prove this. In fact the age-related curve suggests certain properties of the causative factors in Kaposi's sarcoma. It is unlikely to be accumulative and there would seem to be either a steadily increasing sensitivity of cells or an increased exposure in each successive decade. There is little to suggest a hormonal modification of incidence. Other soft-tissue sarcomas as a group showed an even less marked rise with age, but as this in-cluded a large variety of tumour types further analysis would be meaningless.

The proportional rates of connective tissue tumours vary markedly in different parts of the country. Kaposi's sarcoma seems to be relatively more common in the west of the country (Table 3). The highest proportional rate found was among the Bakonjo who live around the Ruwenzori mountains where Kaposi's sarcoma ac-counted for 15.4% of tumours overall and the Karamojong 11.1%. In both these tribes the number of cases is low and registration bias is likely to be considerable. Apart from these, the highest figure was found in the northwest among the Lugbara and the proportional rate falls gradually as one travels south through Toro, Ankole and Kigezi to Ruanda. Nilotic people (Acholi and Lango) seem to be relatively less likely to suffer from Kaposi's sarcoma but Para-Nilotic susceptibility varies very widely indeed. Bantu tribes occupied a median position. The reasons for this variation are not known.

Other forms of connective-tissue tumours show a variation which is much less marked. There did not appear to be either a positive or a negative correlation with Kaposi's sarcoma. The highest rates were seen in Gishu and Kiga people living on opposite sides of the country; both are Bantu and both live at high altitude. This group of diseases includes a wide range of tumour types but no individual tumour showed a strong geographical variation apart from Kaposi's sarcoma.

The Baganda are much the best served in terms of hospitals and transport and they showed the highest incidence of these tumours, though a low proportional rate. It could be suggested on this basis that there is a negative correlation between diagnostic efficiency and the proportion of connective tissue tumours. However, among other tribes there did not appear to be any correlation either negative or posi-tive between the proportion of connective tissue tumours and the diagnostic efficiency (see Chapter 1).

Fibrous-Tissue Tumours

Tumours and tumour-like conditions of fibrous tissue are difficult to classify and to diagnose. There are no sharp distinctions between reactive states, benign neoplasms and malignant neoplasms. There is no sharp distinction between diseases of fibro-blasts, diseases of other cells associated with collagen production and mixtures of the two. A histological appearance diagnosable as malignant in adult life is likely to behave in a benign fashion in infants. These statements are of course true of other entities, but it is probably in the assessment of fibrous-tissue proliferation that the average pathologist is made to realise his inadequacy most acutely. The present author is very much aware of his deficiencies in this field, particularly in connection with the distinction between malignant tumours of fibroblastic and Schwann-cell types. The classification used and the number of cases in each group is shown in Table 4.

Table 4. Tumours and tumour-like conditions of fibrous tissue

Dermatofibroma (sclerosing haemangioma)	42
Fibromas	18
Keloid	131
Nodular fasciitis	13
Fibromatosis Colli (sternomastoid tumour)	4
Plantar and palmar fibromatosis	11
Ainhum	6
Nasopharyngeal fibroma	1
Aggressive musculo aponeurotic fibromatosis	41
Dermatofibrosarcoma protuberans	35
Fibrosarcoma	27
Total	329

A. Fibroma and Dermatofibroma (Histiocytoma)

Sixty cases were diagnosed under this heading. This is a heterogeneous group and almost certainly includes examples of other entities which have become sclerosed and are no longer recognizable as neurofibromas or leiomyomas. Dermatofibroma was diagnosed in 42 cases. One general rule which has proved invaluable in practice in Africa is never to diagnose histiocytoma or dermatofibroma without a Ziehl-Nielsen stain, since lepromatous leprosy is difficult to distinguish on haematoxylin- and eosin-stained material.

B. Fibromatoses

1. Hypertrophic Scars

These are seen regularly in clinical practice but are very seldom sent for histological examination.

2. Keloid Scars

These occur very frequently indeed. They tend to be found most frequently over the ears, neck and upper part of the trunk (DAVEY, 1968). The Department of Pathology received 131 specimens during the period under study but this represents only a fraction of the cases seen in Uganda. Material is submitted only when the diagnosis is in doubt and it is all too often extremely easy. Histologically the characteristic feature of keloid scars are the broad bands of hyalinized collagen which run in haphazard fashion through the mass. Between these there are small numbers of spindle cells, but unless the scar has been excised very early there is little problem in differentiation from other types of fibrous proliferation. The epidermis overlying a keloid scar is usually thin and atrophic and skin accessories are absent.

3. Nodular Fasciitis

In the early period of this survey (1964 and 1965) no cases were noted, but latterly a number of examples were seen, particularly in a group of Ruandan refugees. These people had at that time a high incidence of Buruli ulcer which had made them acutely conscious of the value of prompt excision of all subcutaneous nodules. Four of the 13 cases diagnosed came from this small group within a period of one year, suggesting that this condition is more common than at present appreciated.

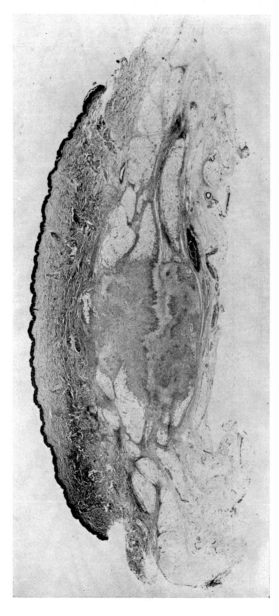

Fig. 2. Photomicrograph of nodular fasciitis

Eight of the 13 patients were male and there were 5 females. The age range was 9 to 50 years (mean 26 years). The commonest site was on the trunk and only in 5 cases were the limbs affected. In two of these cases the lesions were on the forearm, which is probably the commonest site in Caucasian subjects. The lesions were usually located at the level of the superficial fascia (Fig. 2) and extended into the sub-cutaneous fat. The nodules were most often less than 3 cm in diameter but in some cases larger lesions were seen. All cases were solitary.

Histologically the diagnosis was seldom problematic, providing an excisional biopsy had been carried out. There was considerably greater difficulty when previous incision had been carried out, particularly when a marked inflammatory reaction due to super-added infection was present.

4. Fibromatosis Colli

Four examples of sternomastoid tumour were seen. These were all unilateral and differed in no way from experience in other countries. Iron stains were negative and no evidence in favour of traumatic origin was discovered.

5. Plantar and Palmar Fibromatosis

Only 11 cases were seen and in 10 of these the lesions occurred on the plantar region. In view of the high incidence of other fibrosing lesions this low incidence was surprising. It would seem that the incidence of Dupuytrens contracture is genuinely low. This finding was unexpected, since manual work is universal and cirrhosis is common. The cases which did occur were typical and showed mature collagen in the fascial layer of palm and sole. Seven of the 11 patients were male and the age range was from 20 to 55 years.

6. Ainhum

This strange condition, so common in some parts of Africa, was seen only occasion-ally. Cases seem to occur more frequently in the north of the country than in Kam-pala, but specimens were seldom sent to the laboratory and material from only 6 cases was received. A band of mature collagen was seen in the region of the superficial fascia surrounding the toe or finger. No indication of the aetiology of this lesion was found in the histological study. A useful summary of this condition is that of COLE (1968).

7. Nasopharyngeal Fibroma

Only one example of this condition was seen. By far the commonest tumour in teenage males was nasopharyngeal carcinoma which seems to occur at a younger age in Ugandan Africans than in other peoples.

8. Musculoaponeurotic Fibromatosis, Aggressive Fibromatosis, Desmoid

Such lesions appear to be very common in Uganda. Forty-one examples were seen in the five-year period under review (Table 5). There were 17 males and 24 females and the age ranged from 6 weeks to 69 years. In 17 cases the lesions occurred in the anterior abdominal wall and 13 of these patients were female. One male and one female had had previous laparotomies but in the other cases the tumour had developed spontaneously. 5 patients had primary lesions on the foot. Four of these were under the age of 5 years and had had the lesions since birth. In these children the lesions were located on the toes and often more than one digit was involved. Recurrence after local excision was seen once but no long-term follow-up is available. Similar cases have been described by REYE (1956) as "fibromatous tumours" of infancy. All congenital fibromatoses seen in Uganda developed in the sterno-mastoid muscle or the toes. No case of generalized fibromatosis was seen. No patient either in infancy or adult life developed metastases but a large number recurred locally and

Table 5. Showing the distribution of 41 cases
of musculo-aponeurotic fibromatoses

Scalp	1
Neck	1
Arm	4
Shoulder	2
Chest wall	4
Trunk	20
(17 anterior abdominal wall, 3 mesentery)	
Scrotum	1
Lower limb	8
(4 neonatal cases with lesions on the toes)	
Total	41

required repeated excisions. There did not appear to be any geographical variations in the distribution of these tumours.

On histological examination these lesions consist mainly of collagen that maintains a fibrillary structure in contrast with the hyaline appearance of a keloid scar. The intervening fibroblasts are small and regular. Muscle fibres and skin accessories are surrounded and the bizarre appearance of degenerating muscle incorporated in the mass may suggest a highly malignant neoplasm.

C. Dermatofibrosarcoma Protuberans

There were 35 examples of this condition, which appears to be rather more common than in other countries. There were 22 males and 13 females with a mean age of 34 years. Lesions occurred in almost all parts of the body except the hands and the feet, with the majority being found on the trunk and lower limbs (Table 6).

Clinically the subcutaneous lobulated appearance was characteristic unless ulceration had been produced by attempted excisions at home. Histologically the tumour was made up of spindle cells arranged in cartwheel fashion (Fig. 3), which extended from immediately under the epidermis deep into the subcutaneous fat. Mitoses were few and necrosis was not seen. No metastases were recorded but one patient had had 12 recurrences after surgical excision and many others occurred less frequently.

There was a slight tendency for an excess of patients to come from western region (13 out of 35 cases), with a deficiency of patients from the north (5 cases), but this variation was not marked. There is some evidence to suggest that dermatofibrosarcoma protuberans may be more common in negroes than in Caucasians. The

Table 6. Distribution of 35 cases of dermatofibrosarcoma protuberans

Head and neck	4
Shoulder region	6
Upper limb	2
Trunk	10
Pelvis	3
Lower limb	10
Total	35

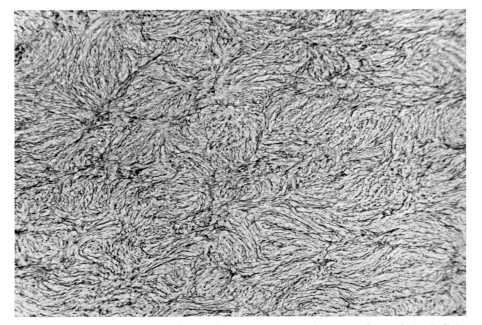

Fig. 3. Dermatofibrosarcoma protuberans showing the cartwheel pattern of growth (Reticulin)

present series of 35 cases compared with 27 fibrosarcomas suggests an increased frequency. KREMENTZ and SCHAUER (1963) in the U.S.A. found 6 out of their 8 cases of dermatofibrosarcoma protuberans occurred in negroes, whereas negro patients provided about half the cases of connective-tissue tumours overall.

D. Fibrosarcoma

The diagnosis of fibrosarcoma is often difficult. Areas of fibrosarcomatous tissue may be found in a wide variety of mesenchymal tumour types. The incidence, therefore, depends to some extent upon diagnostic criteria. Fibrosarcoma and neurogenic sarcoma are extremely difficult to separate and division may be artifical in many instances; some authors do not attempt this distinction (THORBJARNASON, 1961). However, in this study these two entities were separated but it is likely that other pathologists reviewing the same material would have classified the cases differently. The problem of differentiation from pseudosarcomatous conditions was not as commonly met with as in countries where radiotherapy is used and where there are a greater proportion of old people in the population. Some cases of peritoneal infection such as that following gonococcal salpingitis may result in gross reactive proliferation which can easily be confused with a neoplasm. Spindle-cell squamous carcinomas arising from long-standing tropical ulcers mimicked fibrosarcoma closely in some cases but, provided that an adequate biopsy is taken, areas of more obviously squamous derivation can usually be found.

Twenty-seven patients were diagnosed as having fibrosarcoma; there were 14 males and 13 females. The age ranged from birth to 63 with a mean age of

Table 7. Distribution of 27 cases of fibrosarcoma

Head and neck	3
(Palate, nose, temporal region)	
Upper limb	7
(upper arm 2, forearm 4, hand 1)	
Trunk	10
(chest wall 3, groin 2, 1 case each buttock, scrotum, retroperitoneal and axilla)	
Lower limb	7
(thigh 3, lower leg 4)	
Total	27

27 years. Three tumours were present at birth, a proportion very much higher than reported from elsewhere but probably a result of the population distribution. A further three cases were seen in patients under the age of 14 years. The tumours were mainly situated deep to the deep fascia. The anatomical distribution is shown in Table 7. Grading of these tumours showed 17 well differentiated and 10 poorly differentiated tumours. There is no information available on follow-up of these cases.

Smooth-Muscle Tumours

These tumours were by far the most common. The great majority occurred in the uterus and a few in the gastrointestinal tract, but smooth-muscle tumours of the subcutaneous tissues were by no means uncommon. It is generally agreed that subcutaneous solitary leiomyoma arises from vessels in the dermis and such tumours have been more fully described in the section on vascular neoplasms (p. 254).

A. Benign Leiomyomyomata

1. Uterine (816 cases)

Only a very small proportion of such tumours reach the Pathology Department; many are symptomless and most do not bring the patient to hospital. Of patients diagnosed as having fibroids most are not operated upon and since the macroscopic appearance is typical many are not submitted to the laboratory. There is therefore little reliable information as to incidence. It is generally agreed that uterine fibroids occur more commonly in American negroes than in whites (TORPIN et al., 1942). There is some suggestion from our records that women of Nilo-Hamitic tribes develop uterine fibroids less frequently than Nilotic or Sudanic peoples. Bantu women have an intermediate incidence. This possibility requires further investigation. The histological appearance is exactly similar to that seen elsewhere. All the secondary changes, such as infarction, liquefaction, hyalinization and calcification were seen from time to time.

2. Gastrointestinal

Gastrointestinal tumours were diagnosed in 29 cases; 6 in the oesophagus, 8 in the stomach, 12 in the small intestine, one in the colon, and 2 close to the anus.

Tumours of the stomach were usually discovered incidentally at post mortem but in two cases superficial ulceration of tumour nodules had occurred, giving rise to haematemesis. Four of the tumours of the small intestine had caused intussusception

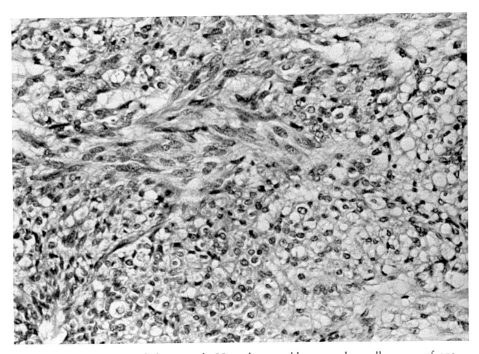

Fig. 4. Leiomyoblastoma of the stomach. Note the resemblance to clear-cell tumour of aponeuroses (Fig. 13) and areas in Kaposi's sarcoma (Fig. 9)

and the remainder were found incidentally at post mortem. In 3 cases it was difficult to distinguish these lesions from neurofibromata since the poor preservation of intussuscepted tissue rendered the PTAH stain negative.

3. Subcutaneous

One hundred four cases were diagnosed and are discussed more fully below in the section on vascular tumours.

4. Leiomyoblastoma (Embryonal Leiomyoma Bizarre Smooth Muscle Tumour)

Two examples were seen, both of which occurred in the stomach (Fig. 4). One was massive and appeared to be attached to the pancreas and spleen. The other was smaller and had given rise to pain following central ulceration. The precise taxonomic position of this tumour is arguable. Stout (1962) maintained that these cells were similar to embryonal smooth muscle. Clear cell areas were found very frequently in leiomyomas and leiomyosarcomas of the bowel in this series. They were absent in uterine tumours and were moderately frequent in subcutaneous lesions. This variation suggests that the cell of origin and pathogenesis of leiomyomas at these various sites might be different.

B. Malignant — Leiomyosarcoma

Sixty-one cases were diagnosed, that is 18% of malignant soft-tissue tumours (excluding Kaposi's sarcoma). The majority of these tumours arose in the abdomen from the uterus or bowel and the incidence at these sites is probably the same as in other countries, although figures are difficult to obtain. Superficial leiomyosarcomas were found in 19 cases a considerably higher proportion than in other parts of the world (Stout and Hill, 1958). Three of these tumours arose in association with

Table 8. Anatomical distribution of leiomyosarcomata

Region	Cases	Site
Subcutaneous	19	9 Lower limb
		4 Head and neck
		4 Trunk
		1 Upper limb
		1 Not stated
Retroperitoneal	11	
Visceral	15	2 Stomach
		7 Small intestine
		3 Colon
		1 Rectum
		1 Bladder
		1 Spleen
Uterine	16	
Total	61	

multiple subcutaneous nodules which might have been Kaposi's sarcoma (in none of these areas was another nodule biopsied). There is probably a close relation between Kaposi's sarcoma and leiomyosarcoma.

The age ranged from 12 to 60 years (mean 44 years). Sixteen cases arose in the uterus. Of the remaining 45 cases 24 occurred in males and 21 in females. The anatomical distribution of lesions is shown in Table 8.

The histopathological appearance was exactly similar to that described in standard textbooks. The diagnosis of leiomyosarcoma depends upon recognition of the square-ended nuclei, the presence of mitotic figures and staining of longitudinal striations with PTAH and trichrome methods. Nuclear pleiomorphism was often marked and mitoses were less frequent than in fibrous tissue tumours of similar degrees of nuclear pleiomorphism.

In the subcutaneous tissues the most difficult differential diagnostic problem was the distinction from an aggressive Kaposi's lesions. In some cases of lesions of Kaposi's sarcoma, the spindle-cell element predominates, the nuclei are more plump and less tapering than usual and mitoses are frequent. Electron microscope studies have shown cytoplasmic fibrils and attachment plates in Kaposi's sarcoma very similar to those of smooth-muscle cells (SMITH and WOLFE, 1970). Some cases of leiomyosarcoma contain clear-cell areas such as are seen in leiomyoblastomas, which may be indistinguishable from vascular capillaries on conventional light microscopy, and a few tumours contain eosinophilic inclusions typical of Kaposi's sarcoma (LEE, 1968). The differentiation of these entities is difficult and it is probable that they are not sharply distinct. In one case (KCR 440/67) the two tumours lay side by side in the same lesion. Leiomyosarcoma with clearly demonstrable longitudinal striations abutted onto typical Kaposi's sarcoma. This patient had multiple other subcutaneous nodules and it seems reasonable to assume that leiomyosarcoma had developed in one of them. This subject is discussed in greater detail elsewhere (TEMPLETON, 1972 b).

Leiomyosarcoma of the uterus usually occurred in association with benign leiomyomata but in no case was there an intermingling of benign and malignant tumour tissue. It seems likely that sarcomas arise de novo rather than from malignant change occurring in a preexisting benign tumour. This conclusion is in direct contradiction to the accepted view of most pathologists that the vast majority of sarcomas arise in benign leiomyomata (WHEELOCK and WARREN, 1942). It is accepted that virtually all cases arose in a uterus which also contained benign leiomyomata but it would seem just as reasonable to postulate that muscle capable of producing benign lesions might also give rise to malignant growths as to suggest that one preceded the other. Areas of softening within a benign leiomyoma may be accompanied by nuclear pleiomorphism in degenerating cells but it seems probable that many such cases diagnosed as malignant tumours are in reality benign (SCHIFFNER et al., 1955). The differential diagnosis from stromal sarcoma is often problematic and depends upon the demonstration of intracellular longitudinal striations.

Tumours of Adipose Tissue

Adipose tissue undoubtedly behaves in a very different fashion in Ugandans than in Caucasians. Whilst not exactly steatopygic, the female Bantu buttock is well endowed and there may be liberal subcutaneous fat. The amount of adipose tissue in the mesentery or retroperitoneal tissues, however, is usually minimal. No explanation for these apparent differences is available but this may relate to the relative rarity of liposarcoma compared with other sarcomata which occur quite frequently.

Mature adipose tissue has a distinctive and rather immobile appearance. It should be recalled, however, that these cells derive directly from primitive mesenchyme and as such are capable of a wide range of appearances and fatty tissue is often intermingled with other connective tissue elements.

Lipoma

Such tumours are extremely common in Uganda; few will be seen by a doctor and even fewer by a pathologist. Two hundred fifty-nine cases were seen in the Department of Pathology. 20% of these were in patients with multiple subcutaneous lipomata. The excess probably merely reflects a greater tendency to send material from cases which are puzzling rather than straightforward. Solitary lesions usually occurred on the trunk, most frequently on the shoulders and buttocks. Histologically these tumours were very seldom composed of pure fat, the majority having a vascular or fibrous component, but no case of myelolipoma was seen.

One lipoma of the gum was seen and 9 cases of submucous lipomas of the bowel. Six of these latter cases occurred in the colon. Three submucosal lipomata in the small intestine were all diagnosed following intussusception.

Liposarcomas

Eighteen cases were seen, that is 5% of malignant soft-tissue tumours. Thus this tumour appears to be rather less common than most types of soft tissue tumours. PACK and ARIEL (1958) noted that liposarcoma accounted for 14.6% of tumours of soft tissues in New York.

Eight cases occurred in the retroperitoneal region and one in the mediastinum. Nine patients had liposarcomas of the limbs, 7 occurred on the leg, 4 of which were in the thigh, and 2 were on the arm. All these tumours occurred deep in the intermuscular septa where fat is usually absent. Only two tumours occurred in superficial tissues, one on the forearm and one overlying the knee. All malignant tumours appeared to be solitary and none arose in association with lipomatosis.

The age ranged from 14 to 70 years (mean 50.9 years). The age of patients with retroperitoneal tumours was exactly similar to those with tumours of the periphery. Eleven male and 7 female patients were recorded. Four cases occurred in each of Buganda, Western and Eastern regions. Six patients came from the north of the country. Although numbers are very small there appeared to be an excess of cases among Nilotic peoples.

Histological examination showed gross pleiomorphism in 2 cases but the majority were well differentiated and showed minimal mitotic activity. Four appeared lipomatous, 5 had a myxomatous appearance and 5 were made up predominantly of spindle cells. Differential diagnosis was often troublesome. Virtually all large soft-tissue sarcomas contained stainable fat and its presence, unless in very large quantities, was therefore of little diagnostic assistance. In many sarcomas areas of myxomatous degeneration occurred, particularly in tumours of neural origin. Differentiation from myxomas of the thigh and the jaw would be extremely difficult if only small amounts of tissue were available for study. Spindle-cell areas were found in many tumours and such lesions should probably be referred to as fibroliposarcomas, but if neoplastic fatty tissue was found such tumours were diagnosed and recorded as liposarcomas. No case was diagnosed as a malignant mesenchymoma in this series. Those cases which might have been so called by other pathologists are mainly included as liposarcomas.

These tumours were usually slow-growing with little tendency to metastasize. The majority of retroperitoneal swellings were huge before patients presented at hospital but none showed evidence of metastases. Three cases were noted to have recurred after attempted excision but distant metastases were not found in these patients. One pleiomorphic liposarcoma on a limb was found to have given rise to pulmonary metastases at the time of presentation.

Rhabdomyosarcoma

Forty-four cases were diagnosed. Even when they contained striped muscle elements, teratomas and multipotential tumours such as Wilm's tumour or mixed mesodermal tumours of the uterus were not included under this heading and are discussed with other tumours at their site of origin. The classification of these tumours into subgroups such as alveolar, embryonal, pleomorphic and botyroid has been suggested. There is considerable overlap between these entities and the correct diagnosis depends upon examination of many blocks of tissue from each tumour. In this series, multiple blocks were often not available for study and the classification is liable to be somewhat arbitrary. Therefore the group has been treated as a whole and comments made as to the distribution of each subtype where pertinent. The distribution of tumours by age, sex, site and histological type was very similar to that seen in Caucasians (BIZER, 1969).

Rhabdomyosarcoma accounts for 12.5% of malignant soft-tissue tumours in Uganda, which is a similar proportion to that found in the U.S.A. (THORBJARNASON, 1961; KREMENTZ and SCHAUER, 1963). Subclassification of tumours in this series showed 14 tumours of embryonal type and 10 each of the alveolar, pleomorphic and botyroid varieties.

The age distribution of patients is shown in Table 9. The mean ages of patients with alveolar and embryonal tumours were 12.4 years and 4.2 years respectively. Pleomorphic types were seen at an older age, the mean being 35.1 years. Seventeen

Table 9. Showing the age of patients with rhabdomyosarcoma

0—4	5—14	15—24	25—34	35—44	45—54	55—64	Unknown
12	17	3	2	1	4	4	1

patients were male and 27 female. The sex distribution showed a slight female excess in all histolgical types. Four tumours arose in the female genital tract and 5 in the male genital tract. The tumours in males were far advanced at the time of presentation and it was impossible to distinguish between tumours arising from bladder and prostate. Males predominated in all histological subgroups except that of pleomorphic tumours, where 7 of the 10 patients were female.

The most common sites of involvement were the head and neck, genitourinary
system and lower limb (Table 10). Embryonal tumours were found mainly in the
head and neck, whereas lesions of the limbs were more frequently of pleomorphic
and alveolar type. This distribution is similar to that reported in Caucasians (ENZIN-
GER and SHIRAKI, 1969). Tumours arising in the bile duct are extremely rare. DAVIS
et al. (1969) were able to find 18 case reports and added 5. One of the present series

Table 10. Showing the anatomical distribution of rhabdomyosarcoma

Head and neck	15	(9 embryonal type)
Upper limb	2	(1 alveolar 1 pleomorphic)
Trunk (chest wall)	2	(2 pleomorphic)
Perineum and rectum	4	(2 alveolar pattern, 1 botyroid 1 pleomorphic)
Paratesticular	2	(1 embryonal 1 pleomorphic)
Cervix	6	(All botyroid)
Bladder/Prostate	3	(All botyroid)
Lower limb	9	(5 alveolar pattern 3 pleomorphic 1 embryonal)
Bile duct	1	(embryonal)
Total	44	

of patients (KCR 1618/68) was a 14-year-old boy who presented with cervical
lymphadenopathy and jaundice. He died shortly after admission and at autopsy was
found to have a tumour in the porta hepatis with widespread involvement of retroperitoneal and mediastinal nodes. No metastases were found elsewhere. Rhabdomyosarcoma of the lower urinary tract occurred in 3 male patients. In these cases it was
impossible to say whether the tumours arose in the bladder or prostate since all were
far advanced at diagnosis. The cases were uniformly fatal and at autopsy in one case
(KCR 1617/66) metastases were found in the lungs and neighbouring nodes. In a
review of sarcomas of the bladder and prostate, MACKENZIE et al. (1968) found that
the majority of cases arose in the bladder. Tumours of the head and neck are common and experience of such cases in Uganda has been reviewed previously (TEMPLE-
TON, 1967 a; ZIEGLER et al., 1971). Differentiation from Burkitt's lymphoma may be
difficult both clinically and histologically.

Histologically, these cases were in every way similar to those described from
other countries. Differential diagnosis on clinical grounds was often problematic,
particularly in tumours of the face which closely mimicked the clinical appearance of
Burkitt's lymphoma or metastatic neuroblastoma (TEMPLETON, 1971). Histologically,
differentiation of a large biopsy seldom presented problems, but diagnosis of a small
biopsy specimen, which often shows traumatic artefact, was sometimes difficult. In
such cases, exfoliative touch preparations were much easier to distinguish from
lymphomas. Distinction of the pleomorphic type of tumour from other soft-tissue
sarcomas, particularly leiomyosarcoma, was often problematic. Cross-striations were

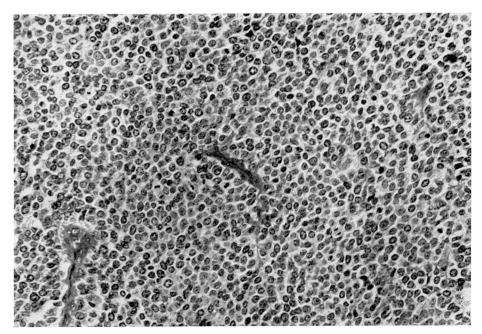

Fig. 5. Alveolar rhabdomyosarcoma. Within the alveoli the constituent cells mimic lymphoma

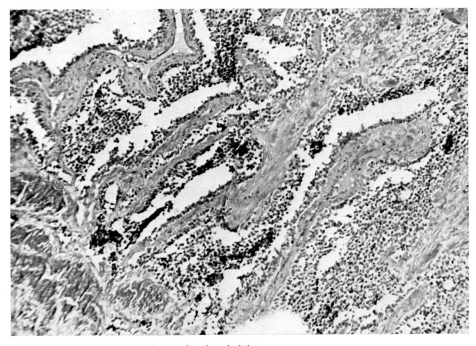

Fig. 6. Alveolar rhabdomyosarcoma

found in only a minority (38%) of embryonal and alveolar tumours but were identified in all but one of botyroid and pleiomorphic types. It is probable that other examples of rhabdomyosarcoma are classified under "unidentified sarcomas" for lack of positive diagnostic features. Alveolar tumours often contained areas of cells which closely resembled histiocytic lymphoma (Fig. 5), but elsewhere more typical areas were always found (Fig. 6).

Seventeen patients were from Buganda, 15 from the Western region, 9 from the Eastern region and only 3 from the North. The deficiency of cases from the north of the country was unexpected and is not due to lack of medical facilities, since patients with Burkitt's tumour who present with very similar signs and symptoms are frequently seen and diagnosed in this area. There was a trend towards a reciprocal relationship between these two conditions in that 5 out of 15 patients with rhabdomyosarcoma of the face came from the southwest of Uganda where Burkitt's tumour is rare, whereas only 2 came from the north where Burkitt's lymphoma is more common. These differences are not statistically significant but deserve attention as more cases are accumulated.

Published series of different types of rhabdomyosarcoma often express surprise that various histological types of rhabdomyosarcoma should have been recognized so late in the course of history. For example, the alveolar pattern was first described in 1956 by RIOPELLE and THÉRIOULT, and yet ENZINGER and SHIRAKI recognized 110 cases in their study in 1969 and a further 10 cases are recorded here. These tumours are therefore not so rare as might have been predicted.

The prognosis in these cases is poor and treatment by various combinations of surgery, chemotherapy and radiotherapy appears to be ineffective in many cases (ENZINGER and SHIRAKI, 1969; SOULE et al., 1968). In Uganda some regression of tumour bulk has been achieved using chemotherapy alone (ZIEGLER, 1971, personal communication) but the majority of patients die within a year of diagnosis.

Vascular Tumours

The interrelationships of these lesions with Kaposi's sarcoma are more fully discussed in papers by LEE (1968) and TEMPLETON (1972 b).

A. Benign

1. Haemangioma

Haemangioma was diagnosed in 131 cases; most of these patients had subcutaneous cavernous lesions on the face and neck but in 40 young adults the lesions were in the mouth. The sex incidence was equal and 54% of cases occurred in children under the age of 15.

The frequency of these lesions appears to be low but it is difficult to be certain whether this is a result of a low rate of presentation or a truly low incidence. Certainly pigmented lesions are much less noticeable under a pigmented skin and are therefore less likely to be brought to hospital. Cavernous haemangiomata were found from time to time in the liver at post mortem. Many patients in this series had multiple subcutaneous lesions and a few were found to have intraosseous involvement. Two patients with Mafucci's syndrome were seen and one patient with multiple haemangiomas of the skin and vertebral bodies developed paraplegia following compression of the spinal cord by tumour extension. The relatively large proportion of patients with multiple lesions probably results from a low rate of biopsy in cases with solitary nodules.

2. Lymphangioma

Seventy-one such tumours were seen. The majority (42 cases) occurred in the neck of young children (cystic hygroma) but lesions were also found on the limbs and in the mesentery. There was a slight male preponderance and 75% of cases occurred in patients under 14 years. Four examples were seen of lymphangioma circumscriptum on the limbs.

3. Granuloma Pyogenicum

Two hundred and forty examples of this entity were seen. In addition to these cases ulcerated tumours, particularly Kaposi's sarcoma, were often surmounted by a layer of proliferative granulation tissue in every way similar to that found in granuloma pyogenicum (Fig. 7). Proliferations in these circumstances have not been included in the total.

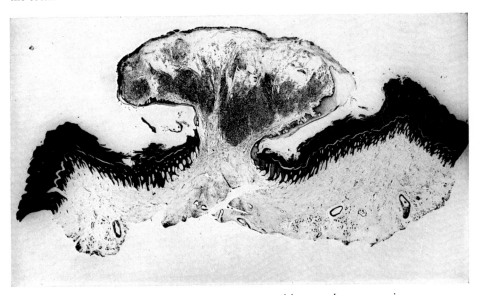

Fig. 7. A nodule of Kaposi's sarcoma surmounted by granuloma pyogenicum

In 46% of cases the lesions occurred on the lower limb but no part of the cutaneous surface was immune. Forty-three examples of granuloma pyogenicum of the gum were found, 28 of these occurring in young adult females 15 of whom were known to be pregnant. In other parts of the body the sex incidence was equal. Many of the patients were young and 71% of lesions occurred in patients under the age of 45.

The incidence of these lesions is rather higher than in many countries but this is probably a result of environmental factors rather than an altered vascular response.

The majority of the population go barefoot and the primary treatment of trauma is usually poor so that many minor abrasions often become infected. The geographical distribution of these lesions showed a slight excess of patients from the West and a diminished proportion from Eastern region. No reason for this variation was readily apparent.

4. Angioleiomyoma

One hundred and four cases of vascular leiomyoma were seen in this five-year period (Templeton, 1972 a). In 1937 Stout presented a paper recording 15 cases and found reference to 85 previous case reports. This lesion is much more common in Caucasians than the paucity of the records would indicate, but the incidence in Uganda none-theless seems to be considerably higher. Ninety-nine patients presented with a solitary subcutaneous nodule. This was usually between 1 and 2 cm in size and was located in the dermis. The patient often reported that the nodule was extremely painful. The presence of spontaneous pain was a characteristic shared with glomus tumours which were much less common in this series. Only 5 patients had multiple lesions. These

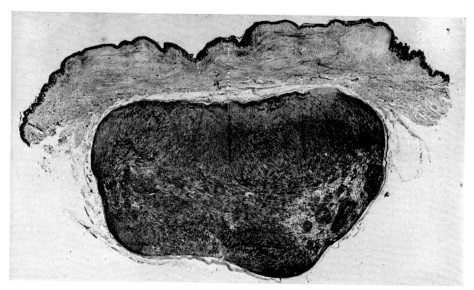

Fig. 8. Subcutaneous leiomyoma. Note the vessels at the lower right hand corner of the nodule

were usually smaller than the solitary type and were usually located more super-ficially just under the epidermis. In Caucasians the multiple form appears to be more common than solitary lesions (Stout, 1937) whereas in Uganda the overwhelming majority were solitary.

The age ranged from 8—70 years with a mean of 38 years. There were 52 male patients and 52 female. There was a slight female excess among patients with lesions of the leg, whereas facial nodules were found more frequently in male patients.

Sixty-five nodules occurred in the leg. The characteristic site was on the anterior aspect of the lower leg slightly above the ankle. The lesion was superficially placed but the skin was moveable over the nodule, contrasting with the lesions of Kaposi's sarcoma over which the skin is usually tethered. All the tumours of the leg were solitary. Forty patients reported that the tumour was spontaneously painful. Solitary lesions occurred in other parts of the body but were not common at any one site. Five patients had multiple nodules, usually on the upper trunk or head and neck. These nodules appeared to be more superficially placed in the upper dermis and were never more than 5 mm in diameter. Solitary lesions were usually between 1 and 2 cm in diameter.

Histologically the nodule is seen to consist of broad sheaves of smooth muscle which flow around numerous vessels amalgamating indistinguishably with the wall. The appearance often suggested that endothelial lined spaces had developed in the nodule. In some cases there was considerable sclerosis in the centre of the nodule and the diagnosis of fibroma was entertained. The presence of large vascular spaces and the recognition of smooth muscle cells at the periphery was always detectable and enabled a correct diagnosis to the made. Solitary nodules occurring in the sub-cutaneous tissue were sharply demarcated and contained many vascular spaces (Fig. 8). The use of silver stains sometimes showed intermingling of nervous tissue in the nodule, but this finding did not correlate well with presence or severity of pain.

Some lesions showed fairly marked nuclear variability particularly prominent in sclerotic nodules but mitoses were never seen and in no case was there a problem in distinguishing malignant lesions.

The geographical distribution of cases showed a slight deficiency of patients from Western region but the frequency in the rest of the country was approximately equal. This geographical pattern was the reverse of that noted in many other vascular tumours but the reasons for this are entirely unknown.

5. Glomus Tumours

Only 7 cases were diagnosed, which suggests that this lesion is less common in Uganda than elsewhere. Six of these 7 cases occurred in adult males, one of whom had multiple tumours, and the other lesions occurred mainly on the feet and hands. The only female had a tumour under a finger nail.

B. Malignant

Kaposi's sarcoma is dealt with separately and this section is concerned with 7 haemangioendotheliosarcomas and 5 haemangiopericytomas.

Table 11. Showing the anatomical distribution of haemangiosarcomas

Head and neck	1 (parotid)
Upper limb	5 (3 in shoulder region
	1 in elbow
	1 wrist)
Trunk	3 (1 in the breast)
Lower limb	3 (1 thigh,
	2 near knee)

Twelve cases were diagnosed, that is 3.5% of soft-tissue tumours (excluding Kaposi's sarcoma). This proportion is similar to that reported from the U.S.A. (PACK and ARIEL, 1958).

The age ranged from 14 to 65 years (mean 36 years), and 6 patients were male and 6 female. The distribution of lesions is shown in Table 11.

Histopathology

The diagnosis of this group of sarcomas depends almost entirely upon the appearance of the reticulin stain. This showed the close relationship of tumour cells to vessels either surrounding or being surrounded by reticulin framework. The most difficult differential diagnosis was from anaplastic variants of Kaposi's sarcoma. In some cases individual tumours from a case of Kaposi's sarcoma exactly mimicked haemangioendotheliosarcoma. In such cases distinction of these two entities could only be made on finding more typical areas of Kaposi's sarcoma elsewhere in the tumour or more readily elsewhere in the patient. A characteristic finding in cases of Kaposi's sarcoma is the presence of eosinophilic inclusions (LEE, 1968); such bodies were found in 3 of the 12 haemangiosarcomas discussed here. These bodies are made up of laminated membrane material which possibly derives from ingested red cells or from lysosomal degeneration. Their presence, though of importance in distinguishing reactive conditions, is of little assistance in differentiating Kaposi's sarcoma from other malignant neoplasms of vascular origin.

Kupffer-cell sarcomas exhibit a very similar morphology to haemangioendotheliosarcomas. Three cases were diagnosed in this period but have been classified separately since the histogenesis appears to be distinct even if the morphology is similar.

Synovial Sarcoma

Seven synovial sarcomas were recognized, that is 1% of malignant soft-tissue tumours. All showed the typical biphasic pattern. No monomorphic tumour was diagnosed and the validity of monophasic synoviomas is a matter for debate. All these tumours occurred on the lower limb and details are discussed under tumours of the bone (p. 229).

Mesothelial Tumours

Three cases were diagnosed, two in males and one in a female. In two cases the tumour involved the peritoneum and in the third it arose in the pleura. One patient presented with a mass in the scrotum and at operation was found to have a mesothelioma of the tunica vaginalis. He returned a few months later with diffuse involvement of the peritoneum by tumour and it is probable that the involvement of the tunica followed a primary tumour of the peritoneum. None of the three patients had any occupational exposure to asbestos.

Tumours of the Peripheral Nerves

Such tumours are very common in Uganda and only a few are biopsied. This applied more especially to benign neoplasms and such instantly recognizable entities as multiple neurofibromatosis.

A. Benign

1. Amputation Neuroma

Only two examples were received in the laboratory.

2. Neurofibroma and Multiple Neurofibromatosis

One hundred and twenty-three such tumours were diagnosed. Their histological pattern ranged across all the well described variations although no lesion was found containing ectopic bone or cartilage. Twenty-six of these cases were known to have multiple nodules but many more were almost certainly associated with Von Reckling-hausen's disease. Examples of some of the diseases associated with neurofibromatosis were seen, such as one patient with phaeochromocytoma and three with deformities of the spine. A significant proportion of these tumours contained scanty pigment-bearing cells, particularly in the case of tumours occurring in young children, an indication of their common origin from neural crest.

3. Neurilemmoma (Schwannoma)

Sharply demarcated tumours composed of spindle cells arranged in a pallisaded fashion were noted in 21 cases. Three occurred on the eighth nerve and presented as cerebello-pontine angle tumours, and one showed the dumbbell appearance of a paraspinal tumour. Eight patients had lesions in the region of the head and neck. The majority of the remaining cases were located more peripherally on the limbs with many cases occurring in the region of the wrist and knee.

The larger lesions often showed considerable nuclear pleomorphism around areas of degeneration but the absence of mitotic activity enabled differentiation from malignant change to be made.

B. Malignant

Neurogenic Sarcoma (Neurofibrosarcoma)

Thirty-five cases were diagnosed, 12 in females and 23 in males. Five patients were known to have multiple neurofibromatosis and in these patients the sarcomas developed on the trunk. In other cases the majority occurred in the sites of flexure. The anatomical distribution is shown in Table 12. The age ranged from 1 to 68 years with a mean of 36 years. The one-year-old child had a tumour of the orbit. No example of the so-called neuroepithelial group of tumours was found. There was no evidence of any geographical or tribal variation in this material.

The histogenesis of these tumours is under dispute. Opinion is divided as to whether they arise from Schwann cells or from neighbouring connective tissue. In the absence of a specific marker for Schwann cells, this problem is unlikely to be resolved by morphological means. Histologically the tumours were composed of spindle cells with a rather loose background which was frequently myxoid. Only minimal collagen production was noted but the reticulin background was often extensive though delicate. Schwann cells have been shown to be facultative fibroblasts in tissue culture (MURRAY, 1942). This fact makes differentiation from fibrosarcomas difficult. Pallisading of nuclei was noted in about 20% of cases and nuclei were elongated and had tapering points. Nuclear variability was marked but the mitotic rate was seldom high. The main diagnostic criteria used were the close relationship to nerve trunks and the frequency of myxoid change. Thus many cases occurred at sites where nerves were easily identified. At other sites pallisading of nuclei was noted more frequently in order that a diagnosis be made. The tendency of cells to anastomose with their neighbours was not found to be a helpful distinguishing feature. Distinction from

Table 12. Showing the anatomical distribution of sarcomas of neural origin

Upper limb	5
(wrist 2, axilla 1, elbow 1, overlying deltoid 1)	
Lower limb	10
(groin 7, popliteal fossa 3)	
Head and Neck	6
(scalp 2, neck 2, orbit and nose 1 each)	
Trunk	13
(breast 3, back 4, abdominal wall 2, 1 each retroperitoneal, sternum, buttock, chest wall)	
Total	34

fibrosarcoma was often difficult and cases with similar morphology but with no known nerve involvement are to be found in the group of undiagnosed tumours. Pallisading of nuclei was regularly seen in leiomyosarcomas as well as neurogenic tumours.

It is very difficult to gain an impression of the relative frequency of sarcomas of nervous origin or of the incidence of malignant change in previously benign lesions. Many series do not differentiate between neural and fibrous sarcomata and whereas papers dealing specifically with tumours of neural origin often do not mention the relative frequency of other entities. KREMENTZ and SHAUER (1963) classified 24 of their 203 cases of soft tissue sarcomas as of neural origin and record a slightly greater proportion in negro patients than in whites. The proportion in this Uganda series is very similar if Kaposi's sarcoma is excluded (11% of cases).

Tumours of Sympathetic Ganglia

A. Benign Ganglion Neuroma

Only two examples were seen. Both occurred in the retroperitoneal tissues in children. Neither biopsy contained neuroblastomatous tissue.

B. Neuroblastoma

Fifteen cases were diagnosed in this period but in more recent years the number of cases seen has increased. The apparently low incidence is therefore probably at least partly a result of failure of diagnosis. Nonetheless, neuroblastoma still accounts for a very small proportion of childhood neoplasms. The diagnosis demands the performance of a laparotomy on children and/or the estimation of catecholamines. Neither facility is widespread in Uganda. A number of cases are mistaken for Burkitt's tumour if they occur in children over the age of two years. Burkitt's lymphoma has not been diagnosed in patients under the age of two years and the age of the child is therefore very useful in distinguishing the two conditions. The age at presentation of children with neuroblastoma in this series ranged from 3 months to 10 years with a mean of 2.8 years. There were 9 males and 6 females.

Seven patients presented with an abdominal mass. Two had enlarged livers and 8 had metastases to the bone, particularly marked in the skull. No information was available as to the site of the primary lesion in most cases but it is presumed most often to have arisen in the adrenal. The history was usually of short duration. There was no evidence of any anomalous geographical variation in these cases. The presenting signs and symptoms are similar to those described in other countries.

Histological diagnosis presented considerable problems. Small dark round-cell tumours are notoriously difficult to diagnose, particularly in bone where microscopic detail is frequently blurred (Chapter 14). Elongation of cells may easily be caused by trauma and in many cases small biopsies were impossible to decipher. The histological picture was identical at different ages. Differential diagnosis from Burkitt's tumour is seldom problematic provided that touch preparations have been made, but on histological section differentiation is more difficult. The edge of the section of Burkitt's lymphoma cases always showed cells with the sharply demarcated amphophilic cytoplasm characteristic of this tumour. Neuroblastoma cells had much less cytoplasm and often appeared as apparently bare nuclei. In none of these cases was there evidence of an associated congenital defect, such as spina bifida or hydrocephalus.

Tumours of Paraganglionic Structures

A. Phaeochromocytoma

Eight examples were seen in the period of this survey. Seven of these produced symptoms and one was discovered incidentally at necropsy. One caused hypertension in pregnancy, and two cases occurred in the bladder of males. Histologically, 7 of the tumours appeared benign but one of the 2 tumours located in the bladder had metastasized to local lymph nodes. One patient also had von Recklinghausen's disease of nerve but the tumour was unilateral and the thyroid appeared normal. One of the patients with phaeochromocytoma of the bladder, a 40-year-old male Mugishu, gave a fascinating history of developing drenching sweats and an occipital headache every time he passed water. This was presumably a result of mechanical disturbance of the tumour due to contraction of the bladder wall.

In a review of phaeochromocytoma from East Africa (TEMPLETON, 1967b) it was noted that the majority of such tumours occurred outside the adrenal gland, for example in the para-aortic region, the mesentery of the bowel, the organ of Zuckerkandl and the bladder wall. This is in marked contrast with experience in Caucasians where 90% of tumours arise in the adrenal medulla. In this series 3 of the 8 cases occurred in the adrenal medulla. Phaeochromocytomata developing outside the adrenal have also been reported from other parts of Africa (COLAS, 1965; KRIBLER, 1966; VAN ZYL et al., 1966) so that this anatomical distribution appears to be a racial characteristic. Tumours of extra-adrenal locations produce virtually exclusively noradrenaline, and this may be why staining with chromaffin methods were often negative. When tumour tissue remains in formalin for many days the chromaffin stains are negative but the strange colouration of the fixative allows a tentative diagnosis to be made on inspection alone. No other material produces quite the same deep brown discolouration of the formalin.

B. Non-Chromaffin Paraganglioma

Six examples of the glomus jugulare tumour were diagnosed. The sex incidence usually shows a marked excess in females not found in this series; there were 3 males and 3 females. Ages ranged from 26 to 55 years with a mean of 40 years. Five patients presented with deafness and aural discharge which the tumour presumably developed from the aural body. This was accompanied by facial palsy in 3 cases. The sixth patient had palsies of the IX to XII cranial nerves, resulting from a tumour of the jugular body. Isolated cases have been described in Africans previously (Erasmus, 1947; Efron, 1957) but there is no indication of the relative frequency in different races.

Histologically these tumours were exactly similar to those found in other countries, and little difficulty was experienced in diagnosis.

Two carotid-body tumours were diagnosed. These had been present for one year and seven years respectively, one in a female of 27 years and the other in a male of 70 years. Hutt and Mody (1963) reported a case of a malignant carotid body tumour in a Ugandan African and suggest that the incidence of these tumours in African is probably similar to that in Europe.

Chordoma

Four examples were diagnosed. Three occurred in the sacral region and one at the mid-lumbar level (see Chapter 14).

Tumours of Uncertain Histiogenesis

A. Benign

1. Granular Cell Myoblastoma

Sixteen cases were diagnosed. Six occurred in infants, 5 of which were situated on the gum; all these patients were female. The cells comprising the neonatal epulis are exactly similar to the other cases but there was no reactive proliferation of the overlying epithelium. A sixth patient, a 9-month-old boy, had a tumour of the anus. The remaining 10 patients were aged between 7 and 54 years and there were 7 females and 3 males. These lesions occurred on the vulva (2 cases), back, clavicle, shoulder, abdominal wall, groin, tongue, and vocal cord. One patient had multiple subcutaneous nodules, two of which were biopsied; both showed a benign appearance. In Caucasians tumours occur more commonly in adults and are often found in the mouth or pharynx.

No example of a malignant granular cell myoblastoma was diagnosed. Many cases so called in the past would probably now be diagnosed as alveolar soft-part sarcoma.

2. Anterior Myelocele

Eight examples were seen. These patients usually presented with a mass in the orbit in early life and connection with CSF is not always demonstrable. In Uganda frontal myelocele is rather more common than sacral defects, a ratio in marked contrast with the findings in Caucasians; the reasons for this are unknown. Six of the patients in this series came from the north of the country, a preponderance which is also unexplained.

3. Myxoma

Three examples of pure myxomas situated deep in the thigh were diagnosed. Myxomatous degeneration of neural tumours was extremely common and if only small biopsies were available the differentiation was impossible.
Three cases of myxoma of the jaw were seen (see Chapter 14).

4. Melanotic Progonoma

One case was seen in a 4-month-old child who presented with a tumour of the zygomatic arch at the margin of the orbit. The histological appearances were typical but the location of the tumour suggests that it has the strongest claim yet advanced for being considered a true retinal-anlage tumour. An interesting racial variation in the distribution of these lesions emerges from a study of the literature. Such tumours in Caucasians arose almost exclusively in the maxilla whereas in negro children the majority of cases have affected different sites such as testes, shoulder or skull (TEMPLE-TON, 1971). This tumour is probably a derivative of the neural crest and the different behaviour of many of the tissues of neural crest origin in negroes is worthy of attention. For example, phaeochromocytoma and melanomas exhibit a very different distribution in Ugandan Africans compared with Caucasians.

5. Fibrous Hamartoma of Infancy

Two examples of this rare entity were noted. Both occurred in the superficial part of the upper arm and showed the typical mixture of dense fibrous tissue, mature adipose tissue, primitive mesenchymal tissue and voluntary muscle (ENZINGER, 1965). It is important to recognize this entity so as to avoid excessive therapeutic measures based on misdiagnosis as sarcoma.

B. Malignant

1. Alveolar Soft-Part Sarcoma

Six cases were seen. There were 4 females and 2 males. Ages ranged from 7 to 35 years (mean 24 years). Five of the 6 tumours occurred on the lower limb and were noted to be extremely large. The sixth patient was a 7-year-old girl with a mass in the right temporal fossa which had been present for a year.

Some authorities consider that the tumour is derived from non-chromaffin para-
ganglia but on the basis of observations on tissue culture, UDEKWU and PULVERTAFT
(1965) showed this to be most unlikely. Electron microscopic studies (FISHER and
REIBORD, 1971) suggest origin from muscle and it is possible that this tumour could
be regarded as a variant of rhabdomyosarcoma.

2. Kaposi's Sarcoma

This is by far the most common malignant tumour of soft tissues in Uganda. During the period of this review 330 cases were diagnosed, that is 8.7% of malignant
tumours in males and 0.6% of tumours in females. Recent papers from Uganda have
covered clinical aspects (TAYLOR et al., 1971 b), therapy (VOGEL et al., 1971), disease
in females and post-mortem findings (TEMPLETON, 1972 c), relationship to other vascular tumours (TEMPLETON, 1972 b), involvement of lymph nodes (BHANA et al.,
1970); rather fuller treatment of different aspects of the disease in Uganda may be
found in these articles. A review of this disease is to be found in Cancer of the Skin
(TEMPLETON, 1973).

Incidence

The crude incidence rate in Uganda is 0.78 cases per 100,000 per year. Calculation of age-specific incidence rates show that the tumour increases in linear fashion
with age (Fig. 1) in a similar way to lymphomas. Carcinomas tend to show an exponential increase with age and it has been suggested that this similarity in increase is
an indication that Kaposi's sarcoma is a tumour of the reticuloendothelial system
(OETTLÉ, 1962).

The true incidence of Kaposi's sarcoma in any country is difficult to derive.
Where statistics are good the tumour is rare, and where the tumour is common statistical evaluation is poor. Some indication of incidence may be obtained from a study
of proportional rates in different countries. In Africa the rates are much higher than
in other parts of the world and the results are summarized in Table 2. Central African countries show a high rate which diminishes if one travels north, south, east or
west. The figures from different registries were collected under widely different
circumstances and are therefore liable to varying bias, but the apparent trend in
incidence is probably genuine. Within Uganda the proportional rates from different
districts also show a variation (Table 3). Western region shows a higher rate than
Eastern district, with Northern and Central areas showing intermediate figures. No
explanation for this variation is available.

Racial Variations

Kaposi's sarcoma is common in Africa. It is rare in American negroes, in whom
it is found about as frequently as in whites in the U.S.A. (HAZEN and FREEMAN,
1950). It was originally described from Vienna (KAPOSI, 1872) and seems to be more
common in Eastern Europeans and Ashkenazic Jews than in other peoples. Isolated
cases have been described from Iraq (PAUTRIER and DISS, 1929), India (YESUDIAN,
1969), Afghanistan (ROUHANI, 1966), Ceylon (ATTYGALLE et al., 1969), Japan
(HASEGAWA, 1962), China (KOCSARD, 1949) and New Guinea (BIGGS et al., 1964),
but in all these areas the disease is an extreme rarity.

In Africans the frequency of the disease appears to be determined by place of residence rather than by ethnic group. Thus close to the western rift valley system in Uganda, Sudanic, Para-Nilotic and Bantu peoples all show a higher frequency than Bantu or Nilotic people living in the east. On the other hand, no case has been described in an Asian subject in Africa, whether resident in a high- or low-incidence area (CHOPRA and TEMPLETON, 1971). It seems probable, therefore, that there is some environmental factor active in central Africa which is only effective in African subjects or possibly to which only African subjects are exposed. The close similarities of Kaposi's sarcoma in structure and behaviour to some virus-induced tumours of animals has led to a search for virus particles or antigen in tumour tissue, so far without success (SMITH and WOLFE, 1970). Cases are described in Europeans in Africa and these patients have usually been Jewish or from Eastern Europe, a fact which argues in favour of some genetic susceptibility.

Clinical Findings

The pattern of disease varies widely but is divisible into three basic groups (TAYLOR et al., 1971 a).

(a) *Nodular disease.* The patient, usually a young adult male, presents with subcutaneous nodules on the limbs. The disease progresses by an irregular appearance of new nodules and regression of others. The prognosis is good and survival for 8 to 10 years or even longer is usual.

(b) *Locally aggressive lesions.* These may arise de novo or from preexisting nodules; the tumour ulcerates and erodes local structures. The capacity for metastasis, however, appears limited (TEMPLETON, 1972 c). This type of lesion is much less common in whites than in Africans. The prognosis is not as good as with nodular disease, but patients may survive for many years.

(c) *Generalized disease.* In this pattern the patient presents with widespread tumours. In children, the lymph nodes are predominantly affected, with little cutaneous or visceral involvement. In young adults widespread lesions in nodes, viscera and skin are seen. The prognosis in untreated cases is very poor and death within two years of onset of the disease is usual.

Histological Features

In the majority of cases the histological appearance is extraordinarily similar, consisting of a mixture of spindle cells and vascular structures in approximately equal proportions (Fig. 9). The characteristic element is the small clear space surrounded by the processes of a single endothelial-like cell. These are probably primitive capillaries and may be seen to contain red cells. Erythrophagocytosis may be noted and some cells contain eosinophilic bodies which may be the end product of phagocytosis. The spindle cell is of medium size with a rather thin, elongated nucleus with tapering rounded ends and is surrounded by an extensive, though delicate, reticulin framework. The production of collagen is minimal except in a regressing nodule. Mature vessels of haematogenous and lymphatic type are seen in the nodule and may be so extensive that differentiation from a cavernous angioma is difficult. More often, however, such vessels are seen in the periphery of the nodule and in the surrounding skin. Inflammatory cells are usually inconspicuous by the time a nodule

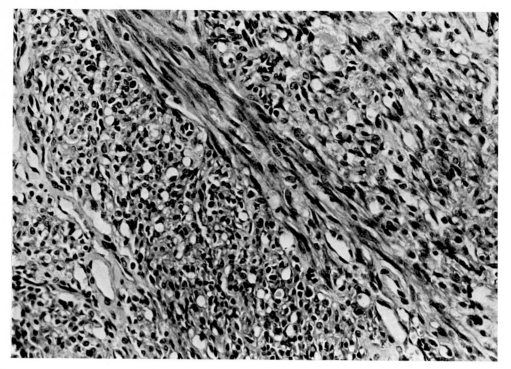

Fig. 9. Kaposi's sarcoma. The classical pattern

has developed but may be seen at the periphery. This mixture of cells is almost instantly recognizable microscopically and with practice is one of the easiest of connective-tissue tumours to diagnose. All cases of generalized disease and the overwhelming proportion of nodules show this pattern but in locally aggressive lesions a rather different histological pattern is seen.

Monomorphic tumour pattern is diagnosed when a single cell type dominates the histological appearance. The most usual pattern seen is that of spindle-cell predominance. The spindle cells in such tumours are shorter and plumper, with a plump nucleus and a higher mitotic index than those seen in mixed cellular nodules (Fig. 10). The amount of vascular tissue present is much reduced, particularly the smallest capillary vessels. Larger vessels are usually present but tumour cells are not intimately related to the wall of these vessels as in other sarcomas. Monomorphic tumours often contain large numbers of plasma cells which are usually seen in large clumps remote from the surface of the tumour. Differential diagnoses from other spindle-cell sarcomas may be difficult. Small areas of more typical Kaposi's sarcoma are usually visible, provided the biopsy is of adequate size, and such prominent clumps of plasma cells are seldom seen in other types of tumour. The gap around blood vessels within the tumour is another distinctive feature (Fig. 11). The most difficult distinction is from leiomyosarcoma. Some leiomyosarcomata contain clear-cell areas such as are found in the so-called leiomyoblastoma and this appearance heightens the resemblance. PTAH-positive longitudinal striations may be visible in leiomyosarcoma and such

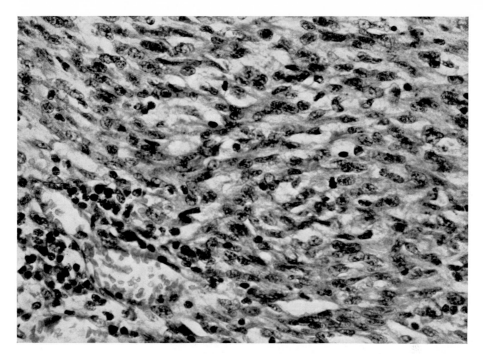

Fig. 10. Kaposi's sarcoma composed almost entirely of spindle cells. There are large numbers of plasma cells in the tumour tissue

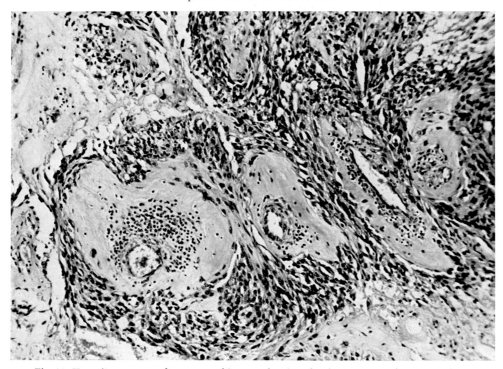

Fig. 11. Kaposi's sarcoma of monomorphic type showing the characteristic clear zone which is found around the vessels in the tumour

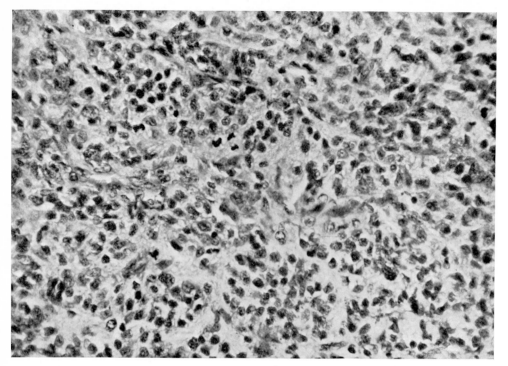

Fig. 12. Monomorphic Kaposi's sarcoma composed mainly of rounded histiocytic cells

striations are exceedingly rare in Kaposi's sarcoma. Only a few leiomyosarcomata
contain phloxinophilic inclusions, which are often found in Kaposi's sarcoma. In one
case in this series areas of leiomyosarcoma were found adjacent to Kaposi's sarcoma
and it is possible that the former developed from a preexisting nodule. If this interpretation is correct then the distinction between leiomyosarcoma and Kaposi's sarcoma may not be a sharp one, a concept supported by recent electron microscopic
studies (SMITH and WOLFE, 1970). In rare cases the monomorphic appearance is made
up of rounded cells and in such cases the distinction from a well-differentiated histiocytic lymphoma may be difficult to make (Fig. 12).

The correlation between histological and clinical characteristics is shown in
Table 13. Nodular disease usually shows a mixed cell appearance. The few cases in
which a monomorphic appearance was found fell into two distinct groups. Patients

A few rapidly growing tumours show a rather different, more pleiomorphic
appearance and have been grouped together as anaplastic variants. These tumours
have in common a high mitotic index and marked cellular pleiomorphism. The
majority of such lesions closely resemble haemangioendotheliosarcoma in appearance
and may be difficult to distinguish unless there are areas of more typical Kaposi tissue
elsewhere in the patient. In a few cases the pattern more closely resembles that of
pleiomorphic rhabdomyosarcoma, an appearance more commonly seen in tumours
which have recurred after treatment.

in which a nodule was regressing either spontaneously or after treatment tend to lose the vascular component and therefore convert to a monomorphic appearance. In others the patient had evidence of aggressive tumour growth elsewhere in the body and though the individual nodule appeared localized it showed the appearance of an aggressive tumour. This was not always the case in that patients might have an

Table 13. The relationship between the clinical and pathologic categories in 314 cases of Kaposi's sarcoma in Ugandan Africans

	Mixed cellular (vascular and spindle)	Monocellular (spindle cell predominance)	Anaplastic variants	Total
Nodular lesions	165	14	—	179
Aggressive lesions	43	63	12	118
Generalized diseases	17	—	—	17
Total	225	77	12	314

aggressive lesion with a monomorphic appearance and a nodule with a mixed cell pattern at the same time. All patients with generalized disease had a mixed pattern and it was not possible to predict from a given cutaneous biopsy whether the patient had nodular disease with a good prognosis or generalized disease which would lead to death within two years. Monomorphic or anaplastic types were almost always associated with an aggressive growth pattern. Conversely, not all aggressive lesions showed this appearance.

Age

Most patients seen in Uganda are aged between 20 and 50 years. Caucasian subjects are usually over the age of 50. This difference is mainly a result of the different populations at risk. Calculation of age-specific incidence rates shows a steadily rising straight line (Fig. 1) which probably also occurs in Caucasians, though numbers are too small to be certain. The fall in incidence after the age of 60 years is probably an artefact.

Ugandans under the age of 5 with Kaposi's sarcoma all showed the lymphadenopathic form of the disease with little or no cutaneous or visceral involvement (SLAVIN et al., 1970). Older children and young adults sometimes showed a nodular distribution but a significant proportion had generalized involvement of nodes, skin and viscera. Generalized disease was sometimes seen in later life but in these cases usually followed a long period of nodular disease. There was little difference in the mean age at presentation of patients with nodular or aggressive lesions.

Sex

There is a marked male preponderance in virtually all parts of the world where series have been accumulated (TEMPLETON, 1973). In Uganda 6% of cases occur in females. The reason for this gross male preponderance is unknown. In a previous survey in Uganda (LOTHE, 1963) females accounted for only 2.1% of cases. It is a general trend in Uganda that as registration rates increase so does the proportion of female patients (TEMPLETON and BIANCHI, 1972 a). This is probably a result of changes in social attitudes. In spite of this effect, it is certain that there is a marked male excess in all countries so far studied, with the exception of a few small series.

Female patients account for a greater proportion of cases of generalized disease (about 25%) than nodular or aggressive forms (5%). Since many patients with generalized disease are children it has been suggested that oestrogenic hormones may exert a protective effect against development of the nodular form of the disease. Hormonal therapy has been ineffective in most cases. If hormones were effective against the disease, it might be predicted that female patients might improve during pregnancy and that the prognosis in women would be better than in men. Neither of these two predictions is correct (TAYLOR et al., 1971 b; TEMPLETON, 1972 c). Alternatively, it might be suggested that some genetic factor protects against the disease, as it appears to in Indians; that this factor is present in higher concentration in females (perhaps therefore sited on the X chromosome) and that only when this is absent do females suffer from the disease. If this were correct females who did develop the disease would suffer earlier and more severely than males. This seems to be the case (TEMPLETON, 1972 c). The nature of this factor is entirely unknown.

Regional Variations in Clinical Appearances

Kaposi's sarcoma is more common in the west of the country than in other areas. The majority (5 out of 8) children with lymphadenopathic forms of this disease came from the east and only one from the west. None of the 14 young adults with generalized disease came from the western region. Very few cases of generalized disease in young adults are recorded in Caucasian subjects but in two cases (KUSNEZOW, 1933; COLLINS and FISHER, 1950) it was noted that the patient had had malaria. Malaria is virtually absent in the Kigezi district of south-west Uganda and generally less common in the higher parts of the country close to the western border than elsewhere. It may be, therefore, that generalized forms develop preferentially in subjects who are suffering or have suffered from malaria. This might help to explain the very different distribution of lesions in African and Caucasian children (DUTZ and STOUT, 1960; SLAVIN et al., 1970).

3. Clear-Cell Sarcoma of Tendons and Aponeuroses

One example of this rare tumour was seen. The patient presented with a mass overlying the patella tendon which was excised. Six months later he returned with involvement of the inguinal and iliac group of glands. These were also excised but the patient died with widespread metastases shortly thereafter. Histologically the tumour consisted of areas of clear cells separated by fibrous septa (Fig. 13). This appearance was seen in the primary tumour and in the secondary deposit.

4. Unclassified Sarcomas

This group includes 43 cases, that is 11% of malignant connective tumours, excluding Kaposi's sarcoma. This compares with 6% in the series of THORBJARNASON (1961) and 36.5% of 717 tumours reviewed by PACK and ARIEL (1958). This group

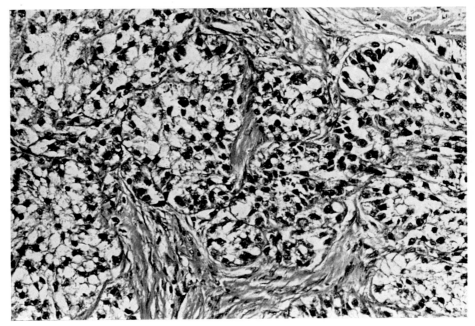

Fig. 13. Clear-cell patellar-tendon tumour

consisted mainly of poorly differentiated spindle-cell neoplasms with marked pleio-morphism and little stroma apart from some collagenous material. The site of origin of these tumours varied widely, as shown in Table 14.

Table 14. Showing the distribution of sarcomas of unclassified type

Lower limb	12 cases
Upper limb	2 cases
Trunk (superficial)	9 cases including one in the breast
Retroperitoneal	4 cases
Uterus	4 cases
Unstated	6 cases

And one case each in the bladder, vulva, heart, liver, maxilla and neck.

One tumour of the abdominal wall had been present since birth and two others occurred in children under the age of 3 years, one in the maxilla and one in the retro-peritoneal tissues. Apart from these three cases the age ranged from 12 to 79 years with a mean value of 51 years. There was therefore a tendency for unclassified tumours to occur at an older age than classified types. There were 28 males and 15 females.

Chapter 16

Lymphoreticular Neoplasms

D. H. WRIGHT

With 18 Figures

Tumours of the lymphoreticular system are common. Burkitt's lymphoma is the most frequent single tumour type. The well known geographical and clinical manifestations of this disease are confirmed. Other tumours show a much less marked geographical variation and the incidence is similar in different parts of the country. Hodgkin's disease often presents in children and is only seldom of the nodular sclerosing or lymphocyte predominant type. Histiocytic medullary reticulosis appears to be much more frequent in Uganda, particularly in Northern district. In other respects the distribution of lymphomas appears to have an essentially similar pattern to those found in other countries.

Neoplasms of the reticuloendothelial system account for a considerable proportion of malignant disease seen in Uganda. Tumours classified under ICD rubrics 200 to 205 inclusive accounted for 14.5% of all malignant tumours in the period 1964—1968. Leukaemia is considered separately in Chapter 17 but mention is made here of cases diagnosed on tissue sections. This chapter is concerned principally with other lymphoreticular neoplasms. These included 304 cases of Burkitt's lymphoma, 167 cases of reticulum cell sarcoma, 134 cases of lymphocytic lymphoma, 131 of Hodgkin's disease and 54 plasma-cell tumours.

Numerous reports have been published on the clinical features, pathology and epidemiology of Burkitt's lymphoma in Uganda (for Summary see BURKITT and WRIGHT, 1970). More recently Hodgkin's disease has been the subject of intensive clinical investigation in this country and there have been several reports on the clinical and pathological aspects of the disease in Uganda (BURN et al., 1971; OLWENY et al., 1971; ZIEGLER et al., 1970). WRIGHT and ROBERTS (1966) compared the geographical distribution of Burkitt's lymphoma with the distribution of other lymphomas in Uganda and showed that the latter did not exhibit the climatic dependence of Burkitt's lymphoma. There have, however, been no reports of the incidence and epidemiology of all types of malignant lymphoma in Uganda.

Paraffin-embedded tissue blocks were available from all biopsy specimens classified as malignant lymphoma. Sections were cut and stained by haematoxylin and eosin, reticulin and methyl green-pyronin. Other staining techniques were used when indicated.

Biopsies were examined without reference to the clinical details or previous diagnosis. They were identified and categorized according to the histological classification of RAPPAPORT (1966). The modified classification recommended by the Nomenclature Committee at the Rye Conference on Hodgkin's Disease was used for the histological typing of Hodgkin's disease. The criteria for the identification of Burkitt's lymphoma have been described in detail elsewhere (BERARD et al., 1969; WRIGHT, 1970; 1971). Whenever they were available, reference was made to May Grunwald-Giemsa-stained imprint preparations of the tumour to confirm the diagnosis of Burkitt's lymphoma.

Results

All Malignant Lymphomas (WHO 200—203)

The age distributions of all malignant lymphomas within the WHO categories 200 to 203 included in the histological series, with the exception of histiocytic medullary reticulosis, are shown in Table 1. The age-incidence rates for tumours in the WHO categories 200 (reticulum-cell sarcoma and lymphosarcoma), 201 (Hodgkin's disease) and 202 (Burkitt's lymphoma) are shown in Figs. 1 and 2 for males

Table 1. Age distribution of malignant lymphomas included in the histological survey

Age	Burkitt's lymphoma	Reticulum-cell sarcoma	Lympho-cytic lymphoma	Plasma-cytoma	Hodgkin's disease
Unknown	1	2	2	—	2
0— 4	37	1	3	—	5
5— 9	144	2	6	—	21
10—14	64	8	9	—	21
15—19	11	6	5	1	12
20—24	4	13	7	3	9
25—29	4	9	6	1	8
30—34	3	12	10	3	9
35—39	2	14	14	1	8
40—44	—	15	7	5	6
45—49	—	10	11	4	4
50—54	1	23	19	11	8
55—59	—	10	6	4	2
60—64	1	11	12	5	6
65—69	—	8	2	1	1
70—74	—	10	2	2	—
75—79	—	1	—	1	—
80—84	—	1	1	—	—
85+	—	1	1	1	1
Adult	—	10	11	3	8
Total	272	167	134	46	131

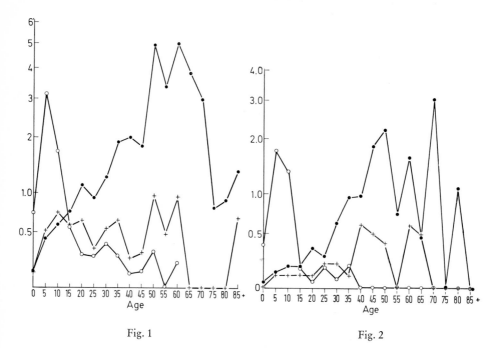

Fig. 1   Fig. 2

Fig. 1. Incidence of malignant lymphoma in Ugandan males (cases per year per 100,000 persons).
    Malignant lymphomas: Uganda 1964—1968
    Rate per 100,000 per year: Males
    ●—● Lymphocytic lymphoma and reticulum cell sarcoma (WHO 200)
    +—+ Hodgkin's disease (WHO 201)
    ○—○ Burkitt's lymphoma (WHO 202)

Fig. 2. Incidence of malignant lymphoma in Ugandan females (cases per year 100,000 persons).
    Malignant lymphomas: Uganda 1964—1968
    Rate per 100,000 per year: Females
    ●—● Lymphocytic lymphomas and reticulum cell sarcoma (WHO 200)
    +—+ Hodgkin's disease (WHO 201)
    ○—○ Burkitt's lymphoma (WHO 202)

and females respectively. The characteristic age distribution of Burkitt's lymphoma in comparison with other malignant lymphomas is clearly evident in these figures.

    Table 2 compares the percentage distribution of tumours of the lymphoreticular system, excluding plasmacytoma, in the sub-groups reticulum-cell sarcoma, lymphosarcoma, Hodgkin's disease and 'others' between Great Britain, U.S.A., Japan and Uganda. The Uganda figures show a relatively high proportion of reticulum-cell sarcomas and a low proportion of Hodgkin's disease in comparison with series reported from Great Britain and the U.S.A. In this respect Uganda shows a similar pattern to that seen in Japan, although the relative paucity of Hodgkin's disease is not so pronounced as in the Japanese reports.

Table 2

	Reticulum-cell sarcoma (% of total)	Lympho-sarcoma (% of total)	Hodgkin's disease (% of total)	Other (% of total)
Great Britain [a]	22.0	26.3	47.2	4.5
U.S.A. [b]	16.2	32.6	49.7	1.7
Japan [c]	64.4	14.3	16.2	5.2
Japan [d]	42.6	32.2	19.8	5.4
Uganda (excluding Burkitt's lymphoma)	38.6	31.0	30.4	0
Uganda (including Burkitt's lymphoma as 'other')	23.7	19.2	18.5	38.6

[a] Based on the reports of: LUMB and NEWTON, 1957; HILTON and SUTTON, 1962; HANCOCK, 1958; SYMMERS, 1958.

[b] Based on the reports of: GALL and MALLORY, 1942; HELLWIG, 1946; JACKSON and PARKER, 1947; WILLIAMS et al., 1959.

[c] Based on the reports of various Japanese authors as quoted by ANDERSON et al., 1970.

[d] Based on Atomic Bomb Casualty Commission survey, ANDERSON et al., 1970.

Lymphosarcoma and Reticulum Cell Sarcoma (WHO 200)

Of the 377 cases originally diagnosed as reticulum-cell sarcoma or lymphosarcoma, 76 were rejected either because the quality of the biopsy precluded an accurate histological diagnosis or placed in another histological category. Table 3 shows the diagnostic categories to which these biopsies were reassigned. These cases represent 20% of the cases originally diagnosed as reticulum-cell sarcoma or lymphosarcoma,

Table 3. Reclassification of 76 biopsies originally diagnosed
as reticulum-cell sarcoma or lymphosarcoma

Diagnosis not possible because of quality of biopsy	14
Anaplastic tumour	27
Secondary carcinoma	26
Amelanotic melanoma	3
Chloroma	2
Hodgkin's disease	1
Reactive hyperplasia	3

although many cases had originally been placed in this category on a tentative basis only. The most common problem encountered was the differentiation between metastatic tumour in lymph nodes and reticulum-cell sarcoma. This was made more difficult by the lack of clinical information in many cases. Some of the cervical tumours were probably metastases from post-nasal space carcinomas. These often have a similar cytological morphology to reticulum-cell sarcoma and the primary tumour may be clinically silent, although the trabecular, cohesive nature of the tumour growth often gives a clue to the true histogenesis (see Chapter 4). Periodic acid-

Schiff staining may help in differentiating carcinomas from lymphomas since the carcinoma cells, or clumps of cells, may be surrounded by PAS-positive basement membrane material or show PAS-positive cytoplasmic staining. Apart from probable non-neoplastic histiocytes in the tumour, the cells of reticulum cell sarcomas are usually PAS-negative.

Lymphocytic lymphomas are sub-divided into well differentiated and poorly differentiated types. This distinction can be obscured by fixation artefacts which cause cell shrinkage and may cause poorly differentiated lymphoid cells to take on the appearance of small lymphocytes. The methyl green-pyronin stain is of assistance in such cases since the majority of cells in a well differentiated lymphocytic lymphoma are only weakly pyroninophilic whereas the reverse is true of poorly differentiated lymphocytic lymphomas.

These biopsies were further divided into those showing a nodular pattern (follicular lymphomas) and diffuse lymphomas. Seven of the 31 cases of lymphocytic lymphomas, well differentiated, and 11 of the 103 cases of lymphocytic lymphomas, poorly differentiated, showed a nodular pattern.

The anatomical location of lymphocytic lymphomas at presentation is shown in Table 4. The majority presented with enlargement of one or more lymph-node

Table 4. Lymphocytic lymphomas: Main presenting site

Site	Total	PDL	WDL
Lymph nodes			
Cervical	22	16	6
Axillary	1	1	0
Inguinal	19	15	4
Generalized	46	35	11
Unspecified	3	2	1
Retroperitoneal	12	9	3
Spleen	4	3	1
Parotid	1	1	0
Mouth and pharynx	3	3	0
Stomach	1	0	1
Caecum and ascending colon	2	2	0
G1 tract unspecified	2	2	0
Urinary tract	1	1	0
Gonads	2	2	0
Lung	1	0	1
Jaw	2	2	0
Head and neck unspecified	1	1	0
Breast	1	1	0
Buttock	1	1	0
Others or unspecified	9	6	3
	134	103	31

PDL = Poorly differentiated lymphocytic
WDL = Well differentiated lymphocytic

Table 5. Reticulum-cell sarcoma: Main presenting site

Site	Total	SC	HL
Lymph nodes			
Cervical	35	17	18
Axillary	4	1	3
Inguinal	18	8	10
Generalized	29	18	11
Retroperitoneal	17	8	9
Unspecified	1	1	0
Spleen	4	1	3
Parotid	1	1	0
Mouth and pharynx	5	2	3
Stomach	1	0	1
Small intestine	5	2	3
Large intestine	3	2	1
G1 tract unspecified	1	0	1
Liver	2	2	0
Urinary tract	2	2	0
Gonads			
Scalp	2	0	2
Cheek	1	1	0
Chin	1	0	1
Nasal sinuses	1	0	1
Jaw	1	1	0
Breast	1	1	0
Buttock	2	1	1
Anterior thorax	4	2	2
Deep trunk unspecified	4	1	3
Unspecified	22	8	14
(skin, bone, muscle, limbs)			
Total	167	80	87

SC: Stem cell lymphoma
HL: Histiocytic lymphoma

groups. Those that presented at extranodal sites might have been primary extranodal lymphomas but in the majority of cases it was not possible to exclude the likelihood that they were the presenting feature of a widespread lymphoma.

Cases diagnosed as reticulum-cell sarcoma were sub-classified as histiocytic lymphomas if they showed clear-cut morphological evidence of differentiation towards histiocytes and as stem-cell lymphomas if such differentiation was not apparent. This division is obviously to some extent arbitrary and perhaps artificial since there is a continuous spectrum between these two sub-types and pathologists' opinions as to what constitutes histiocytic differentiation vary. The site distribution of the cases diagnosed as reticulum-cell sarcoma are shown in Table 5. A higher proportion of these cases (59 out of 167) than of lymphocytic lymphomas (27 out of 134) presented with tumour in extranodal or extralymphatic sites. Hoever, as in the case of the lympho-cytic lymphomas, the information available does not make it possible to determine whether these are primary extranodal lymphomas or are local manifestations of a widespread disease.

Twenty-nine cases in the WHO 200 category were not available for histological study. These have been added to the 301 cases included in the histological survey in the analysis of the overall incidence and the geographical distribution within Uganda. Most of these cases had been seen previously by the author.

The incidence rates for lymphosarcoma and reticulum-cell sarcoma in males and females for Uganda as a whole and for Kyadondo County separately are shown in Table 6 and compared with the rates for Ibadan, Natal, Denmark and two regions

Table 6. Incidence of reticulum-cell sarcoma and lymphosarcoma (WHO 200).
Rate per 100,000 per year

	Males			Females		
	Eur.	World	African	Eur.	World	African
Ibadan [a]	10.3	9.7	8.0	9.3	8.3	6.9
Natal (African) [a]	3.7	2.8	2.2	2.5	2.1	1.9
Denmark [a]	4.0	3.0	2.1	2.4	1.8	1.2
U.K. (Birmingham) [a]	4.5	3.5	2.5	2.6	2.0	1.4
U.K. (Oxford) [a]	4.7	3.6	2.7	2.9	2.2	1.7
Uganda	1.8	1.5	1.3	0.8	0.7	0.6
Kyadondo	5.9	4.7	4.0	2.1	1.6	1.6

[a] DOLL, PAYNE and WATERHOUSE, 1971
Eur.: Based on standardized European population
World: Based on standardized World population
African: Based on standardized African population

in Great Britain. The rates for Kyadondo are higher than those for the European registries, though not as high as that reported from Ibadan, Nigeria. In Uganda as a whole, the incidence is approximately one-third of that in Kyadondo, indicating the probable degree of under-reporting in most districts. Figs. 3 and 4 show the incidence rates for males and females respectively at all ages in Uganda as a whole, in East and West Mengo, and in four regions of England and Wales (DOLL, PAYNE and WATERHOUSE, 1967). For both sexes the incidence in Uganda is similar to that in England and Wales up to the age of 50. Thereafter the Ugandan incidence falls at a time when the rate in England and Wales is rising steeply. However, this fall is undoubtedly due to under-diagnosis and the incidence rates for East and West Mengo (86 males, 33 females) are comparable with those in England and Wales, at least up to the age of 65. These figures suggest that under-reporting affects the older age groups in the districts with poor medical services to a greater extent than the younger ages.

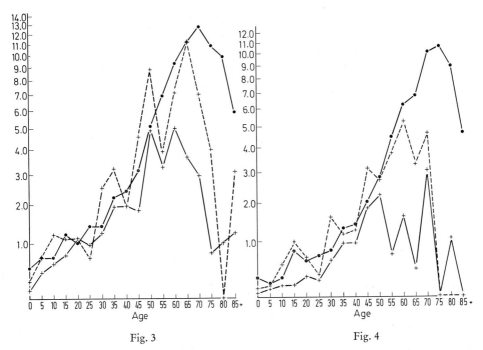

Fig. 3   Fig. 4

Fig. 3. Incidence of reticulum-cell sarcoma and lymphosarcoma in Uganda and England
(males).
Lymphocytic lymphoma and reticulum cell sarcoma
Rate per 100,000 per year: Males
●—● England and Wales (four regions)
+—+ Uganda
+----+ East and West Mengo

Fig. 4. Incidence of reticulum-cell sarcoma and lymphosarcoma in Uganda and England
(females).
Lymphocytic lymphoma and reticulum cell sarcoma
Rate per 100,000 per year: Females
●—● England and Wales (four regions)
+—+ Uganda
+----+ East and West Mengo

The incidence rates for lymphosarcoma and reticulum-cell sarcoma in males and
females in each district of Uganda are shown in Fig. 5. The total number of cases in
each district is shown in Table 7, compared with the number expected on a population
basis and also the number expected in proportion to all tumours diagnosed in that
district. There are no marked discrepancies between the number of tumours observed
and those expected in any one district on the basis of all tumours diagnosed. Differences between the number observed and those expected on a population basis can be
explained by variations in the quality of the medical services between the districts.
No district variations in incidence comparable to those seen with Burkitt's lymphoma
are present.

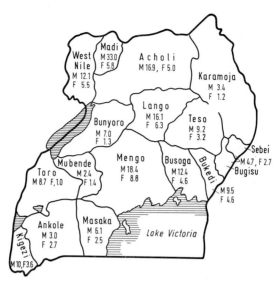

Fig. 5. Incidence of reticulum-cell sarcoma and lymphosarcoma in different districts of Uganda
(crude incidence per million per year)

Table 7. Lymphosarcoma and reticulum-cell sarcoma (WHO 200).
Distribution in districts of Uganda — 1964—1968

	Males			Females		
	Ob	EL	ET	Ob	EL	ET
Ankole	5	18.7	13.0	5	8.5	4.8
Acholi	17	10.8	12.7	5	4.5	5.8
Bugisu and Sebei	5	12.6	8.3	3	4.9	3.6
Bukedi	11	13.0	8.2	6	5.6	3.4
Bunyoro	5	7.6	7.1	1	2.7	2.0
Busoga	29	25.6	20.7	10	9.5	6.9
Karamoja	2	6.5	3.6	1	2.7	1.0
Kigezi	11	12.8	10.3	5	6.5	6.1
Lango	17	12.0	13.9	7	5.0	5.7
Madi	6	2.0	2.3	1	0.9	0.5
Masaka	10	17.8	14.5	4	6.5	4.9
East and West Mengo	86	52.2	91.5	33	17.2	37.0
Mubende	2	8.5	3.3	1	2.8	1.2
Teso	14	17.0	11.6	6	7.7	5.1
Toro	11	14.2	10.9	1	5.4	3.8
West Nile	13	12.4	12.0	7	5.5	3.9
Kyadondo	30	11.2	32.8	7	3.3	14.8

Ob = observed cases.
EL = expected cases assuming a uniform incidence throughout Uganda.
ET = expected cases based on registration of neoplasms of all types from each
district assuming lymphomas form a fixed percentage of total neoplasms.

Hodgkin's Disease (WHO 201)

Histological sections and Cancer Registry cards were available from 166 cases with a provisional diagnosis of Hodgkin's disease. In three cases the tissue sections were of insufficient quality for histological diagnosis. Thirty-two other cases were assigned to disease categories other than Hodgkin's disease. These cases are listed in Table 8. This represents a misdiagnosis rate in the region of 20% in the original

Table 8. Diagnosis given to 32 cases originally diagnosed as Hodgkin's disease

Reactive lymphadenopathy	8
Anaplastic metastatic tumour	9
Histiocytic lymphoma (reticulum cell sarcoma)	7
Lymphocytic lymphoma	4
Metastatic amelanotic melanoma	2
Myeloid metaplasia in lymph node	1
Hypocellular lymph node ? cause	1

material, a figure that is considerably inflated by the inclusion of cases in which Hodgkin's disease was given only as a possible diagnosis.

Extrapolation of these figures gives an incidence rate of 0.5 per 100,000 for males and 0.2 per 100,000 for females for Hodgkin's disease in Uganda. This compares

Table 9. Hodgkin's disease: distribution in districts of Uganda 1964—1968

	Males			Females		
	Ob	EL	ET	Ob	EL	ET
Acholi	6	4.8	6.8	3	1.6	2.4
Ankole	6	8.5	4.6	1	3.0	1.5
Bugisu and Sebei	2	5.0	3.4	2	1.7	1.3
Bukedi	1	5.2	3.6	1	1.9	1.0
Bunyoro	3	2.9	2.4	0	0.9	0.6
Busoga	9	9.9	8.4	4	3.3	2.4
Karamoja	1	3.0	1.5	0	1.0	0.4
Kigezi	6	6.2	4.2	1	2.3	2.0
Lango	9	5.2	8.1	1	1.8	2.4
Madi	0	0.9	1.3	0	0.3	0.2
Masaka	7	7.0	5.4	3	2.2	1.5
East and West Mengo	32	20.2	33.1	13	5.9	12.1
Mubende	2	3.1	0.9	0	0.9	0.3
Teso	8	5.8	5.4	1	2.4	1.8
Toro	6	6.2	3.8	0	1.9	1.2
West Nile	2	5.8	6.8	3	2.0	1.9
Kyadondo	12	4.8	12.7	4	1.2	4.5

Ob = observed cases.
EL = expected cases assuming a uniform incidence throughout Uganda.
ET = expected cases based on registration of neoplasms of all types from each district assuming lymphomas form a fixed percentage of total neoplasms.

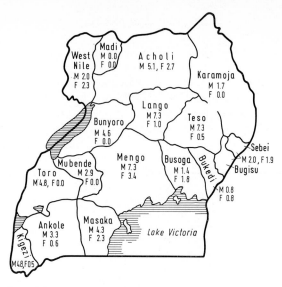

Fig. 6. Incidence of Hodgkin's disease in different districts of Uganda (crude incidence per million per year)

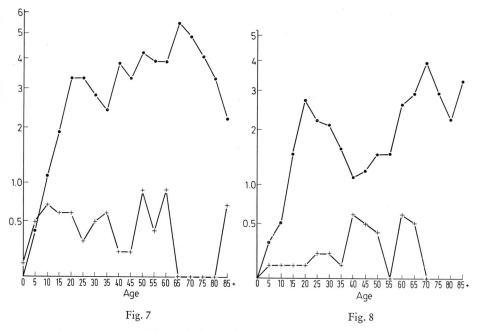

Fig. 7   Fig. 8

Fig. 7. Incidence of Hodgkin's disease in Uganda and England and Wales (males).
Hodgkin's disease
Rate per 100,000 per year: males
●—● England and Wales (four regions)
+—+ Uganda
Fig. 8. Incidence of Hodgkin's disease in Uganda and England and Wales (females).
Hodgkin's disease
Rate per 100,000 per year: females
●—● England and Wales (four regions)
+—+ Uganda

with rates of 2.8 and 1.5 for males and females respectively in England and Wales (DOLL, PAYNE and WATERHOUSE, 1967) and 3.2 and 2.4 for Ibadan, Nigeria (DOLL, MUIR and WATERHOUSE, 1970). These low rates in Uganda are undoubtedly due in part to under-diagnosis. The difference between the incidence rate in Kyadondo and that in Uganda as a whole suggests an approximately three-fold under-reporting factor for the whole country. However, even the rates for Kyadondo County are only 1.5 for males and 0.7 for females, i. e., approximately half the rates for England and Wales and Ibadan. Kyadondo has the best medical services in Uganda and the total cancer-incidence rate for this area is similar to that in Denmark (DAVIES, KNOWELDEN and WILSON, 1965). Thus, it would appear that the low incidence of Hodgkin's disease in Uganda is not entirely due to under-diagnosis of cases.

Table 10. Hodgkin's disease:
Main presenting site of tumour

Lymph nodes:	
Cervical	50
Mediastinal	1
Axillary	3
Retroperitoneal	2
Inguinal	12
Multiple	11
Generalized	33
Unspecified	2
Anterior thorax	1
Liver	5
Spleen	4
Retroperitoneum (unspecified)	1
Intestine	1
Bone	1
Unspecified	4
Total	131

Table 9 shows the number of cases of Hodgkin's disease seen in each of the districts of Uganda compared with the number expected on a population basis. These figures are similarly compared with the expected number of cases calculated from the total number of cancers reported in each district. These latter figures compensate for under-diagnosis in those areas with poor medical services. The incidence rates per million per year for males and females for each district are shown in Fig. 6. There are, in fact, no major discrepancies between the number of cases observed and the number expected in any one district and there is no evidence of any geographical variation in the incidence of Hodgkin's disease comparable to that seen with Burkitt's lymphoma.

Fig. 7 and 8 show graphs of the age-incidence rates for Hodgkin's disease in Uganda compared with England and Wales (Four Regions) for males and females respectively. The rate for Ugandan males is in excess of that seen in England and Wales for the age groups 0 to 5 and 5 to 10 years. If one assumes a three-fold factor for the under-diagnosis of Hodgkin's disease in Uganda as a whole, the rate in

Table 11. Hodgkin's disease: Histological type

Histological type	Male	Female	Not known	Total	M : F ratio
LP	20	3	—	23	6.7 : 1
NS	11	4	—	15	2.7 : 1
MC	46	18	1	65	2.6 : 1
LD	19	6	—	25	3.1 : 1
Total	96	31	1	128	3.1 : 1

Histological typing not possible: 3 cases
LP: Lymphocyte predominance
NS: Nodular sclerosing
MC: Mixed cellularity
LD: Lymphocyte depletion

Table 12. Hodgkin's disease:
Age distribution of various histological types

Age	LP	NS	MC	LD	Total
0—4	1	0	4	0	5
5—9	4	4	11	1	20
10—14	7	1	10	2	20
15—19	1	3	5	3	12
20—24	2	2	4	1	9
25—29	0	1	4	3	8
30—34	0	0	4	5	9
35—39	1	1	5	1	8
40—44	0	0	5	1	6
45—49	1	0	2	1	4
50—54	1	0	4	3	8
55—59	1	1	0	0	2
50—64	3	0	1	2	6
65—69	0	0	1	0	1
85+	0	0	1	0	1
Adult	1	1	3	2	7
Not known	0	1	1	0	2
Total	23	15	65	25	128

Not classified: 3
LP: Lymphocyte predominance
NS: Nodular sclerosing
MC: Mixed cellularity
LD: Lymphocyte depletion

Ugandan males exceeds that in England and Wales at all ages under 15 years. However, the Ugandan males do not show the young adult peak between 15 and 30 years that is seen in England and Wales and other Western countries. Nor yet do they show the late adult peak seen in these countries.

The incidence rates for Ugandan females are low at all ages but particularly in the first three decades of life. If these rates are multiplied by three to allow for underdiagnosis, it is only in the 40- to 50-year age group that the incidence would exceed that in females in England and Wales. The sex incidence for Hodgkin's disease in Uganda shows an overall male-to-female ratio 3.3 : 1, the most marked male preponderance being in the first two decades of life.

The main presenting sites of the tumour are shown in Table 10. The predominance of superficial lymphadenopathy as a presenting feature is probably related to the unsophisticated nature of the medical services and the relative ease of biopsy of superficial lymph nodes.

Histological typing was not possible on three biopsies because of the small size of the specimen. The modified classification recommended by the Nomenclature Committee at the Rye Conference on Hodgkin's disease was used to type the remaining 128 cases. The sub-division into the four histological categories for each sex is shown in Table 11. Table 12 shows the histological sub-types at each age. There is a deficit of the nodular sclerosis sub-group in the Ugandan patients when compared with series reported from the U.S.A. (Table 13), though this is not so marked in comparison with most reports from Britain.

Table 13. Histological classification

Author	Country	Number of cases	Age	LP (%)	NS (%)	MC (%)	LD (%)
Present series	Uganda	128	All ages	18	12	50	20
OLWENY et al., 1971	Uganda	100	Adults	8	7	47	38
BURN et al., 1971	East Africa	133	< 15 yrs.	19.5	10.5	31.6	38.4
BURN et al., 1971	U.K.	53	< 15 yrs.	30.2	11.3	49.1	9.4
GOUGH, 1970	U.K.	96	All ages	20	15	29	36
FARRER BROWN et al., 1971	U.K.	50	All ages	14	56	30	0
LUKES and BUTLER, 1966	U.S.A.	377	All ages	16	40	26	18
KADIN et al., 1971	U.S.A.	117	All ages	11	73	16	0

The Ugandan patients show a deficit of the lymphocyte predominance sub-group and an excess of mixed cellularity and lymphocyte depleted groups when compared with patients reported from Britain and the U.S.A. This paucity of cases showing lymphocyte predominance does not appear to be due to the relatively young age of the Ugandan patients since in this series most patients with this histological sub-type were under the age of 20 years.

Burkitt's Lymphoma (WHO 202)

In the histological survey there were 272 cases diagnosed as Burkitt's lymphoma. These cases had been reviewed several times in the past few years by the author and by other workers interested in this tumour. The sections were classified into three categories according to the quality of the histology and the degree of confidence with which a diagnosis of Burkitt's lymphoma could be made on histological criteria alone. Two hundred cases were classified as 'confident Burkitt's lymphoma,' 47 as probable cases and 25 as possible cases. Problems in the diagnosis of Burkitt's lymphoma have been discussed in detail elsewhere (WRIGHT, 1970; 1971).

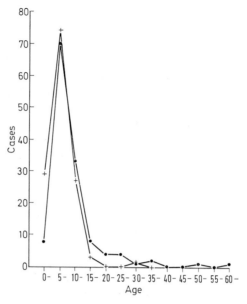

Fig. 9. Age distribution of patients with Burkitt's lymphoma.
Burkitt's lymphoma
+—+ Jaw cases
●—● "Non-jaw" cases

A further 32 cases of Burkitt's lymphoma were diagnosed during the years 1964 to 1968 inclusive but not included in the histological survey. This was because the diagnosis was based on cytological preparations, post-mortem examination, or a combination of characteristic clinical features. These 32 cases are included with the 272 cases in the histological series in the analysis of Burkitt's lymphoma by district, giving a total of 304 cases.

The cases of Burkitt's lymphoma have not been analyzed to show the presenting features or sites of tumour distribution since these features have been presented in detail elsewhere (WRIGHT, 1970; 1971) and are best obtained from patients studied more intensively than was possible with many cases in this series. Fig. 9 shows a graph of the age distribution of those cases with jaw tumours and those without jaw involvement. The number of cases in each category is approximately equal. There is a preponderance of cases with jaw involvement in the first five years of life, confirming the observation previously made by BURKITT and WRIGHT (1966) that the percentage of cases with jaw involvement is highest at 3 years of age and falls progressively thereafter. Fig. 9 show the high relative proportion of 'non-jaw' cases in the late teens and adult life compared with the younger age groups.

Fig. 10 shows the distribution of Burkitt's lymphoma in the five- to ten-year age group in Uganda. The highest rate in males, 13.3 per 100,000, seen in the West Nile district, is similar to the rate reported by EDINGTON and MACLEAN (1964) for males aged five to nine years in Ibadan. High rates are seen also in the northern and central districts of Madi, Acholi, Lango and Teso. Toro, in the West, has a moderately high incidence, most of the cases in this district coming from the Semliki valley and other

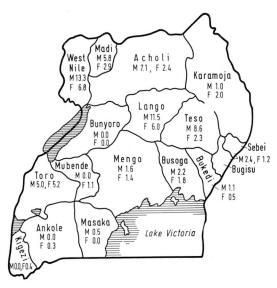

Fig. 10. Incidence of Burkitt's lymphoma in the age group 5—10 years in different districts
(all figures per 100,000 children per year)

Table 14. Burkitt's lymphoma: Distribution in districts of Uganda 1964—1968

	Males			Females		
	Ob	EL	ET	Ob	EL	ET
Acholi	27	11.0	18.5	14	6.0	10.5
Ankole	1	20.1	6.4	2	11.5	3.6
Bugisu & Sebei	9	11.0	7.7	7	6.0	4.7
Bukedi	8	11.9	7.9	3	6.5	3.5
Bunyoro	1	5.9	4.3	1	3.0	1.5
Busoga	16	20.4	14.8	7	10.9	9.3
Karamoja	2	6.8	2.9	2	3.8	2.0
Kigezi	0	15.9	9.5	1	9.1	5.1
Lango	35	11.7	24.3	14	6.4	12.7
Madi	6	2.2	2.8	3	1.2	1.3
Masaka	10	14.4	8.4	3	7.6	3.1
East & West Mengo	38	38.5	58.3	21	20.2	32.5
Mubende	1	6.0	1.0	1	3.2	1.5
Teso	21	11.3	16.4	11	6.1	5.7
Toro	4	13.2	6.9	3	6.8	4.5
West Nile	36	13.9	24.9	23	7.5	14.5
Kyodondo	10	8.1	20.2	2	4.3	11.2

Ob = observed cases.
EL = expected cases assuming a uniform incidence throughout Uganda.
ET = expected cases based on registration of neoplasms of all types from each
      district assuming lymphomas form a fixed percentage of total neoplasms.

low-lying areas. Ankole and Kigezi districts in the South West and Bunyoro in the West show very low incidence rates. These rates closely reflect the endemism of malaria in Uganda, high rates of Burkitt's lymphoma occurring in those districts in which many localities show hyper- or holoendemic malaria (KAFUKO et al., 1969; KAFUKO and BURKITT, 1970).

The number of cases of Burkitt's lymphoma diagnosed in each district of Uganda is shown in Table 14. These are compared with the number of cases expected on a population basis assuming random distribution of the tumour. Such an analysis would show a higher incidence than this "expected" one in those areas with good medical services compared with the less developed districts. It has been shown that the number of patients coming to a given hospital in Uganda decreases logarithmically with the distance of the patient's home from the hospital (KING, 1965). The expected numbers of lymphomas have therefore also been calculated on the basis of all neoplasms diagnosed in each district. Significantly more cases than expected were seen in Acholi, Lango, Teso and West Nile districts. Fewer cases than expected were seen in Ankole, Bunyoro and Kigezi districts. East and West Mengo showed the number of cases expected on the basis of population but fewer than expected on the basis of all cancers diagnosed in the district. This reflects the good medical services and communications in this district.

Plasmacytoma (WHO 203)

The material in this survey is biased in favour of lesions that are readily biopsied. Plasmacytomas (multiple myeloma) are often diagnosed on radiological and biochemical features, together with bone-marrow examination, and these investigations are not always available in district hospitals. There is therefore probably marked under-diagnosis of this tumour in this series. This is emphasized by the fact that the highest rate for plasmacytoma outside Kyadondo County was seen in Acholi district. This distribution is related to the presence within Acholi district of a mission hospital with facilities for performing serum electrophoresis.

Figs. 11 and 12 show the age-incidence rate for plasmacytoma in Uganda compared with England and Wales (four regions). The rates in Uganda for males and females remain at low levels at all ages and although there is a rise after the age of 40, this is small compared with that seen in the population of England and Wales.

The tumours were predominantly osseous in their distribution; 36 occurred in the skeleton, often as part of multiple myelomatosis. Four tumours involved lymph nodes and had to be distinguished from extreme plasma-cell hyperplasia. Those that were diagnosed at this site showed effacement of the normal nodal architecture and varying degrees of cytological atypia. The site of tumour was not clearly specified in four patients.

Leukaemia

Most cases of leukaemia were diagnosed on the basis of haematological investigations and were not therefore included in the histological survey. Sections were available from a small number of bone-marrow, lymph-node, liver or spleen biopsies

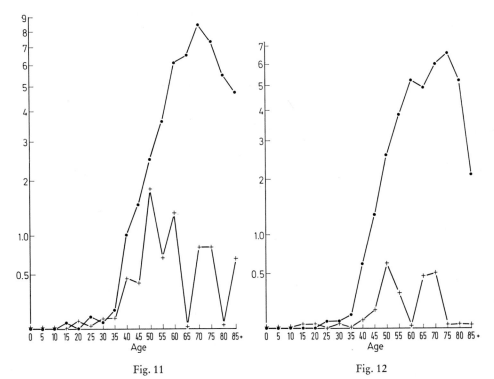

Fig. 11

Fig. 12

Fig. 11. Incidence of plasmacytoma in Uganda and England and Wales (males).
Plasmacytoma
Rate per 100,000 per year: Males
●—● England and Wales (four regions)
+—+ Uganda

Fig. 12. Incidence of plasmacytoma in Uganda and England and Wales (females).
Plasmacytoma
Rate per 100,000 per year: Females
●—● England and Wales (four regions)
+—+ Uganda

from patients with leukaemia. Three sections were from chloromatous tumours in patients with granulocytic leukaemia. Two of these involved lymph nodes and were originally diagnosed as reticulum cell sarcomas. The presence of eosinophil myelocytes in the tumour often gives a clue to its true identity which can be confirmed by the naphthol-AS-D-chloroacetate esterase stain.

Discussion

The study of epidemiology of tumours of the lymphoreticular system is beset with problems. The first is that this group of tumours is amongst the most difficult for histopathologists to diagnose, in part due to the fragility of the cells of these tumours and the range of appearances that can be induced by fixation and histological artefacts. Diagnosis is dependent to a large extent on the morphology of the individual tumour cells with no overall structural pattern to aid the pathologist. SYMMERS (1968 a and b) has shown the high rate of misdiagnosis for Hodgkin's disease and reticulum-cell sarcoma in material referred to him. Similarly, in the series reported here, approximately 20% of cases originally designated as Hodgkin's disease or reticulum-cell sarcoma were subsequently re-allocated to other histological categories. It has already been pointed out that the original designation may have been only tentative and that the relative lack of clinical information accentuates these diagnostic problems in much of the Ugandan material. However, these figures do illustrate the need for caution in interpreting 'raw' cancer registry information.

The second major problem in the study of the epidemiology of tumours of the lymphoreticular system is the semantic and conceptual problems that beset the classification of lymphomas. In the WHO coding, reticulum-cell sarcoma and lymphosarcoma are grouped together, whereas these are distinct histological and clinical entities. What is usually designated lymphosarcoma also consists of two separate entities: lymphocytic lymphoma poorly differentiated and lymphocytic lymphoma well differentiated. In comparing lymphoreticular tumours in Uganda with those in other areas of the world, it is logical to regard Burkitt's lymphoma as a separate tumour and not to amalgamate it with any other category of lymphoma.

The incidence of lymphosarcoma and reticulum sarcoma together (WHO 200) in Uganda as a whole is slightly less than that in England and Wales up to the age of 50 years. Thereafter the rate in Uganda levels off, then falls, whereas the rate in England and Wales rises steeply to reach a peak at the age of 70. The incidence rate for this group of tumours in East and West Mengo is higher than that in England and Wales up to the age of 50 and reaches a peak at 65 years. Reticulum-cell sarcomas form a larger proportion of this group in Uganda than in series reported from Britain and the U.S.A., in this respect resembling series reported from Japan. It can be deduced from this that the incidence of reticulum cell sarcoma in Uganda is higher than in England and Wales, at least in age groups below 50 and probably up to the age of 65. A similarly high incidence of reticulum-cell sarcoma has been reported from Ibadan (DOLL, MUIR and WATERHOUSE, 1970). It should be stressed that this high incidence is not due to inclusion of Burkitt's lymphoma cases, which have different clinical and pathological features and a markedly different age distribution. This increased incidence of reticulum-cell sarcoma might be related to stimulation of the lymphoreticular system by infective disease or possibly to immune depression associated with malnutrition or infectious diseases.

DORFMAN (1963) found a low incidence of nodular lymphomas among the Bantu in South Africa, and in the series of 253 cases of nodular lymphoma reported by RAPPAPORT, WINTER and HICKS (1956) from the Armed Forces Institute of Pathology, only 2% were in negroes. In this series, 21 of 301 (7%) of the cases diagnosed as lymphosarcoma or reticulum-cell sarcoma showed a nodular pattern. This compares with 11.2% in the series of GALL and MALLORY (1942); 22% in the series reported by LUMB and NEWTON (1957); and 12.7% in the series of ROSENBERG et al. (1961). The incidence in this series is low in comparison but not as low as might be expected from the reports of DORFMAN and RAPPAPORT, WINTER and HICKS. Approximately 75% of cases of nodular lymphoma progress to diffuse lymphoma before the death of the patient (RAPPAPORT, 1963), so that delayed diagnosis may account for the low incidence of nodular lymphoma in Uganda. The young age of the Ugandan population would also tend to reduce the proportion of nodular lymphomas.

If the age-standardized rates for Hodgkin's disease in Kyadondo County are not grossly affected by under-reporting, the incidence of this disease is approximately half that seen in England and Wales and Ibadan, both for males and females. The lower rate in the rest of Uganda would indicate that only one case in three comes to histological diagnosis throughout the country as a whole. Low incidence rates for Hodgkin's disease have been reported from Japan and India (DOLL, PAYNE and WATERHOUSE, 1966; DOLL, MUIR and WATERHOUSE, 1970), although the incidence in Ibadan, as noted above, is recorded as being of the same order of magnitude as that in Western Europe and North America.

The proportion of Ugandan patients under the age of 15 years with Hodgkin's disease (47 out of 131) is much higher than that seen in Western Europe and North America. This is in part due to the difference in age structure of the population in Africa compared with Western Europe and North America. However, when age-specific incidence rates are calculated and allowance is made for under-reporting, it is seeen that the incidence of Hodgkin's disease in males in Uganda exceeds that in England and Wales for the first 15 years of life. However, the Ugandan males do not show the incidence peaks in young and late adult life that are seen in Europe and North America. CORREA and O'CONOR (1971) noted a similar age pattern for Hodgkin's disease in Colombia, although in their series there was a more definite late adult peak than seen in Uganda.

There is a low incidence of Hodgkin's disease in females in Uganda at all ages of life. They do not show the high incidence in childhood that is shown by males, and the male-to-female ratio in the first fifteen years of life in Uganda is 5.7:1. FRAUMENI and LI (1969) noted a similar marked male excess in Hodgkin' disease in childhood in the U.S.A. If the rates in Ugandan females were multiplied by three to bring them up to the rate in Kyadondo and to compensate for under-reporting, the only age at which the incidence would exceed that in females in England and Wales would be between 40 and 50 years. This corresponds to the trough between the two adult peaks in the English and Welsh series.

Several authors have reported a relative excess in Africans of the mixed cellularity and lymphocyte depletion sub-types with a corresponding decrease in the lymphocyte predominance and nodular sclerosis groups in comparison with series reported from Western Europe and North America. This series shows a similar pattern. CORREA and O'CONOR noted a similar distribution of histological sub-types in Colombia. The excess of those histological sub types with a poor prognosis is not directly related to the age distribution of the Ugandan series. When patients under 15 years are compared with those over 15 years, it is seen that the lymphocyte predominance sub-type occurs in 27% of the former and only 14% of the latter. Conversely, the lymphocyte depletion sub-type occurs in 7% of the under-15 age group but in 27% of the over-15 age group. The relative incidence of nodular sclerosis and mixed cellularity is the same in both age groups.

CORREA and O'CONOR postulated a relationship between socioeconomic status, age susceptibility and host response in Hodgkin's disease. In communities with poor

socioeconomic standards, exposure to an hypothetical infectious aetiological agent
occurs at a young age, giving rise to a high incidence of the disease in young males
who, because of an immature or defective host response, develop those histological
sub-types of Hodgkin's disease characterized by lymphocyte depletion. In more highly
developed countries children are protected from infectious disease and exposure to the
agent or agents of Hodgkin's disease does not occur until young adult life when the
better host response is reflected in the predominance of histological sub-types with a
favourable prognosis. However, CORREA and O'CONOR noted that the majority of
young adults who develop the disease in Colombia display the less favourable sub-
types of mixed cellularity and lymphocyte depletion and in this series these sub-types
formed a larger proportion of the adult cases than of the childhood cases. Thus the
younger age distribution of Hodgkin's disease in the underdeveloped countries could
be due to earlier contact with an infectious agent, but the predominance of those
histological sub-types with a poor prognosis is not due to an age-dependent host
response alone.

Any analysis of the epidemiology of Hodgkin's disease in Africa in comparison
with Europe and North America must take into account the high incidence of
infectious disease in many parts of Africa. The ravages of hyperendemic malaria in
particular have a profound influence on the population. Repeated exposure to malarial parasites from birth results in eventual death of immunity. The survivors are
thus selected and have a highly stimulated lymphoreticular system. Such a background might be expected to influence the incidence and behaviour of Hodgkin's
disease which may, in some patients, be associated with impairment of certain types
of immunity. This background of holoendemic and hyperendemic malaria might be
invoked to explain the low incidence of Hodgkin's disease in Uganda. However, it
should be noted that the incidence is no greater in the mountainous districts of southwestern Uganda, where malaria is not endemic, than in central and northern
Uganda. Also the incidence of Hodgkin's disease reported from Ibadan, where
malaria is hyperendemic, is as high as that reported from Western Europe. The low
incidence of Hodgkin's disease in Uganda, as in Japan, is unexplained.

Burkitt's lymphoma is the commonest malignant lymphoma in Uganda, accounting for 36% of all solid tumours of the lymphoreticular system. The highest incidence
rate is in the five- to ten-year-old age group for both males and females. The age
distribution based on incidence rates (Figs. 1 and 2) is similar in shape to that based
on total number of cases, with a peak between five and ten years of age and a rapid
fall in the late teens to a low level in adult life.

EDINGTON and MACLEAN (1964) reported a crude age-specific incidence rate of
15 per 100,000 per year for the five- to nine-year-old age group in Ibadan, where
Burkitt's lymphoma accounts for 70% of all malignancies in childhood. The overall
incidence of Burkitt's lymphoma in Uganda reaches a peak of 3.1 per 100,000 per
year in males in this age group; however, in the West Nile district the incidence in
males is 13.3 per 100,000, a figure approaching that seen in Ibadan.

Fig. 10 clearly illustrates the wide variation in the incidence of Burkitt's lymphoma throughout Uganda. High rates are seen in the districts north of Lake Kyoga
and the River Nile, notably West Nile, Madi, Acholi, Lango and Teso. Low rates are
seen around Mount Elgon in Bugisu and Sebei and Bukedi. Very low rates are found

in southwestern and western Uganda with the exception of Toro. Those cases that were seen in Toro came from the Semiliki Valley and other low-lying areas in the district. Mengo and Busoga districts, despite their good medical services, have a low incidence of Burkitt's lymphoma compared with the northern districts of Uganda. The relationship of this geographical distribution to climatic parameters and possible aetiological agents has been discussed elsewhere (BURKITT, 1970). There is a parallel between the incidence of Burkitt's lymphoma in Uganda and the endemism of malaria (KAFUKO and BURKITT, 1970), the tumour being most prevalent in those districts in which malaria is holo- and hyperendemic.

The incidence of plasmacytoma in this series is low at all ages in comparison with England and Wales. As has been explained above, this is almost certainly due to under-diagnosis or under-reporting. OETTLÉ (1963) noted that the incidence of plasmacytoma in the Bantu in South Africa was equal to that in whites, and in view of the greater chance of tumours being missed among the Bantu he suggested that this could indicate a higher incidence of this tumour in this group. In view of the exposure of Africans to infectious diseases and the marked proliferation of plasma cells often seen in lymph nodes and bone marrow, it would be interesting to know if they develop a high incidence of plasmacytomas. Until there is an improvement in the haematological, biochemical and radiological services in the district hospitals in Uganda, the true incidence of this tumour will remain unclear. Obviously these investigations will need to be sophisticated enough to discriminate between plasmacytoma and the reactive plasma-cell proliferations and polyclonal increase in gamma globulins frequently seen in Africans.

Previous reports have suggested that leukaemia is rare in children in East and West Africa (DAVIES, KNOWELDEN and WILSON, 1965; EDINGTON and MACLEAN, 1964). O'CONOR and DAVIES (1960) postulated that the reversed ratio between malignant lymphoma and leukaemia in African children compared with American children might be due to a different host response in the two groups. This hypothesis was further elaborated by DALLDORF (1962) and DALLDORF et al. (1964). However, VANIER and PIKE (1967) and LOTHE (1967) have presented evidence that the apparent low incidence of childhood leukaemia in Africa may be due mainly to under-reporting. VANIER and PIKE noted that improvement in the paediatric haematology service in Mulago Hospital increased the incidence rate for leukaemia in children in Kyadondo County to 6.6 per 100,000 per year. Lothe noted a similar increase in the number of cases of leukaemia diagnosed when a pathologist reported the blood films. He also noted that the cytology of some of the childhood leukaemias in African children resembled chronic lymphatic leukaemia although the clinical course was that of the acute disease.

One of the arguments against the hypothesis that there is a substitution of Burkitt's lymphoma for acute leukaemia in children in tropical Africa is that the incidence of Burkitt's lymphoma in some areas of African is much higher than the incidence of childhood leukaemia in temperate climates. The age incidence of the two diseases is also different, with the maximum incidence of childhood leukaemia in the first five years of live and of Burkitt's lymphoma between five and ten years. This study also shows that there is no corresponding increase in the incidence of leukaemia in those areas of Uganda that have a low incidence of Burkitt's lymphoma (p. 298).

Histiocytic Medullary Reticulosis

A. Serck-Hanssen

Histiocytic medullary reticulosis (HMR) was defined as a distinct pathological entity within the lymphoma group by Robb-Smith (1938). It is a rare condition, only 64 cases having been reported by 1969, although there is undoubtedly marked under-reporting in the literature.

During the period of this survey (1964—1968) 23 cases, 18 males and 5 females, were diagnosed as dying from this disease in Uganda. This constitutes three percent of all malignant lymphomas (including plasmacytoma) diagnosed histologically during the same period. Fourteen of these cases have previously been described in some detail (Serck-Hanssen and Purohit, 1968).

Age and Sex

The age distribution is shown in Table 15.

Table 15. Age distribution of 23 cases of histiocytic medullary reticulosis

Age group (years)	5—9	10—19	20—29	30—39	40—49	Total
Number of cases	1	9	4	7	2	23

Post-mortem Findings

There were no specific gross findings. All cases showed hepatosplenomegaly with the splenic enlargement dominating, some spleens weighing as much as 2000 g.

Histology

The basic histology is remarkably constant, characterized by the presence of large numbers of histiocytes diffusely throughout the reticuloendothelial system, many of them with malignant features. Erythrophagocytosis is always seen, but varies in degree and is mainly observed in the more normal-looking histiocytes.

In the majority of cases the histological diagnosis is made most easily on the liver, where a diffuse sinusoidal histiocytic infiltration is observed (Figs. 13 and 14), either alone or in conjunction with well demarcated peri-portal infiltrates. In addition Kupffer cell hyperplasia is usually marked.

In the lymph nodes, even when these are not enlarged, the most striking feature is the medullary sinusoidal infiltration by histiocytes with preservation of the general architecture of the node (Fig. 15). Erythrophagocytosis is commonly rather more pronounced in the lymph nodes than in the liver.

The spleen (Figs. 16 and 17) is characterized by partial or complete loss of Malpighian corpuscles and total loss of germinal centres. Histiocytic infiltration occurs primarily in the red pulp and may vary considerably from area to area and from case to case. It is frequently obscured by marked congestion.

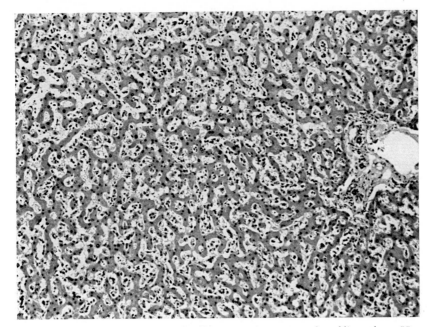

Fig. 13. Liver showing diffuse sinusoidal infiltration and some atrophy of liver plates. Haematoxylin and eosin (HE) ×85

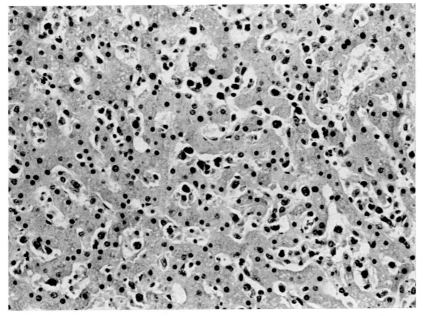

Fig. 14. Liver showing sinusoids infiltrated by large numbers of mononuclear cells, many of which are abnormal. There is also some degree of Kupffer-cell hyperplasia. HE ×225

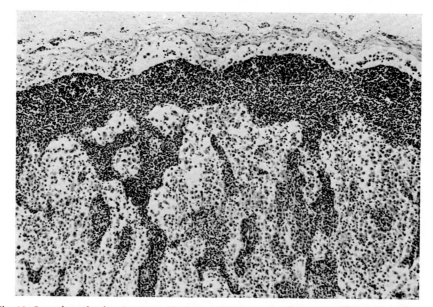

Fig. 15. Lymph node showing a marked sinusoidal, mainly medullary, infiltration of histiocytes. HE ×85

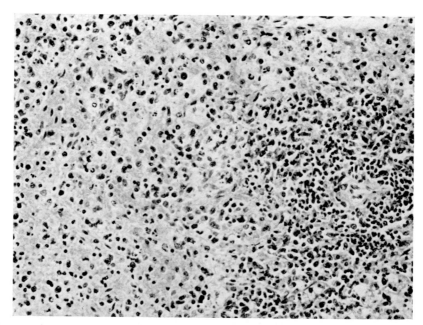

Fig. 16. Spleen showing marked atrophy of Malpighian corpuscle and large numbers of mononuclear cells in red pulp. HE ×150

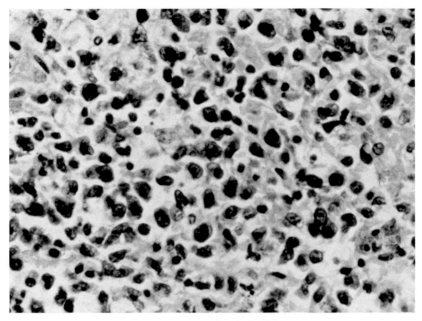

Fig. 17. Higher-power photomicrograph of spleen showing large number of abnormal histiocytes in red pulp. HE ×300

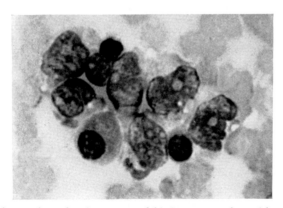

Fig. 18. Imprint from spleen showing group of histiocytes together with a plasma cell and
lymphocytes: May-Grunwald/Giemsa. ×900

The bone marrow is usually normoblastic and moderately hypoplastic, and contains abnormal histiocytes in varying numbers. Interpretation of the marrow sections
is usually more difficult than that of any of the above-mentioned organs, but smears
from marrow or imprints from other organs (Fig. 18) may give good cytological
details (VAITHIANATHAN, FISHKIN and GRUHN, 1967).

Occasionally infiltrates of abnormal histiocytes may be seen in other organs or tissues such as the skin, lungs and kidneys, or intravascularly in sections from any organs.

Stainable iron (haemosiderin) is found in all organs infiltrated by erythrophagocytic histiocytes.

Differential Diagnosis

The most important and sometimes most difficult differential diagnosis is from cases with a reactive histiocytosis such as may be encountered during various types of infection, particularly typhoid, where widespread histiocytic infiltration accompanied by erythrophagocytosis is common. The differentiation between typhoid and HMR may be very relevant as the clinical manifestations of the two diseases may be similar. In typhoid, however, the histiocytes found, sometimes in large numbers in the sinusoids of the liver, are morphologically normal. Moreover, focal areas of liver-cell necrosis are nearly always present in typhoid.

Extramedullary haematopoiesis may be difficult to differentiate, particularly when associated with a haemolytic process. The megakaryocytes may be mistaken for abnormal histiocytes, and erythrophagocytosis may be present. Usually, however, the present of other myeloid and erythroid elements will help to distinguish the two conditions.

"Big-spleen disease" (MARSDEN et al., 1965) does not usually cause difficulties, as the hepatic sinusoids are infiltrated by small mature lymphocytes. Occasionally, however, these are replaced by larger, more immature lymphocytes that may be mistaken for histiocytes. Additional difficulties may be encountered if the condition is complicated by a haemolytic episode associated with erythrophagocytosis which is sometimes the case (HUTT, 1968, personal communication). However, undoubted malignant histiocytes are not a feature of "big-spleen disease."

HMR should also be distinguished from 3 other types of malignant histiocytosis:

1. Visceral, fulminant Hodgkin's disease which may have a very similar clinical course to HMR. In this condition tumour-formation, the pleomorphic nature of the infiltrates and the presence of Sternberg-Reed cells will usually serve to distinguish it from HMR.

2. Malignant lymphoma of histiocytic type (reticulum cell sarcoma) will usually show circumscribed tumour masses if the liver and spleen are involved and affected lymph nodes do not retain their general architecture, a feature characteristic of HMR.

3. Letterer-Siwe's disease is characterized by infiltration of the viscera and skin by histiocytes lacking the malignant morphological features seen in HMR and the patients are nearly always below the age of 3 years.

Clinical Behaviour and Prognosis

The disease runs a fulminant course. Many patients die within 12 weeks, and few survive longer than 6 months. Fever, anorexia, wasting and abdominal pain are usually present. Jaundice is commonly seen and haemorrhagic episodes may occur in the terminal stages.

Aetiological Factors

The aetiology is unknown, but the condition appears to be more common in Uganda than in temperate climates. It has been suggested that the high degree of stimulation of the reticuloendothelial system by various parasitic and bacterial agents may be a factor in its development (SERCK-HANSSEN and PUROHIT, 1968).

Further studies are required to establish the true incidence of HMR in Uganda and other tropical countries. The entity is not well known and unless a post-mortem examination is performed on all patients dying with fulminant febrile illnesses associated with hepatosplenomegaly for which no other cause is found, these cases will be missed. If the rate of diagnosis of these cases could be improved, a study of the tribal distribution might well reveal genetic or environmental factors of importance in the understanding of the pathogenesis and aetiology of this condition.

Chapter 17

Leukaemia

A. C. TEMPLETON

Information on the incidence of leukaemia is inferior to that regarding solid tumours. This is partly a result of the methods of case collection and partly due to the peculiar difficulties in diagnosis, particularly of acute leukaemia. The overall incidence of acute leukaemias appears to be low but it is difficult to be certain. Myeloid forms predominate and patients often presented with solid aggregations of tumour cells (chloromas), frequently around the eyes. Chronic leukaemias were seen fairly frequently and showed no particular differences from experience in other countries.

Leukaemia was diagnosed in 200 cases in the period 1964 to 1968, that is 2.7% of all cases of cancer. There were 83 females and 114 males. The sex of three patients was not stated. The numbers of cases recorded in each calendar year were 38, 40, 45, 45 and 32. This is a considerable underestimate of the true frequency of this group of diseases. Many patients with leukaemia probably do not seek medical aid. Symptoms and signs may be minimal and, particularly in children, the course may be rapid. Patients with leukaemia are very susceptible to infections and may die before manifesting the disease. Patients coming to dispensaries will often not be diagnosed and the proportion of missed cases, even among those admitted to hospital, is high. This underdiagnosis results from a number of factors including shortage of trained personnel, the frequency of anaemia associated with an enlarged spleen due to other causes and the fact that many films are examined with different objects in mind, for example, malarial parasites, under which circumstances white cell abnormalities are likely to be missed.

Table 1. The diagnosis of childhood leukaemia in each year
(A special survey of childhood haematological problems was carried out in 1966)

	1962	1963	1964	1965	1966	1967	1968	1969	1970	1971
Mulago	4	1	7	8	16	6	3	7	8	5
Others	0	2	1	1	2	4	5	4	4	1
Total	4	3	8	9	18	10	8	11	12	6

It is difficult to obtain a reliable indication of the extent of underdiagnosis of leukaemia. This group of diseases accounts for 4.8% of all malignant disease seen at Mulago Hospital compared with 1.7% at other hospitals in the country. Moreover,

21 of the 85 cases referred from other hospitals were diagnosed at a single mission hospital (St. Mary's Hospital, Lacor) and a number of larger hospitals did not submit a single case. If St. Mary's Hospital is excluded then the proportional rate for leukaemia diagnosed outside Mulago Hospital falls to 1.3%. This proportion is less than one-third of the Mulago figure, suggesting that the diagnosis of leukaemia in most up-country hospitals underestimates the incidence by about $3^1/_2$ times compared with Mulago, and cases are undoubtedly missed in Mulago. If the incidence of leukaemia in Kyadondo County is applied to the country there should be some 150 cases occurring annually instead of the 40 cases presently diagnosed, a ratio of 3.75 to 1. Under-registration is unlikely to be the same in all the many different types of leukaemia since the signs, symptoms and cause of the disease vary so widely. The different types of leukaemia found are shown in Table 2. Myelomonocytic cases are included under myeloid and lymphosarcoma-cell leukaemia is included under lymphatic types.

Table 2. Showing the age distribution of different types of leukaemia

	Cases	Age range (years)	Mean age (years)
Acute myeloid	54	$3^1/_2$ months—50	19.4
Acute lymphatic	33	3 months—65	16.9
Chronic myeloid	53	12—80	39.8
Chronic lymphatic	46	10—78	49.7
Monocytic	4	18—23	20.5
De Guiglielmos	2	6 and 30	18
Unspecified	8	24—55	34.5

The incidence of leukaemia in childhood has attracted considerable attention (DAVIES, 1965), particularly compared with the increased incidence of lymphoma. In 1966 a special survey of childhood haematological problems was carried out and the effect upon registration is shown in Table 1. In that year the incidence of childhood leukaemia in Kyadondo and Busiro counties was not significantly lower than in other countries (VANIER and PIKE, 1967) although calculations were based on very small samples. The registration rate in 1966 was so much higher than in other years that it suggests that rather less than half the cases of childhood leukaemia that reach Mulago Hospital in an average year are being diagnosed and registered. By implication, therefore, only one case in seven is diagnosed in the rest of the country. A similar estimate of under-diagnosis is obtained by comparing proportional rates from St. Mary's Hospital, Lacor, with other up-country hospitals. The indications are that childhood leukaemia is probably not significantly less common than in other countries. An alternative explanation is that leukaemoid reactions are being confused with true leukaemia at Mulago and Lacor and that the true incidence is indeed low. In European countries acute lymphatic leukaemia is considerably more common than myeloid forms, whereas in Uganda, acute myeloid leukaemia accounted for 56% of childhood leukaemias. Lymphatic leukaemia was diagnosed in only one child seen outside Mulago Hospital whereas granulocytic leukaemia was referred much more frequently

(8 cases). Chronic leukaemia seemed to be equally distributed across the country but acute leukaemia showed some interesting variations (Table 3). Acute myeloid and lymphatic leukaemia appeared with equal frequency in all areas except the north of the country where there was an excess of myeloid types. The absolute number of cases diagnosed is, of course, dependent upon facilities available for diagnosis but the relative proportions suggest a deficiency of acute lymphatic leukaemia. That this

Table 3. Showing the distribution of leukaemia in different regions of Uganda

	Acute lymphatic leukaemia	Acute myeloid leukaemia	Chronic lymphatic leukaemia	Chronic myeloid leukaemia	Total
Buganda	24	32	20	35	111
North	2	11	19	5	37
East	4	2	4	1	11
West	3	4	—	12	19
All Uganda	33	49	43	53	178

apparent deficiency should occur in that part of the country where Burkitt's lymphoma is most common is of great interest. This could be regarded as evidence in favour of the hypothesis that these two entities are alternative forms of one another (O'CONOR and DAVIES, 1960) although this hypothesis was later abandoned by DAVIES (1965). In Kyadondo County proportional rates of leukaemia of all types combined were similar in all tribes (TEMPLETON, BUXTON and BIANCHI, 1972). The surprisingly high proportion of cases coming from Busiro County noted by previous authors (LOTHE, 1967; VANIER and PIKE, 1967) was found to persist, but no explanation is apparent.

The presentation of patients with leukaemia was very similar to that seen in other countries with the exception of acute myeloid leukaemia. This disease was seen in 28 children, 11 of whom presented with chloromatous masses which were particularly common in the orbit. The proportion of children with chloromas was much smaller among the Baganda (3 out of 15) than in other tribes (8 out of 13). This difference may be a result of failure of diagnosis of non-chloromatous cases outside Kampala or of a relatively greater proportion of patients who had myeloid forms of disease among other tribes. The high proportion of patients with chloromata has been commented on previously (DAVIES and OWOR, 1965) and is still found in 1971. Eight of the 17 children who did not have a chloroma were noted to have prominent lymphadenopathy. This proportion is also distinctly higher than that found in other countries. There were 21 children with lymphatic forms of leukaemia. A number of these undoubtedly had lymphosarcoma-cell leukaemia but in many cases films were not available for review so that it is impossible to be certain of the proportion. One of the children with acute lymphatic leukaemia suffered from Down's syndrome. Postmortem examinations were performed on 8 children with myeloid leukaemia and 2 with lymphatic leukaemia. No case of meningeal leukaemia was found though 3 patients had died of cerebral haemorrhage. This is probably a result of the short survival time of these patients.

Leukaemia in adults was similar to that reported elsewhere except that the mean age at presentation (Table 2) was younger than in many countries. This is in part a function of the age structure of the population at risk. It has been suggested that some cases of chronic lymphatic leukaemia develop from the lymphocytic proliferation associated with tropical splenomegaly syndrome or "Big-Spleen Disease" (LOWENTHAL and HUTT, 1968). Certainly patients have been seen with anaemia, a big spleen and hepatic sinusoidal lymphocytosis, who later developed a particularly slowly progressing form of lymphatic leukaemia. Some of these patients seem to have a neoplastic disease from the outset and these cases can be differentiated from reactive lymphocytosis by the fact that neoplastic lymphocytes do not transform following exhibition of phytohaemagglutinin (SAGOE, 1970).

Chapter 18

Tumours of Unknown Origin

A. C. TEMPLETON

An analysis of tumours of unknown primary site indicates that many probably derived from the stomach, pancreas, ovary or bronchus. The influence of this upon the incidence rates of tumours of different sites is examined.

Regrettably there were 301 tumours of unknown origin, 4.1% of all the tumours registered. This high figure is a result of many factors. Patients often present late in the course of disease when tumour masses involve many organs at the time that the patient is first seen. Disseminated intra-abdominal tumours, or tumours involving bladder, uterus and rectum are examples of difficulties in this respect. In many Ugandan hospitals facilities for diagnosis and treatment are limited. For example, if a patient presents with a node in the neck it is only of interest to diagnose a malignant neoplasm in order to exclude some more readily treatable condition. If the node contains a secondary tumour the patient is likely to be beyond curative therapy, whatever the primary site, so further investigation is largely academic. A third group of cases are those in which request forms and case notes were not adequately filled in. This was particularly true of patients seen in outpatient clinics in advanced stages of malignant cachexia; such phrases as "fungating tumour of face, refused therapy", "massive nodular tumour in abdomen with ascites" were fairly frequently seen on request forms. This is particularly a problem when patients are unwilling to submit to diagnostic procedures or to surgery.

Secondary Tumours in Lymph Nodes

In 151 patients who presented with lymph node enlargement biopsy revealed secondary cancer. In none of these cases was there adequate evidence of a primary site of origin; however, in a few there was some suggestion of a possible site or origin. The distribution of cases by sex and possible site of origin is shown in Table 1. There was no excess of cases from a particular tribal group or district. The age of patients ranged from 12 to 80 years (mean 44 years).

In 23 cases there was division of opinion as to whether a biopsy was to be interpreted as lymphoma or anaplastic carcinoma. In all such cases the tumour was classified as cancer of unknown type but the possibility must be allowed that some of these cases in fact were lymphomas, a total of perhaps 10 cases in all.

Table 1. Tumour deposits in lymph nodes

Site	Males	Females	Possible diagnosis
Cervical	38	34	15 adenocarcinoma (3 thyroid, 2 breast, 2 prostate, 1 bronchus, 2 stomach, 2 colon) 14 squamous (1 larynx, 2 bronchus, 4 maxillary sinus) 44 anaplastic (14 lymphoma, 8 naso-pharynx, 4 bronchus, 2 stomach)
Axilla	7	5	(5 ? lymphoma, 3 bronchus, 1 thyroid, 1 breast)
Retro-peritoneal	7	7	(1 pancreas, 1 prostate, 1 colon, 4 ? lymphoma)
Groin	28	16	8 adeno (4 prostate, 1 bile duct, 1 ovary, 1 rectum) 16 squamous (6 cervix, 7 bladder) 20 anaplastic (1 melanoma, 1 hepatoma, 1 cervix)
Generalized [a]	5	4	
Total	85	66	

[a] There were 2 patients with generalized lymph node enlargement of unstated sex.

Tumour Deposits in Bones

Fifty-four patients presented with lesions of the skeleton which on biopsy proved to be due to secondary deposits. In 28 cases the histology of the tumour or subsequent information was sufficient for an accurate diagnosis of the primary site. The commonest primary sites in descending order of frequency were thyroid, liver, prostate

Table 2. Tumours of unknown origin not in lymph nodes

Site	Males	Females	Possible diagnosis
Facial	3	3	2 parotid, 2 sinus, 1 orbit, 1 mandible
Pleura	11	6	3 bronchus, 1 stomach, 1 thyroid
Peritoneal	31		2 colon, 5 stomach, 4 pancreas
		50	9 ovary, 11 stomach, 4 colon, 1 bladder, 1 fallopian tube, 1 small intestine
Retro-peritoneal	5	1	6 ? sarcoma
Pelvic		13	7 cervix, 3 ovary, 2 uterine body, 1 rectum
Subcutaneous	6	3	1 breast
Bones	15	13	5 bronchus, 4 liver, 2 thyroid, ? G.I.T., 1 each kidney, nasopharynx, prostate, breast
All sites	71	89	

and neuroblastoma. These results are discussed more fully elsewhere (Templeton, Hutt and Dodge, 1972). Among the remaining 26 cases some tentative suggestions as to a likely primary site could be made but not proved (Table 2). A significant number of these were thought to arise in the bronchus. If this suggestion is correct then it indicates that carcinoma of the bronchus is a major cause of bone secondaries in Uganda in spite of the relative rarity of the primary tumour.

Secondary tumours of bone occur at different sites from primary tumours. Virtually all secondary tumours involved either the skull, vertebrae, ribs or pelvic and shoulder girdles. Primary tumours were frequently localized in the region of the knee (Chapter 14).

Extensive Involvement of the Abdomen or Pelvis

A large group of 100 patients are included under this title. There were 64 females and 36 males. This female excess would suggest that about 30 cases in females were derived from genital organs. In fact 22 were strongly suspected as being of genital origin but a number of other cases in which evidence of origin was even less strong were probably also of genital origin. In addition to these cases there were 14 patients in whom a diagnosis of diffuse intra-abdominal malignancy was made without biopsy, 8 of them in women; at least some of these were probably derived from the genitalia. There were 13 cases, all in women, where tumour was found only in the pelvis. Many of these cases were thought clinically to be a result of tumours of the cervix (Table 2), although the histology showed adenocarcinoma. Diffuse abdominal involvement was probably more often a result of ovarian cancer but there was no proof of ovarian origin as opposed to the gastrointestinal tract. Out of the total of 50 abdominal tumours in women it is probable that about 10 were a result of stomach cancer, perhaps 5 were due to colonic tumours and a further 4 to pancreatic or biliary tract tumours. The remaining 29 cases probably derived from the female genitalia, the majority from the ovary.

Other Sites

A few extensive carcinomas of the head and neck were seen, probably derived either from the parotid or maxillary antrum. Nine patients presented with malignant pleural effusions and 9 had subcutaneous swellings which were often multiple estimates of likely primary sites and, where possible, are shown in Table 2.

Discussion

Some estimate of a primary site was possible in 155 out of 301 cases. If the estimated primary sites are accepted as correct, then statistics of relative tumour frequencies require some slight revision. The sites which show most marked change (Table 3) are bronchus, pancreas, stomach and ovary.

It is highly likely that carcinoma of the bronchus is underdiagnosed in Uganda. It is known to be unusual so rigid criteria are demanded for its diagnosis and the diagnosis is often not considered in a country where tuberculosis is common. Thus carcinoma of the bronchus is unusual but not as rare as it might appear. In spite of this, carcinoma of the bronchus is a significant cause of metastatic disease in bones and brain.

Carcinoma of the pancreas is difficult to diagnose with certainty in advanced cases; underdiagnosis is therefore likely, particularly when the tumour is in the tail of the pancreas. In the cancer registry returns cancers of the bile duct appear to be almost as frequent as pancreatic tumours. It is likely that this aparent relative excess is not as great as it appears to be.

Table 3. Possible diagnoses among tumours of unknown origin compared with confirmed cases

	Registered cases	Possible additions	% increase
Bronchus	49	18	37
Pancreas	30	7	23
Stomach	18	24	14
Ovary	219	26	12
Colon	58	6	10
Uterine body	49	5	10
Nasopharynx	88	9	10
Thyroid	82	7	9

Carcinoma of the stomach spreads widely and early and in a number of cases the primary tumour may remain inconspicuous. The additional cases of possible gastric tumours showed a similar distribution by sex and geography to tumours certainly of gastric origin.

Ovarian tumours account for a large proportion of genital tumours in Uganda (see Chapter 6). If anything, this proportion is an underestimate, since about 10% of cases may be included under the heading of tumours of unknown origin. The proportion of undiagnosed cases at other sites within the female genitalia, with the possible exception of the fallopian tube, is much lower.

The addition of possible extra cases at other sites produced negligible differences to their proportional rate.

Chapter 19

Childhood Tumours

J. N. P. DAVIES

Almost half the population of Uganda are less than 15 years old and tumours of childhood account for just over 10% of total malignancy. Burkitt's lymphoma accounted for 36% of all childhood cancer across the country but this proportion varied in different districts. Other tumours seen frequently included retinoblastoma, nephroblastoma and Hodgkin's disease. Tumours which appeared to be rather less common than in many countries included Ewing's tumour, glioma and neuroblastoma. The true incidence of acute leukaemia of childhood is still unfortunately unknown, registration over the country is undoubtedly deficient but whether this is a result of deficient diagnosis or a true reduction in incidence is disputed. There appears to be a relative deficiency of lymphatic varieties, particularly in the northern parts of the country. Other differences in the relative proportion of tumour types are discussed.

If childhood is defined as terminating on the 15th birthday, then 46% of the population of Uganda are children. Almost 20% are aged 4 years or less, thus falling into the age group particularly vulnerable to several specific forms of childhood cancer as well as to malnutrition and various infectious and parasitic diseases. By sheer weight of numbers all childhood diseases achieve very considerable importance in Uganda, as in other tropical and subtropical countries, but there are very few areas where the attention devoted to childhood neoplasms has been commensurate with the number seen. Yet they are of extreme importance, not only individually because of the increasing frequency of successful therapy, but to the community, because exposure to carcinogenic stimuli is likely to be of shorter duration and of less varied nature in the child than in the adult. For this reason it is likely that the aetiological factors important in human carcinogenesis will be easier to define, categorize, and hopefully, to eradicate in children than in adults. Comparisons of the incidence and relative frequency of tumours of childhood in different parts of the world have therefore been undertaken, most recently under the aegis of the International Union against Cancer. Some of the results have been discussed elsewhere (DAVIES, 1968; 1973).

The duty of all professionally concerned with a child exhibiting a tumour must be first to the child and his or her interests, and then to the family, including the parents, the sibs and more distant relatives. But with all this the interests of the community and the world as a whole should not be overlooked. A childhood cancer may be indicative of congenital or acquired disease in the other members of the family or of some carcinogenic hazard to them or to other members of the community. The primary interests of the affected child demand the speediest possible accurate diagnosis and institution of such appropriate treatment as is available. Accurate diagnosis depends on histology, and biopsy is mandatory in every case because of the increasingly favourable responses to treatment, especially chemotherapy. This is likely to become increasingly successful; the excellent results in some childhood cancers, e. g. nephroblastomas, are already beginning to affect the death rates (FRAUMENI et al., 1972) and we must increasingly expect chemotherapy to be tailored to match the histopathology. Because there is so much variation in childhood cancer from country to country no norm of childhood cancer biopsy is universally accepted. Thus in Uganda, where Burkitt's lymphoma is very common, can involve many sites and responds so well to treatment, every childhood tumour must be biopsied and it is never safe to assume that a kidney tumour in a young child, whether uni- or bilateral, is a nephroblastoma, for it might well be a lymphoma or a renal carcinoma.

Occurrence of Childhood Cancers in Uganda

In the period 1964—1968 a total of 766 tumours regarded as malignant or potentially malignant were histologically diagnosed in Kampala. A further 157 were diagnosed in patients aged 15—19 years. Data has been collected on childhood neoplasias in Uganda since 1948 and this has been supplemented by the help of colleagues in other East African countries who have generously contributed slides and information so that the data recorded in 1964—1968 can be interpreted against a far greater number of childhood neoplasms from East Africa.

Table 1. Childhood cancers. Selective comparisons. Uganda and Manchester

	Manchester (MARSDEN and STEWARD, 1968)	Uganda (present series)
Total childhood cancers	994	766
Leukaemia. All types	29.5%	7.1%
Non-leukaemic reticuloendothelial	8.7%	49.2%
Tumours		
Burkitt's	—	36.2%
Hodgkin's disease	2.5%	6.3%
Other lymphomas	7.3%	6.8%
Gliomas and intracranial	17.0%	1.3%
Sympathetic system	7.5%	2.2%
Retinoblastoma	3.1%	7.4%
Nephroblastomas	5.4%	7.3%
Epithelial tumours	3.8%	2.7%
Connective tissue	11.7%	14.75%

The distribution of some of the cases seen in 1964—1968 is shown in Table 1 compared with the distribution in the population-based Manchester children's Tumour Registry (MARSDEN and STEWARD, 1968) for certain tumour categories only. Table 2 shows the comparisons with the Ugandan patients in the 15—19 year age group. In the Kyadondo Survey of 1954—1960 the incidence rates in children were approximately the same overall as in the U.S.A. but the distribution in the three quinquennia

of childhood was different with relatively more cases in the third quinquennium
(DAVIES, 1964; DAVIES et al., 1965). This was also noted in Nigeria (EDINGTON and
MACLEAN, 1965) where, as in Uganda, a major factor was the low incidence of
leukaemia diagnosed in the early years of childhood as against the higher frequency
diagnosed in the later years. Similarly very few gliomas were diagnosed. In both areas
there was a high incidence of solid lymphomas, especially Burkitt's lymphoma.

Table 2. Tumours of Ugandans in the first two decades of life

	0—14 years	15—19 years
Leukaemia	54	10
Solid reticuloendothelial	377	44
Glioma and intracranial	10	—
Sympathetic system	17	6
Retinoblastomas	57	1
Nephroblastomas	56	1
Soft-tissue and bone	116	40
Ovary	14	2
Testes	6	2
Teratomas (extragenital)	10	0
Epithelial. nasopharynx	6	11
Liver	12	12
Others	26	28
Totals	766	157

This immediately raises the question as to how far underdiagnosis or unwillingness
to seek medical attention accounts for these discrepancies, especially in leukaemia and
gliomas. There was little evidence in the Kyadondo survey to suggest either factor
was important in the area immediately continguous to Kampala and there was no
overall scarcity of childhood cancer. The situation does not seem to have changed
since (TEMPLETON et al., 1972). But the figures for 1964—1968 are based on the whole
of Uganda and there is every reason to believe that serious underdiagnosis is occurring, though it is difficult to assess the extent of this. In other chapters estimates based
on various tumour types have suggested that perhaps only about one-third of the
cancers that occur are registered. This is supported when we estimate the extent of
underdiagnosis in childhood cancers on the basis of nephroblastomas. Recent evidence
(MILLER, 1968) suggests that this tumour is distributed throughout the world remarkably evenly; a small proportion of cases are associated with aniridria and hemihypertrophy or some other recognized congenital defects but these do not seem to affect the
general even distribution.

In virtually every country where reliable statistics are available (DOLL et al.,
1966; 1970) the incidence of nephroblastoma is about one case per year for every
200,000—250,000 children under 14 years of age. In Uganda there are two areas
where cancer registration has been carried out locally and where resonably reliable
statistics are available. These are the Kyadondo area and the West Nile District
(WILLIAMS, 1972; TEMPLETON et al., 1972) and the incidence is close to the above
figure in both, though the number of cases is small. This is probably significant. Thus

if nephroblastomas are used as the long-sought index cancer (DAVIES, 1967) and the registration rate of nephroblastomas in one area is found to be half that in another we may presume that only half the cases are being registered in the first area and that this probably applies to other deep-seated childhood neoplasms, though it may be less true of more superficial neoplasms. In Uganda as a whole nephroblastoma is registered at a rate of one case per 400,000 children per year. This implies that only about half the childhood cancers that occur are being registered; if the East and West Mengo districts are excluded it would appear that only about one-third of nephroblastomas, and by implication, of other childhood tumours are being registered in the rest of the country.

The figures in Tables 1 and 2 have to be assessed in the light of this estimate of underdiagnosis in Uganda. It is quite evident that this cannot explain the differences, particularly the excesses, and indeed it only exaggerates the differences. It is obvious that the pattern of childhood neoplasia in Uganda is widely different from that seen in Manchester. Thus Burkitt's lymphoma accounts for 36% of all cases of childhood neoplasia in Uganda, and solid reticuloendothelial neoplasms form 49% of childhood neoplasms, as opposed to 8.7% in Manchester. It is of some interest to note that leukaemias of all sorts, Wilm's tumours, retinoblastomas and Hodgkin's disease are all being registered with approximately equal frequency in Uganda.

The two tumour types in which the Uganda series is grossly deficient are the leukaemias and the gliomas. Underdiagnosis is suspected in both types, and there are many factors that might contribute to this, such as shortage of medical staff, lack of neurosurgical units, registries operating primarily on tissue diagnoses, less efficient registration of cases diagnosed by blood smears or cytology, and inexpert examination of these perhaps directed only at the evaluation of parasitemia. There may be other reasons for underdiagnosis, especially in the case of acute leukaemia, e. g. inadequate parental and medical awareness, the frequency of anaemia, in which it may be overlooked, and its rapid evolution and high mortality. These and other factors could lead to a considerable degree of underdiagnosis, particularly of leukaemia and gliomas. However, over the last 25 years large numbers of autopsies have been performed on children in Kampala (BROWN and WRIGHT, 1967), there has been active cancer registration for the last 15 years particular interest has been shown in childhood neoplasia and in leukaemia and gliomas in the light of their apparent deficiency (DAVIES, 1960; 1965) and this has been true of other areas in Africa (WATSON-WILLIAMS and ALLEN, 1963).

Moreover, the basis of the controversy has not always been understood. It has never been claimed that leukaemias did not occur in African children but that they differed in frequency, types, and manifestations from those seen in western countries, notably by the lack of an early age peak due to a low number of cases of acute lymphatic leukaemia. There has been no suggestion that leukaemia in adults was different in frequency or in form in Africa from that seen in western countries. Similarly, gliomas have long been recorded in African children and adults; indeed one of the first autopsies recorded in Uganda (LOW and CASTELLANI, 1903) was that of a patient with a glioma producing symptoms confused with those of sleeping sickness; all types are recorded but with a frequency far below that seen in caucasian children or adults. It is evident from Table 1 that if leukaemias and gliomas were occurring in Uganda with a frequency comparable to that of Manchester an enormous number were missed.

Leukaemia in Children in Uganda

The question of the precise frequency with which leukaemia occurs in children in Uganda has been discussed elsewhere (Davies, 1960; 1965. Vanier and Pike, 1967; Lothe, 1967; Davies et al., 1972). Clearly much further study of leukaemia in children is necessary. Whatever the true incidence there are obviously features about childhood leukaemia in Uganda and elsewhere in Africa which are peculiar to these areas. Firstly, acute lymphatic leukaemia is diagnosed far less commonly than in caucasian children and a peak at the end of the first quinquennium is barely apparent. Secondly, relatively more cases of myeloid leukaemia are diagnosed (O'Conor and Davies, 1960); while the majority of these are acute myeloid leukaemia, a fair proportion of chronic myeloid leukaemias are seen and quite a few of the acute myeloid leukaemias progress in a subacute fashion. Allied to this is the frequency with which either chloromas (Davies and Owor, 1965) or other solid deposits of myeloblastomatous cells are seen. Such deposits are also seen in some cases of lymphatic leukaemia. These may cause orbital masses producing exophthalmos or extra-orbital masses. Occasionally a chloroma may be biopsied at a stage when there are no changes in the blood or the bone marrow although these soon develop. A high frequency of solid orbital masses has been noted in children with leukaemia in Turkey (Cavdar et al., 1971). In lymphatic leukaemia there may be little or no lymphadenopathy when there is marked splenomegaly.

Essien (1972) and Barr et al. (1972) have described the signs and symptoms of acute leukaemia; the main changes are fever, symptomatic anaemia, purpuric lesions, bone pain, and proptosis. About half the children will show some severe manifestation other than anaemia.

Templeton and Viegas (1970) sum up the situation by remarking that their low incidence figure for leukaemia in childhood in Uganda (0.5/100,000 per annum) is partly due to underdiagnosis, but that there would seem to be a genuine 2—3 fold deficiency as compared with the incidence in western communities. Certainly leukaemia is an important field of study in Uganda; its true incidence is unknown but it appears

Table 3. Childhood tumours. Some inter-tribal differences

Tribe	Total	Burkitt's (%)	Leukaemia	Hodgkin's	Renal	Ocular	Other lymph.
Ganda	142	23 (16%)	30	7	17	10	9
Kiga	39	1 (3%)	—	3	8	7	1
Toro	13	1 (8%)	1	1	1	2	—
Lugbara	53	41 (77%)	—	2	1	1	2
Acholi	70	34 (49%)	3	7	7	3	4
Lango	82	46 (55%)	4	7	3	2	8
Teso	52	31 (60%)	1	4	3	1	4
Soga	49	21 (43%)	—	2	1	3	2
R/R	29	9 (30%)	2	—	1	3	2
Ankole	37	5 (13.5%)	2	4	6	6	—
Other tribes	200	55 (27%)	11	11	8	21	20
Total	766	277	54	48	56	59	52

to be increasing (LOTHE, 1967; VANIER and PIKE, 1967; DAVIES et al., 1972). There may be factors in Uganda which tend to localize neoplastic processes which tend to diffuse in children in other countries (DAVIES, 1965); this suggestion is supported by the frequency of Burkitt's lymphoma, and of solid tumour lesions in leukaemia, and also by the occurrence of the splenomegaly without lymphadenopathy in lymphatic leukaemia. The localizing factor may be related to malaria. The relationship of malaria to Burkitt's lymphoma is evident but the connection, if any, with leukaemia, remains obscure. There does not seem to be any tendency (see Table 3) for the tribes with a low incidence of Burkitt's lymphoma to have higher leukaemia rates than those tribes where this lymphoma is common; indeed the reverse seems possible.

Solid Reticuloendothelial Tumours

As Burkitt's lymphoma has been discussed at length in a recent monograph (BURKITT and WRIGHT, 1970) only a few aspects will be discussed here. Its frequency makes it the dominant paediatric cancer problem in Uganda, and the multiplicity of sites at which it can develop, comparable to neuroblastoma in caucasian children, and its remarkable response to chemotherapy make it mandatory that every tumour in an African child should be biopsied. But the incidence varies widely in different parts of the country so that it accounts for a varying proportion of childhood cancers in different tribes, the proportion being highest in the Lugbara and lowest in the Bakiga (Table 3), which is as would be expected in view of its dependence on geographic and climatic factors. The role of malaria in determining both the limits and the features of Burkitt's lymphoma has been accepted as important but the exact role of the EB virus has yet to be determined. Both malaria and EB virus infection are virtually ubiquitous in Burkitt's lymphoma cases (ZIEGLER et al., 1972) and are very frequent in early childhood in Uganda. Explanation of the occurrence of a rare phonomenon by the interaction of two common and widely distributed factors is not easily accepted, and does not account for the epidemic drift of Burkitt's lymphoma described in the West Nile District (WILLIAMS et al., 1969) or the time-space clusters seen in Bwamba (MORROW et al., 1971). Some other, at present undetermined, factor must be important in the aetiology. It was long ago suggested that Burkitt's lymphoma might be the biological equivalent of lymphatic leukaemia elsewhere (O'CONNOR and DAVIES, 1960) and that malaria might be one possible factor in keeping the lesions localized rather than letting the cells diffuse as in leukaemia. It is very uncommon for Burkitt's lymphoma to terminate in leukaemia in a Ugandan child. It will be of interest to see how these diseases vary in relation to malaria.

The Non-Burkitt Lymphomas

It is a notable feature of Burkitt's lymphoma that it often spares the peripheral lymph nodes and is localized in extranodal sites. The other lymphomas chiefly affect the peripheral nodes, liver and spleen, and in many cases in children the gastrointestinal tract. The other lymphomas are discussed generally in Chapter 16. Lymphosarcomas occur relatively uncommonly in children in Uganda but the few cases seen presented with a peripheral lymphadenopathy and solid lymphosarcomatous tumours developed but a terminal leukaemic state rarely supervened. Histiocytic sarcomas also occur, not infrequently with small-intestine involvement and these have a similar course. One lymphomatous process seen repeatedly in children and adults in Uganda, with a frequency far exceeding that recorded elsewhere is Robb-Smith's histiocytic medullary reticulosis (Serck-Hanssen and Purohit, 1968). While it is most often seen in children in the later years of childhood in Uganda one patient was a girl aged only 2 years. Peripheral lymphadenopathy may be marked and dominate the clinical picture together with hepatosplenomegaly and bone pains. Deterioration is rapid with no response to any treatment, and pyrexia, jaundice with haemolytic anaemia, and ascites, are often marked features. A bone-marrow examination may be diagnostic if active erythrophagocytosis by histiocytes can be seen; it may also be recognized in lymph-node, spleen or liver biopsy specimens, but even at autopsy the condition may not be easily recognized, and many cases are thought to be acute Hodgkin's Disease. It is curious how few cases of Letterer-Siwe Disease or other storage reticuloendo-theliosis have been recorded in African children. Cases occur but they seem relatively more common in Asian and European children living in Africa.

Hodgkin's Disease

Hodgkin's disease is the second most common lymphoma seen in children in Uganda and where Burkitt's lymphoma is uncommon it is the most frequently encountered lymphoma, developing in children with a frequency perhaps three times that seen in western countries (see Chapter 16). Indeed the age-specific incidence peak in Uganda is unimodal with a single peak in childhood (Correa and O'Conor, 1971). Thus in Uganda, as in other tropical and less affluent societies, Hodgkin's disease is predominantly a paediatric problem with an aggressive presentation (Ziegler et al., 1970; Olweny et al., 1971) and a short history, often involving generalized polylymphadenopathy with hepatosplenomegaly, bone lesions, pyrexia, severe constitutional symptoms, and on histological examination a preponderance of the histologic subtypes associated with a poor prognosis; in one series (Burn et al., 1971) 38% were of the lymphocyte-depleted type. This is the common pattern in East African children and the disease used to progress rapidly to death. Happily it has now been shown that, despite the severity of the disease and the ominous histo-logy, children in Uganda respond superbly to chemotherapy, and early diagnosis with lymph-gland biopsy is essential so that treatment can be started as early as possible.

In other countries it has been noted that with socioeconomic improvement the maximum incidence of Hodgkin's disease shifts into adult life to produce one age peak in young adults and another in elderly adults (Correa and O'Conor, 1971). Neither development is currently discernible in East Africa. The reasons for this change are not understood but no other childhood cancer seems to exhibit this be-haviour, which seems more suggestive of an infectious disease. While it has been suggested that the distribution of Hodgkin's disease is uniform over Uganda the figures in Table 3 would suggest a slight tendency for the disease to appear more commonly in tribes who show a high rate of Burkitt's lymphoma. Thus if the latter and the leukaemias are excluded, Hodgkin's disease accounts for between 9 and 21% of the remaining cases of lymphoproliferative diseases of childhood. But in the Lango, Acholi, Teso, and Lugbara (see Table 3) Hodgkin's disease accounted for 20 of 105 cases (19%) as compared with only 3 of 36 such tumours (9%) in Bakiga children. In a previous survey of childhood cancers in Uganda (O'CONOR and DAVIES, 1960) the ratio of Hodgkin's disease to Burkitt's lymphoma was 1 : 19, whereas in this series it is less than 1 : 6. In a country with serious problems of underdiagnosis it is difficult to be certain if these differences are real and not artefactual. It may be that the incidence of the Burkitt lymphoma is decreasing; there is some evidence of this in the increasingly urbanized Kyadondo county and in other areas where children are given antimalarials.

Kaposi's Sarcoma

There are two conditions which can clinically mimic Hodgkin's disease to perfection in children. One is disseminated glandular tuberculosis (TROWELL, 1960). The other is Kaposi's sarcoma when it takes, as it so often does in young children, the polylymphadenopathic form with either absent or sparse and anomalously sited skin lesions (LOTHE and DAVIES, 1962; SLAVIN et al., 1970). With advancing age the frequency of skin nodules on the extremities increases and nodules may occur in the ocular tissues or produce orbital lesions. Kaposi's sarcoma is discussed in more detail under soft-tissue tumours in Chapter 15. Lymph-node lesions occur even in African adults, but it is most unusual for these lymphadenopathies to dominate the clinical picture as they do in young children, in whom the clinical course may be one of rapid progression to death with venous compression syndromes. Response to chemotherapy may be excellent. There were 14 cases of Kaposi's sarcoma in children, 11 of them in males. Though the course may be rapidly progressive in childhood it still runs true to type and the child dies with disseminated lesions of Kaposi's sarcoma but without concurrent Hodgkin's disease or other lymphoma lesions such as are sometimes seen in adults.

Neural Tumours

The frequency of all types of neural tumours also varies widely, and as always where a low incidence is recorded the question of underdiagnosis is raised, especially in regard to gliomas and other intracranial tumours. These have been sought for many years in Uganda, where virtually all types of intracranial tumour have been seen in children, but they do not occur with anything like the frequency, or with the same type distribution, that is found in caucasian children. It has been claimed by some that the commonest cause of intracranial space-occupying lesions in Africans are infectious, e. g. tuberculomas or granulomas, abscesses or helminthic tumours such as hydatids. There is no clinical or autopsy evidence to support this in Uganda. In the period 1964—1968 experience was much the same as in previous years, a variety of types of intracranial tumour seen in very low frequency compared with experience elsewhere. Meningeal or other intracranial involvement by Burkitt's lymphoma is the cause of the vast majority of intracranial neoplastic lesions.

Of the primary neural-tissue tumours one neuro-fibrosarcoma developed in the orbit and gave rise to intracranial masses, as did two aesthioneuroblastomas arising in the nasal tissues. This leaves 10 primary intracranial neoplasms. One of these was a primary leptomeningeal melanoma, two were craniopharyngiomas and only 7 were primary neural tumours (Table 4). Half the intracranial neoplasms seen were diagnosed in the third quinquennium and 7 cases came to autopsy. The majority of tumours diagnosed occurred in Baganda children. This very clearly points to overall underdiagnosis and some degree of underdiagnosis in Ganda children especially in the early years of life. The percentage of intracranial primary neoplasms in Ganda children is 3.5% including Burkitt's lymphoma, 4.2% excluding Burkitt's lymphoma,

Table 4. Primary intracranial neoplasms
Occurring in children

Case	Sex	Tribe	Age	Diagnoses
1	F	Ganda	4 yrs.	Medulloblastoma
2	M	Gishu	4^1/$_2$ yrs.	Astrocytoma. Grade II 3rd ventricle
3	F	Ganda	7 yrs.	Leptomeningeal melanoma
4	M	Ganda	8 yrs.	Poorly differentiated glioma
5	F	Ganda	9 yrs.	Craniopharyngioma
6	F	Ganda	10 yrs.	Astrocytoma. Grade III
7	F	Ganda	11 yrs.	Astrocytoma. Grade II
8	M	Ganda	11 yrs.	Craniopharyngioma
9	M	Longo	12 yrs.	Ependymoma
10	M	Ganda	13 yrs.	Medulloblastoma. Cerebellum

figures far below those of the Manchester Registry (see Table 1). In this series there were four astrocytomas to two medulloblastomas. In the overall series of over 50 intracranial neoplasms in East African children medulloblastomas were rather more frequent than astrocytomas. This rarity of intracranial neoplasms in childhood is seen in both Nigeria and Kenya. The opening of neurosurgical units will lead to many more cases being diagnosed. It will be of considerable interest to see whether there is an actual rise in the incidence rates or a mere harvesting of cases from wider areas.

Sympathetic-System Tumours

These include the neuroblastoma, the ganglioneuroblastoma and the ganglio-neuroma. All appear exceptionally uncommon in Ugandan children, and in African children generally, though they were much overdiagnosed before the peculiarities of Burkitt's lymphoma were recognized. The lack of chemical studies of catecholamine excretion and of good radiographic facilities means that they are often diagnosed on rather tenuous evidence. However, their notorious tendency to produce bizarre metastases, often superficially located or involving bone (see Chapter 15), means that the diagnosis has to be considered whenever an anaplastic small-cell tumour is encountered. Very often such a tumour is called a neuroblastoma on quite inadequate evidence. In this series, besides the two aesthioneuroblastomas, 17 patients were classified as suffering from sympathetic-system tumours; one was a body of three who had a ganglioneuroblastoma with extensive calcification producing an abdominal mass. One female of five years came to autopsy with a primary adrenal neuroblastoma; 12 others were diagnosed on a single biopsy and two had repeat biopsies. Only four were Ganda and a total of 13 tribes were represented in the 17 cases. Three cases were diagnosed at less than one year of age, a total of 11 before five years of age, four more under the age of 10 years and only two in the third quinquennium. Only one was diagnosed from an apparent bone metastasis (see Chapter 15), and on re-assessment it was felt that an assumed diagnosis could only be maintained in three cases and the remainder could only be regarded as presumptive. The rarity of neuroblastomas in Ugandan children has been noted previously (O'CONOR and DAVIES, 1960) and these tumours seem to be rare all over tropical Africa. Recent calculations (DAVIES et al., 1972) have suggested that as compared with England and Wales, childhood neoplasias in Ibadan, Kampala and Nairobi are 85% deficient in leukaemias and 89% deficient in neuroblastomas and cerebral tumours, for children under five years the figures are 93% and 90% respectively and for children over 10 years, 71% and 90% respectively. It has been suggested that these deficiencies may be related to malaria exposure and it will be of interest to see how this alters with diminution in malaria.

In contrast, there is no shortage whatsoever of retinoblastomas. These accounted for 57 of 59 tumours of the eye proper. Occasional conjunctival squamous carcinomas and melanomas occur and very rarely retinal gliomas but for practical purposes retinoblastomas are the only intraocular tumours of African children and occur with a frequency comparable to that seen elsewhere, about 1 per 23,000—25,000 live births (TEMPLETON, 1967). Because of the severe ocular signs and symptoms produced these tumours come more readily to medical attention and it is probable that the registration rate is closer to the actual incidence in Uganda than is the case with other childhood neoplasms. Unhappily the early evidence of the presence of a retinoblastoma is often ignored by the parents and too often children are brought to medical attention when the eye globe has ruptured and the orbit is full of tumour growth. This raises difficult diagnostic problems in the differentiation from other orbital tumours of childhood which currently vary widely in their response to chemotherapy, e. g. Burkitt's lymphoma, chloroma or other leukemic orbital mass, rhabdomyosarcoma or other cancers of the nose, sinuses or adjacent areas which can produce proptosis and eyeball destruction, or even benign orbital tumours. Examination of the opposite eye may produce diagnostic evidence, e. g. another retinoblastoma, blood or bone-marrow examination may distinguish a leukaemic process, and x-ray of the bony tissue or of the orbital soft tissue may help. Often only histology will decide and even then the diagnosis may be difficult when necrosis and infection are present. The best clue to a retinoblastoma may be the diffuse spotty calcification, often appreciable by x-ray or by a gritty feel on sectioning. It does not seem to be a feature of tumours of the orbit other than retinoblastomas. Unhappily, in the absence of radiotherapy, treatment is not presently very effective and local recurrence and intracranial involvement develop rapidly. The distinction of lymphomatous tumours of the facial region in childhood is discussed elsewhere (ZIEGLER et al., 1970).

Nephroblastomas

As previously noted the frequency with which these tumours occur seems very uniform throughout the world. There are known associations of these tumours with aniridia, with hemihypertrophy and with certain other developmental anomalies (MILLER, 1968) but these have been little studied in non-western countries and seem to be important factors in only a small minority of cases. While predominantly a tumour of the early years of childhood, indeed often occurring in the first months of life in Ugandan children, its appearance is often delayed to later in childhood (Table 5). The Ugandan material has not been analyzed in terms of laterality but

Table 5. Age at presentation of patients with nephroblastoma

Age (years)	0—1	1—4	5—9	10—15
Male	4	15	7	1
Female	5	18	6	0
Total	9	33	13	1

there seems no evidence of differences from that recorded elsewhere in Africa (DAVEY, 1964). In view of the now dramatic responses noted to chemotherapy the importance of establishing the true diagnosis in a renal tumour in childhood cannot be over-estimated. In this series there was one tumour, apparently arising primarily in the bladder that had the structure of a Wilm's tumour.

Ovarian and Testicular Tumours in Children

While there is no evidence that these occur overall with greater frequency in African children, when they do occur they present some peculiar features. Testicular tumours are remarkably infrequent in African adults (see Chapter 7), particularly seminomas. Only six testicular tumours were diagnosed in children in this study. One remains unclassified as the biopsy specimen was very small, one was a teratomatous embryonal carcinoma and all four others were cases of orchioblastoma, the clear-cell adenocarcinoma of the infant testes, which has a relatively good prognosis.

Nearly three times as many ovarian tumours were noted. This total excludes ovarian involvement seen in Burkitt's lymphoma. GINSBERG and DAVIES (1972) studied a series of 119 cases of ovarian tumours occurring in East Africa, which accounted for over 5% of malignancies in girls. They found 67 cases of Burkitt's lymphoma, 24 dysgerminomas, 12 embryonal carcinomas, 6 granulosa cell tumours and 2 adenocarcinomas. This experience is somewhat comparable in the Ugandan cases registered in 1964—1968, which included 5 dysgerminomas, 5 embryonal carcinomas, 1 granulosa cell tumour, 1 serous cystadenocarcinoma and 2 unclassified anaplastic malignancies. The main difference is in the embryonal carcinomas. In both series embryonal carcinomas were the only malignant teratomas seen. When this malignant element is seen, as it often is, as part of a dysgerminomatous, or other developmental tumour, it determines the outcome and so this minor difference between the series may be no more than a difference of emphasis. However, it is clear that dysgerminomas and embryonal carcinomas are the most common and important.

The dysgerminomas in other countries are often associated with developmental malformations of the genitalia but these, and the more complicated cytogenetic states in such children have regrettably not been explored in African children. While they are often tumours that behave benignly the prognosis in African children seems rather poor and the malignancy appears much higher. The prognosis with embryonal carcinomas is appalling and few children survive more than a few weeks; with granulosa cell tumours it is very variable.

The embryonal carcinomas therefore need to be distinguished and the histologic pattern, the lacey clear-cell pattern with intra- and extracellular eosinophilic hyaline bodies is distinctive even if there are none of the "glomerular-like" structures to be seen. Exactly the same histologic patterns are to be seen in the embryonal carcinomas that develop in the sacrococcygeal teratomas which seem to occur quite commonly in Uganda.

Teratomatous Growths

Ten teratomatous growths arising extragenitally were seen. One epignathus, one thyroid teratoma in a girl of 13 years, one teratoma of the liver (KIRYABIRWE and MUGERWA, 1967) and seven teratomas of the sacro-coccygeal region. In six of these the tumour was present at birth, but in the seventh it did not become apparent until the sixth year. Five such tumours occurred in girls, two in boys.

Connective-Tissue Tumours

These have been discussed in detail elsewhere, soft-tissue tumours in Chapter 14, bone tumours in Chapter 15, where the difficulties of diagnosis have been emphasized and the problems of some special tumours, e. g. Kaposi's sarcoma, delineated. Here only a few aspects of these tumours in childhood will be noted.

Bone Tumours

Sixteen of the osteogenic sarcomas developed in children, eleven of these, as would be expected, in the third quinquennium, and a further eleven in the late teens, most of which were in the knee region. A chondrosarcoma developed in the ankle region in a girl of 10. Three ameloblastomas of the jaw were seen and two chordomas of the lower spine and one synoviosarcoma of the hip were registered. Diagnosis was uncertain in the other cases; there were four bone tumours of the small round-cell type, two of the jaw, one of the humerus, 1 of the knee region. No clear differentiation was possible between neuroblastoma, Ewing's tumour or some other anaplastic malignancy. The evidence that these were Ewing's sarcoma is unsatisfactory and African experience would seem to concur with American in the infrequency of Ewing's sarcoma in persons of African descent (FRAUMENI and GLASS, 1970).

The circumstances under which bone tumours are diagnosed in Africa are not conducive to accurate diagnosis in either adults or children, at least outside the largest centres. Simple diagnostic guidelines are therefore particularly helpful. All that can be said is that Ewing's sarcoma and neuroblastoma seem to be very uncommon tumours of bone in African children; in long bones one should first consider lymphoma and osteogenic sarcoma, in flat bones, lymphomas, chloromas and non-osteogenic sarcomas.

Soft-Tissue Tumours

A multiplicity of sites and types makes any general statements about soft-tissue malignancies difficult (Tables 6 and 7). The histological diagnoses made are shown in Table 6. Kaposi's sarcoma has been referred to already. Fibrous-tissue tumours usually occurred on the extremities (Table 7) and rhabdomyosarcomas in the facial region or in the pelvis. When occurring in the face rhabdomyosarcoma was sometimes difficult to differentiate from Burkitt's lymphoma (Ziegler et al., 1970). Botryoid sarcoma of the bladder or prostate in males and of the uterus or cervix in females accounted for 7 cases, and alveolar rhabdomyosarcoma of the pararectal area was also seen.

Table 6. Soft-tissue tumours of childhood

	M	F	Total
Kaposi's sarcoma	11	3	14
Rhabdomyosarcoma	10	12	22
Fibrosarcoma	5	3	8
Musculo-aponeurotic fibromatoses	13	6	19
Others	17	9	26
All cases	56	33	89

Table 7. Anatomical distribution of soft-tissue tumours

	Fibromatous tumours	Soft-tissue sarcomas
Head	4	15
Trunk	3	18
Arm	6	4
Leg	10	5

Epithelial Tumours

Epithelial tumours are relatively unusual in children, accounting for a much lower proportion of total cases than among adults. It is of particular interest to note whether children are affected by a tumour known to be common among adults in a particular area. Thus in those parts of the world where oesophageal cancer is common children are only rarely affected. Hepatocellular carcinoma, however, is not uncommon in children in high-incidence areas such as Mozambique (Doll et al., 1966). This relative frequency of tumours would be influenced by the length of the incubation period and the exposure of children to the relevant carcinogenic hazard. The commonest epithelial tumours of childhood in Uganda were of the nasopharynx, liver and skin.

There is no doubt of the frequency of hepatocellular cancer in adults in Uganda and no less than 7 cases of this cancer were seen in children, all of which occurred in the later years of childhood. Conversely four children were seen with hepatoblastoma; all of these were young as corresponds with experience elsewhere. There is no evidence that hepatoblastomas are especially frequent in African children.

Integumentary-tissue cancers are common in adults in Uganda and this series included three children with malignant melanoma of the skin and six with squamous carcinomas of the skin. In previous series melanomas and squamous carcinomas of the conjunctiva were recorded in children (DAVIES et al., 1968) but none were seen in this period. One child developed a squamous carcinoma of the tongue at the age of six years, the only epithelial cancer of the alimentary tract seen in a child though a carcinoma of the ascending colon was seen in a boy of 16 years. The boy with the tongue cancer and at least three of the six with squamous skin cancers were sufferers from xeroderma pigmentosa, an association often noted in the past and of great theoretical interest (CLEAVER, 1969).

Nasopharyngeal carcinoma is unduly common in Ugandan adults and occurs mainly in the northern parts of the country (SCHMAUZ and TEMPLETON, 1972) (see Chapter 4). Six children were seen, all from northern tribes, making this the commonest childhood cancer arising in surface epithelium in this series. It often presented with bilateral cervical lymph-node swelling in childhood, as it does in adults (TEMPLETON and SCHMAUZ, 1970).

The only other epithelial tumours which occurred in children with any frequency were mucoepidermoid carcinomas of the salivary glands or mucous glands in the mouth; four muco-epidermoid carcinomas and one anaplastic carcinoma of the major salivary glands were seen, equally distributed by sex and all occurring around 10—12 years of age. One mucoepidermoid carcinoma and one adenoid cystic carcinoma were seen in the oral mucous glands at ages 12 years and 8 years in a boy and a girl respectively. All other tumours were single and isolated examples.

Examination of the situation in the later teens (see Table 2) reveals that the proportion of nasopharyngeal and liver cancers continued to increase but that the proportions of virtually all other tumours seen in childhood decreased. This applies even to Hodgkin's disease which might on western experience be expected to increase. No intracranial tumours were seen and leukaemias diminished. There were a few childhood tumours that carried over, these included nephroblastoma, neuroblastoma and retinoblastoma, all of which occasionally present in adult life.

Retrospect

Though we know from the Mengo Hospital records (DAVIES et al., 1964) that childhood cancers, especially Burkitt's lymphoma, have been occurring in Uganda for the past 70 years, it is only recently that attention has been paid to them. In the period 1931—1947 only 5 childhood cancers were autopsied at Mulago Hospital, including one medulloblastoma (DAVIES, 1948), out of 144 cancer cases autopsied. In 1947 only 8 childhood tumours were submitted for histology and 9 in 1948, including 3 retinoblastomas, several lymphomas and a chloroma. Except from the point of view of scientific interest it was not important since even if radiotherapy had been available, nothing effective could have been done for the children. Radiotherapy is still not available in Uganda but everything else is changed. The commonest childhood cancer in Uganda, Burkitt's lymphoma, responds remarkably to chemotherapy, as do Hodgkin's disease, nephroblastomas and Kaposi's sarcoma. Almost 60% of the approximately 200 childhood cancers diagnosed each year in Uganda, perhaps only one-third to one-half of those that occur, can be treated with a good chance of success. Childhood cancer in Uganda needs to be investigated much more fully, but these figures provide the justification for studies such as these.

References

ABELEV, G. I.: In: "Liver Cancer". I.A.R.C. Scientific Publications No. 1, Lyon, 1971.

ABELEV, G. I., PEROVA, S. D., KHRAMKOVA, N. I., POSTNIKOVA, Z. A., IRLIN, I. S.: Production of embryonal a-globulin by tranplantable mouse hepatomas. Transplantation 1, 778 (1963).

ACHONG, B. G., MANSELL, P. W. A., EPSTEIN, A., CLIFFORD, P.: An unusual virus in cultures from a human nasopharyngeal carcinoma. J. nat. Cancer Inst. 46, 299—307 (1971).

ACKERMAN, L. V.: Verrucous carcinoma of the oral cavity. Surgery 23, 670—678 (1948 a).

ACKERMAN, L. V.: Malignant melanoma of the Skin. Amer. J. clin. Path. 18, 602—604 (1948 b).

ACKERMAN, L. V., MURRAY, J. F. (Eds.): Symposium on Kaposi's Sarcoma, Makerere College, Kampala, 1961. Basel: S. Karger 1963.

ACOSTA-SISON, H.: Trophoblastic or chorionic Tumours as observed in the Philippines. In: Choriocarcinoma, p. 33. (See HOLLAND, J. F., HRESHCHYSHYN, M. M.) 1967.

ADELOYE, A., ODEKU, E. L.: Metastatic neoplasms of the brain in Nigeria. Brit. J. Cancer 23, 340—348 (1969).

AFFLECK, D. H.: Melanomas. Amer. J. Cancer 27, 120—138 (1936).

AHMED, N.: Geographical incidence of eosophageal cancer in West Kenya. E. Afr. med. J. 43, 235—248 (1966).

AHMED, N., COOK, P.: The incidence of cancer of the oesophagus in West Kenya. Brit. J. Cancer 23, 302—312 (1969).

AKINOSI, J. O., WILLIAMS, A. O.: Ameloblastoma in Ibadan Nigeria. Oral Surg. 27, 257—265 (1969).

ALI, M. Y.: Distribution and Character of the Squamous Epithelium in the Human Nosopharynx. In: Cancer of the Nasopharynx U.I.C.C. Monograph Series, Vol. 1, p. 138—146, 1967.

ALLEN, A. C., SPITZ, S.: Malignant Melanoma — A Clinico-Pathological Analysis of the Criteria for Prognosis and Diagnosis. Cancer (Philad.) 6, 1—45 (1953).

ALLEN, N. C., WATSON-WILLIAMS, E. J.: A Study of Leukaemia Among Nigerians. Proc. 9th Congr. Europ. Soc. Hemat. 906—915 (1963).

ALPERT, M. E., HUTT, M. S. R., DAVIDSON, C. S.: Hepatoma in Uganda. A study in geographic pathology. Lancet 1968 I, 1265—1267.

ALPERT, M. E., HUTT, M. S. R., DAVIDSON, C. S.: Primary Hepatoma in Uganda. A prospective clinical and epidemiologic study of 46 patients. Amer. J. Med. 46, 794—802 (1969).

ALPERT, M. E., HUTT, M. S. R., WOGAN, G. N., DAVIDSON, C. S.: Association between aflatoxin content of food and hepatoma frequency in Uganda. Cancer (Philad.) 28, 253 (1971).

ALPERT, M. E., URIEL, J., DE NECHAUD, B.: Alpha-fetoglobulin in the Diagnosis of human hepatoma. New Engl. J. Med. 218, 984—986 (1968).

American Cancer Society: Manual on Tumour Nomenclature and Coding. American Cancer Society, 1956.

ANAND, S. V., DAVEY, W. W., COHEN, B.: Tumours of the jaw in West Africa. Brit. J. Surg. 54, 901—917 (1967).

ANDERSON, R. E., ISHIDA, K., LI, Y., ISHIMARU, T., NISHLYAMA, H.: Geographic aspects of malignant lymphoma and multiple myeloma. Amer. J. Path. 61, 85—98 (1970).

ANTHONY, P. P.: Primary carcinoma of the liver. A study of 282 cases in Ugandan Africans. 1973 (in press).

ANTHONY, P. P., DRURY, R. A. B.: Elastic vascular sclerosis of mesenteric blood vessels in argentaffin carcinoma. J. clin. Path. 23, 110—118 (1970).

ANTHONY, P. P., McADAM, I. W. J.: Helminthic pseudotumours of the bowel (helminthomas). A study of 34 cases. Gut 13, 8 (1972).

ANTHONY, P. P., VOGEL, C. L., SADIKALI, F., BARKER, L. F., PETERSON, M. R.: Hepatitis-associated antigen and antibody in Uganda: correlation of serological testing with histopathology. Brit. med. J. 1, 403—406 (1972).

APT, A.: Circumcision and prostatic cancer. Acta med. scand. 187, 493—504 (1965).

ARIES, V., CROWTHER, J. S., DRASAR, B. S., HILL, M. J., WILLIAMS, R. E. O.: Bacteria and the aetiology of cancer of the large bowel. Gut 10, 334—335 (1969).

ASADOURIAN, L. A., TAYLOR, H. B.: Dysgerminoma: an analysis of 105 cases. Obstet. and Gynec. 33, 370—379 (1969).

ASHLEY, D. J. B.: On the incidence of carcinoma of the prostate. J. Path. Bact. 90, 217—224 (1965).

ATTYGALLE, D., RATNEIKE, V. T., SUNTHARALINGAM, M.: A case of Kaposi's sarcoma. Ceylon Med. J. 14, 196—199 (1969).

AURE, J. C., HOEG, K., KOLSTAD, P.: Clinical and histologic studies of ovarian carcinoma. Obstet. and Gynec. 37, 1—9 (1971).

BAGSHAWE, A. F., PARKER, A. M.: Age-distribution of alpha-fetoprotein in hepatocellular carcinoma. Lancet 1970 II, 268.

BAGSHAWE, A. F., PARKER, A. M., JINDANI, A.: Hepatitis-associated antigen in liver disease in Kenya. Brit. med. J. 1, 88—89 (1971).

BAILEY, I. C.: The Pattern and Presentation of Intracranial Tumours in Uganda. E. Afr. med. J. 48, 565—575 (1971).

BAILEY, I. C., THOMAS, J. D.: Pituitary Tumours in Uganda. E. Afr. med. J. 48, 90—99 (1971).

BAIRD, I. M., DODGE, O. G., PALMER, F. J., WAWMAN, R. J.: The tongue and oesophagus in iron deficiency anaemia and the effect of iron therapy. J. clin. Path. 14, 603—609 (1961).

BANK, S., MARKS, I. N., SEALY, R., LOUW, J. H., SILBER, W.: Malignant Zollinger-Ellison syndrome in a Bantu woman with a prolonged remission after gastric radiotherapy. Gut 6, 279—285 (1965).

BARR, R. S., MEHTA, S.: E. Afr. med. J. 1972 (in press).

BARTSICH, E. G., BOWE, E. T., MOORE, J. G.: Leiomyosarcoma of the uterus: a 50 year review of 42 cases. Obstet. and Gynec. 32, 101—106 (1968).

BARTSICH, E. G., O'LEARY, J. A., MOORE, J. G.: Carcinosarcoma of the uterus: a 50 year review of 32 cases (1917—1966). Obstet. and Gynec. 30, 518—523 (1967).

BAUDART, M.: Le goitre endemique dans la région de l'Ebola. Ann. Soc. belge Méd. trop. 19, 129—155 (1939).

BAXTER, H.: A review of malignant melanoma of the mouth. Amer. J. Surg. 51, 379—386 (1941).

BECK, R. P., LATOUR, J. P. A.: A review of 1019 benign ovarian neoplasms. Obstet and Gynec. 16, 479—482 (1960).

BECKER, B. J. P., CHATGIDAKIS, C. B.: Primary carcinoma of the liver in Johannesburg. Acta Un. int. Cancr. 17, 650—653 (1961).

BECKER, S. W.: Dermatological investigation of melanin pigmentation in the biology of Melanoma. Ann. N. Y. Acad. Sci. 4, 82—100 (1948).

BEISCHER, N. A., FORTUNE, D. W.: Significance of chromatin patterns in cases of hydatidiform mole with an associated fetus. Amer. J. Obstet. Gynec. 100, 276—282 (1968).

BELL, E. T.: Classification of renal tumours with observations on frequency of various types. J. Urol. (Baltimore) 39, 238 (1938).

BENNETT, F. J.: Social determinants of gonorrhoea in an East African town. E. Afr. med. J. 39, 332—342 (1962).

BENNETT, F. J.: Gonorrhoea: a rural pattern of transmission. E. Afr. med. J. 41, 163—167 (1964).

BENNINGTON, J. L., FERGUSON, B. R., HABER, S. L.: Incidence and relative frequency of benign and malignant ovarian neoplasms. Obstet. and Gynec. 32, 627—632 (1968).

BERARD, C., O'CONOR, G. T., THOMAS, L. B., TORLONI, H.: Histopathological definition of Burkitt's tumour. Bull. Wld. Hlth Org. 40, 601 (1969).

BERMAN, C.: Primary carcinoma of the Liver. London: Lewis 1951.

BHAMARAPRAVATI, N., VIRRANUVATTI, V.: Liver diseases in Thailand. An analysis of liver biopsies. Amer. J. Gastroent. **45**, 267—275 (1966).

BHANA, D., TEMPLETON, A. C., MASTER, S. P., KYALWAZI, S. K.: Kaposi's sarcoma of lymph nodes. Brit. J. Cancer **24**, 464—470 (1970).

BIGGS, B., COOKE, R. A., McGOVERN, V. J.: Kaposi's sarcoma. Report of a case from New Guinea. Austr. J. Derm. **7**, 131 (1964).

BILLINGHURST, J. R.: Intracranial space-occupying lesions in African patients at Mulago Hospital, Kampala. E. Afr. med. J. **43**, 385—393 (1966).

BILLINGHURST, J. R., WELCHMAN, J. M.: Idiopathic Ulcerative Colitis in the African: a Report of 4 cases. Brit. med. J. **1**, 211—213 (1966).

BIZER, L. S.: Rhabdomyosarcoma (a review). Amer. J. Surg. **118**, 453—458 (1969).

BLOOM, H. J. G., DUKES, C. E., MITCHLEY, B. C. V.: Hormone dependent tumours of the kidney. 1. The oestrogen-induced renal tumour of the Syrian hamster. Hormone treatment and possible relationship to carcinoma of the kidney in man. Brit. J. Cancer **17**, 611—645 (1963).

BLUMBERG, B. S., ALTER, H. J., VISNICH, S.: A "new" antigen in leukaemia serum. J. Amer. med. Ass. **191**, 541—546 (1965).

BODIAN, M., RIGBY, C.: In: Tumours of the kidney and ureter. Ed. by: Sir Eric Riches. Edinburgh and London: E. & S. Livingstone Ltd. 1964.

BÖCK, J., FEYRTER, F.: Die Tumoren der Tränendrüse. Ophthalmologica (Basel) **151**, 331—348 (1966).

BOLDT, W.: Über erste Erfahrungen mit der routinemäßigen Beschneidung des Neugeborenen in Deutschland und Gedanken zur Krebsprophylaxe. Geburtsh. u. Frauenheilk. **19**, 624—626 (1959).

BOOTH, K., COOKE, R., SCOTT, G., ATKINSON, L.: Cancer in the Territory of Papua — New Guinea. In Cancer in Africa. Nairobi: East African Publishing House 1968.

BORGES, E. J., PAYMASTER, J. C., BHANSALI, S. K.: Primary Malignant Tumours of the Bone. Clinical Study of 330 Cases. Amer. J. Surg. **113**, 225—231 (1967).

BOUTSELIS, J. G., ULLERY, J. C.: Sarcoma of the uterus. Obstet. and Gynec. **20**, 23—35 (1962).

BOYLAND, E.: The biochemistry of bladder cancer. Springfield (Illinois): Thomas 1963.

BRADLEY, D. J.: Schistosomiasis: In: Uganda Atlas of Disease Distribution, p. 71—74. Kampala: Makerere University College 1968.

BRAS, G.: Nutritional aspects of cirrhosis and carcinoma of the liver. Fed. Proc. **20** (Suppl. 7), 353 (1961).

BRAS, G., WATLER, D. C.: Cancer Incidence in the West Indies. In: DOLL et al., 1970.

BREMNER, C. G., ACKERMAN, L. V.: Polyps and Carcinoma of the large bowel in the South African Bantu. Cancer (Philad.) **26**, 991—999 (1970).

BREWER, J. I., GERBIE, A. B.: Early Development of Choriocarcinoma, p. 45. (See HOLLAND, J. F., HRESHCHYSHYN, M. M.: Choriocarcinoma.) 1967.

British Medical Journal: Leading Article. Circumcision and cervical cancer. Brit. med. J. **2**, 397—398 (1964).

British Medical Journal: Leading Article. Genital Herpes and Cervical Cancer. Brit. med. J. **4**, 256 (1970).

BROOMHALL, C., LEWIS, M. G.: Malignant melanoma of the oral cavity in Ugandan Africans. Brit. J. Surg. **54**, 581—584 (1967).

BROWN, R., WRIGHT, B.: Malignancies in African Children. How do these differ from malignancies in the United States. Clin. Pediat. **6**, 106—115 (1967).

BUCKLEY, R. M.: Patterns of cancer of Ishaka Hospital in Uganda. E. Afr. J. **44**, 465—468 (1967).

BURKITT, D.: A sarcoma involving the jaws in African children. Brit. J. Surg. **46**, 218—223 (1958).

BURKITT, D.: Determining the climatic limitations of a children's cancer common in Africa. Brit. med. J. **2**, 1019—1023 (1962).

BURKITT, D.: Chemotherapy of jaw lymphomata. E. Afr. med. J. **42**, 244—248 (1965).

BURKITT, D. P.: Surgical pathology in the course of the Nile. Ann. roy. Coll. Surg. Engl. **39**, 236—247 (1966).

BURKITT, D. P.: Etiology of Burkitt's lymphoma — an alternative hypothesis to a vectored virus. J. nat. Cancer Inst. 42, 19—28 (1969).

BURKITT, D. P.: Geographical distribution. In: Burkitt's Lymphoma. Ed.: BURKITT, D. P., WRIGHT, D. H. Edinburgh and London: Livingstone 1970, pp. 186—197.

BURKITT, D. P.: Epidemiology of Cancer of the Colon and Rectum. Cancer (Philad.) 28, 3—13 (1971).

BURKITT, D. P., BUNDSCHUH, M., DAHLIN, K., DAHLIN, L., NEALE, R.: Some cancer patterns in W. Kenya and N.W. Tanzania. E. Afr. med. J. 46, 188—193 (1969).

BURKITT, D. P., HUTT, M. S. R., SLAVIN, G.: Clinico-Pathological Studies of Cancer Distribution in Africa. Brit. J. Cancer 22, 1—6 (1968).

BURKITT, D. P., NELSON, C. L., WILLIAMS, E. H.: Some geographical variations in disease pattern in East and Central Africa. E. Afr. med. J. 40, 1—6 (1963).

BURKITT, D., O'CONOR, G. T.: Malignant lymphoma in African children. I — a clinical syndrome. Cancer (Philad.) 14, 258—269 (1961).

BURKITT, D., WRIGHT, D.: Geographical and tribal distribution of the African lymphoma in Uganda. Brit. med. J. 1, 569—573 (1966).

BURKITT, D. P., WRIGHT, D. H.: Burkitt's Lymphoma. Edinburgh and London: Livingstone 1970.

BURN, C., DAVIES, J. N. P., DODGE, O. G., NIAS, B. E.: Hodgkin's disease in English and African children. J. nat. Cancer Inst. 46, 37 (1971).

BUTTERWORTH, T., KLAUDER, J. V.: Malignant melanoma arising in males (Report of 50 cases). J. Amer. med. Ass. 102, 739—745 (1934).

CAFFEY, J.: Pediatric X-ray diagnosis. Chicago: Yearbook Medical Publishers 1961.

CAMAIN, R., TUYNS, A. J., SARRAT, H., QUENUM, C., FAYE, I.: Cutaneous Cancer in Dakar. J. nat. Cancer Inst. 48, 33—50 (1972).

CASE, R. A. M.: Cohort analysis of cancer mortality in England and Wales 1911—1954, by site and sex. Brit. J. prev. soc. Med. 10, 172—199 (1956).

CASE, R. A. M.: Some observations on the alleged causal relationship between infestation with Schistosoma (Bilharzia) haematobium and cancer of the urinary bladder in man. U.I.C.C. Symposium on Bladder Cancer, Cairo (Egypt) 1962.

CASE, R. A. M.: In: Tumours of the Kidney and Ureter. Ed. by: Sir ERIC RICHES. Edinburgh and London: E. & S. Livingstone Ltd. 1964.

CASE, R. A. M.: Tumours of the urinary tract as an occupational disease in several industries. Ann. roy. Coll. Surg. Engl. 39, 213 (1966).

CAVDAR, A. O., ARCASOY, A., GOZDASOGLU, S., DEMIRAG, B.: Chloroma like Ocular Manifestations in Turkish Children with Acute Myelomonocytic Leukemia. Lancet 1971 I, 680—682.

CHAPMAN, D. S.: Cancer of the Penis. A Study of 41 Cases. Med. Proc. 4, 814—820 and 837—845 (1958).

CHARLES, A. H.: Carcinoma of the vulva. Brit. med. J. 1, 397—402 (1972).

CHESTERMAN, C.: Three cases of Malignant Melanoma of the Foot from Congo, with Crab Yaws. Lancet 1, 183—184 (1931).

CHOPRA, S., TEMPLETON, A. C.: Cancer in East African Indians. Int. J. Cancer 8, 176—183 (1971).

CHOU, S. T., GIBSON, J. B.: The histochemistry of biliary mucins and the changes caused by infestation with *clonorchis sinensis*. J. Path. Bact. 101, 185—197 (1970).

CHUANG, J. T., VAN VELDEN, D. J. J., GRAHAM, J. B.: Carcinosarcoma and Mixed Mesodermal tumour of the uterine corpus. Obstet. and Gynec. 35, 769—780 (1970).

CHUTTANI, H. K., SIDHO, A. S., WIG, K. L., GUPTA, D. N., RAMALINGASWAMI, V.: Follow-up study of cases from the Delhi epidemic of infectious hepatitis of 1955—56. Brit. med. J. 2, 676 (1966).

CLEAVER, J. E.: Xeroderma Pigmentosum: A Human Disease in which an initial stage of DNA repair is defective. Proc. nat. Acad. Sci. (Wash.) 63, 428—435 (1969).

CLEMMESEN, J., Ed.: Symposium on tumours of the liver. Acta Un. int. Cancr. 13, 515—860 (1957).

CLEMMESEN, J.: Statistical studies in the aetiology of malignant neoplasms. 1. Review and results. Copenhagen: Munksgaard 1965.

CLEMMESEN, J.: Statistical studies in malignant neoplasms — III. Testis cancer and Basic Tables. Acta path. microbiol. scand. suppl. **1969,** 209.

CLEMMESEN, J., MAISIN, J., GIGASE, P.: Cancer in Kivu and Ruanda-Urundi. A preliminary report. Institut du Cancer, Université de Louvain, 1962.

CLEMMESEN, J., NIELSEN, A., LOCKWOOD, K.: Mortality rates for cancer of the urinary bladder in various countries. Brit. J. Cancer **11,** 1—7 (1957).

CLIFFORD, P.: Malignant disease of the nasopharynx paranasal sinuses in Kenya in "Cancer of the Nasopharynx". U.I.C.C. Monograph Series, no 1: Cancer of the nasopharynx. Copenhagen: Munksgaard, **1967,** pp. 82—94.

CLIFFORD, P.: On the epidemiology of nasopharyngeal carcinoma. Int. J. Cancer **5,** 287—303 (1970).

CLIFFORD, P., BEECHER, J. L.: Nasopharyngeal cancer in Kenya. Clinical and environmental aspects. Brit. J. Cancer **18,** 25—43 (1964).

COLAS, J. L.: Paroxysmal hypertension with haemoptysis due to a retroperitoneal paraganglioma. E. Afr. med. J. **42,** 535—540 (1965).

COLE, G. J.: Ainhum. Chapter 7 of Davey W. W. Companion to Surgery in Africa. Edinburgh: Livingstone 1968.

COLLINS, D. H., PUGH, R. C. B.: The Pathology of Testicular Tumours. Edinburgh and London: E. & S. Livingstone Ltd. 1965.

COLLINS, M. D., FISHER, H.: A case of generalised haemangiosarcomatosis erroneously considered as generalised tuberculosis. Amer. Rev. Tuberc. **61,** 257—262 (1950).

COLLOMB, H., COURSON, B., PHILIPPE, Y., CARAYON, A., CAMAIN, P., DUMAS M.: Tumeurs cerebrales chez l'Africain (a propos de 43 cas). Bull. Soc. méd. Afr. Noire Langue Frse **8,** 261—278 (1963).

CONNERY, D. B.: Leukoplakia of urinary bladder and its association with carcinoma. J. Urol. (Baltimore) **69,** 121 (1953).

CONNOR, D. H., FOLLIS, R. H.: Thyroid hyperplasia at autopsy in Mulago Hospital. E. Afr. med. J. **43,** 107—113 (1966).

CONSTABLE, W. C., BIRRELL, W. R. S., TRUSKETT, I. D.: Cancer of the ovary. Obst. and Gynec. **128,** 294—300 (1969).

COOK, A. R.: Disease patterns in Uganda. J. trop. Med. Hyg. **4,** 175—178 (1901).

COOK, PAULA, BURKITT, D. P.: An Epidemiological Study of Seven Malignant Tumours in East Africa. Cyclostyled booklet, Medical Research Council, January 1970.

COOK, PAULA J., BURKITT, D. P.: Cancer in Africa. Brit. med. Bull. **27,** 14—20 (1971).

COOKE, R. A.: Verrucous Carcinoma of the Oral Mucosa in Papua, New Guinea. Cancer (Philad.) **24,** 397—402 (1969).

COPPLESON, M., REID, B.: Preclinical carcinoma of the cervix uteri, p. 274. Oxford: Pergamon Press 1967.

CORREA, P., CUELLO, C., DUQUE, E.: Carcinoma and intestinal metaplasia of the stomach in Colombian migrants. J. nat. Cancer. Inst. **44,** 297—306 (1970).

CORREA, P., O'CONOR, G. T.: Epidemiologic patterns of Hodgkin's disease. Int. J. Cancer **8,** 192 (1971).

CRAWFORD, E. J., TUCKER, R.: Sarcoma of the uterus. Amer. J. Obstet. Gynec. **77,** 286—291 (1959).

CRAWFORD, M. A.: Excretion of 5 hydroxyindolylacetic acid in East Africans. Lancet **1962 I,** 352.

CUELLO, C., CORREA, P., EISENBERG, H.: Geographic pathology of thyroid carcinoma. Cancer (Philad.) **23,** 230—239 (1969).

CZERNOBILSKY, B., SILVERMAN, B. B., ENTERLINE, H. T.: Clear cell carcinoma of the ovary. Cancer (Philad.) **25,** 762—772 (1970).

DAHLIN, D. C.: Bone Tumours. Springfield (Illinois): Charles C. Thomas 1957.

DALLDORF, G.: Lymphomas of African children. J. Amer. med. Ass. **181,** 1026—1028 (1962).

DALLDORF, G., LINSELL, C. A., BARNHART, F. E., MARTYN, R.: An epidemiological approach to the lymphomas of African children and Burkitt's sarcoma of the jaws. Perspect. Biol. Med. **7,** 435—449 (1964).

DALTON, A. J., MORRIS, H. P., DUBNIK, C. S.: Morphologic changes in the organs of female C₃H mice after long-term ingestion of thiourea and thiouracil. J. nat. Cancer Inst. **9**, 201—223 (1948).

DAOUD, E. H., EL HASSAN, A. M., ZAK, F., ZAKOVA, N.: Aspects of Malignant disease in the Sudan. p. 43 in "Cancer in Africa". Eds.: CLIFFORD, P., LINSELL, C. A. and TIMMS, G. L. East African Publishing House 1968.

DAVEY, W. W.: Companion to Surgery in Africa. Edinburgh: Livingstone 1968.

DAVEY, W. W.: Renal Tumours in Nigeria. Brit. J. Urol. **36**, 340—346 (1964).

DAVIES, A. G. M., DAVIES, J. N. P.: Tumours of the Jaw in Uganda Africans. Acta Un. int. Cancr. **16**, 1320—1324 (1960).

DAVIES, J. N. P.: Pathology of Central African Natives. Mulago Hospital Post-Mortem Studies, No. 6 — Cancer in Africans. E. Afr. med. J. **25**, 117—122 (1948).

DAVIES, J. N. P.: History of syphilis in Uganda. Bull. Wld. Hlth Org. **15**, 1041—1055 (1956).

DAVIES, J. N. P.: Collection of statistical data on cancer in Africa. Acta Un. int. Cancr. **13**, 904—910 (1957).

DAVIES, J. N. P.: Cancer in Africa. Modern Trends in Pathology. Ed.: COLLINS, D. H. (London), p. 132—160, 1959.

DAVIES, J. N. P.: Leukaemia in children in tropical Africa. Lancet **1965 II**, 65—67.

DAVIES, J. N. P.: Leukemia in Trans-Saharan Africa. Acta Un. int. Cancr. **16**, 1618—1622 (1960).

DAVIES, J. N. P.: Lymphomas and Leukemias in Uganda Africans. Ed.: ROULET, F. C. Symposium on Lymphoreticular Tumours in Africa, 1964.

DAVIES, J. N. P.: Retinoblastoma as Possible Index Cancer. Lancet **11**, 1039 (1967).

DAVIES, J. N. P.: Tumours in Children. Some variations in childhood cancers throughout the world. Ed.: MARSDEN, H. B., STEWARD, J. K.: Springer 1968.

DAVIES, J. N. P., DODGE, O. G., BURKITT, D. P.: Salivary-gland tumors in Uganda. Cancer **17**, 1310—1322 (1964).

DAVIES, J. N. P., ELMES, S., HUTT, M. S. R., MTIMAVALYE, L. A. R., OWOR, R., SHAPER, L.: Cancer in an African Community, 1897—1956. An analysis of the records of Mengo Hospital, Kampala, Uganda. Brit. med. J. **1**, 259—264 (1964).

DAVIES, J. N. P., KNOWELDEN, J., WILSON, B. A.: Incidence rates of cancer in Kyadondo County, Uganda, 1954—60. J. nat. Cancer Inst. **35**, 789—821 (1965).

DAVIES, J. N. P., LOTHE, F.: Kaposi's Sarcoma in African Children. Acta Un. int. Cancr. **18**, 394—399 (1962).

DAVIES, J. N. P., OWOR, R.: The diagnosis of primary carcinoma of the liver. E. Afr. med. J. **37**, 249—254 (1960).

DAVIES, J. N. P., OWOR, R.: Chloromatous tumours in African children in Uganda. Brit. med. J. **2**, 405—407 (1965).

DAVIES, J. N. P., STEINER, P. E.: Cirrhosis and primary liver carcinoma in Uganda Africans. Brit. J. Cancer **11**, 523—534 (1957).

DAVIES, J. N. P., STEWART, A., DALLDORF, G., BARNHARD, F.: In Course of Publication, 1972.

DAVIES, J. N. P., TANK, R., MEYER, R., THURSTON, P.: Cancer of the integumentary tissues in Uganda Africans: The basis for prevention. J. nat. Cancer Inst. **41**, 31—51 (1968).

DAVIES, J. N. P., WILSON, B. A.: Cancer in Kampala, 1952—53. E. Afr. med. J. **31**, 394—416 (1954).

DAVIES, J. N. P., WILSON, B. A., KNOWELDEN, J.: Cancer in Kampala: A survey in an underdeveloped country. Brit. med. J. **2**, 439—443 (1958).

DAVIS, G. L., KESSONI, J. M., ISHAK, K. G.: Embryonal Rhabdomyosarcoma of the biliary tree. Report of 5 cases and a review of the literature. Cancer (Philad.) **24**, 333—342 (1969).

DAVIS, N. C., HERRON, J. J., McLEOD, G. R.: Malignant Melanoma in Queensland. Analysis of 400 skin lesions. Lancet **1966 II**, 407—410.

DEO, M. G., DAYAL, Y., RAMALINGASWAMI, V.: Aflatoxins and liver injury in the rhesus monkey. J. Path. **101**, 47—56 (1970).

Department of Obstetrics Annual Report: 1966—1967. Makerere University College, Kampala 1967.

DIMETTE, R. M., SPROAT, H. F., SAYEGH, E. S.: The classification of carcinoma of the urinary bladder associated with schistosomiasis and metaplasia. J. Urol. (Baltimore) 75, 680 (1956).

DINNERSTEIN, A. J., O'LEARY, J. A.: Granulosa-theca cell tumors: a clinical review of 102 patients. Obstet. and Gynec. 31, 654—658 (1968).

DIXON, F. J., MOORE, R. A.: Tumours of the male sex organs. p. 45. Atlas of human pathology. Section 8, Fascicles 31 and 32. Armed Forces Institute of Pathology, Washington 1952.

DOBBIE, B. M. W., TAYLOR, C. W., WATERHOUSE, J. A. H.: A study of carcinoma of the endometrium. J. Obstet. Gynaec. Brit. Cwlth. 72, 659—673 (1965).

DODGE, O. G.: Tumours of the bladder in Uganda Africans. Acta Un. int. Cancr. 18, 548 (1962).

DODGE, O. G.: Carcinoma of the prostate in Uganda Africans. Cancer (Philad.) 16, 1264—1268 (1963).

DODGE, O. G.: Bone Tumours in Uganda Africans. Brit. J. Cancer 18, 627—633 (1964 a).

DODGE, O. G.: Tumors of the bladder and urethra associated with urinary retention in Uganda Africans. Cancer (Philad.) 17, 1433—1436 (1964 b).

DODGE, O. G.: Carcinoma of the penis in East Africans. Brit. J. Urol. 31, 223—226 (1965 a).

DODGE, O. G.: Tumors of the jaw, odontogenic tissues and maxillary antrum (excluding Burkitt lymphoma) in Uganda Africans. Cancer (Philad.) 18, 205—215 (1965 b).

DODGE, O. G., KAVITI, J. N.: Male circumcision among the peoples of E. Africa and the incidence of genital cancer. E. Afr. med. J. 42, 98 (1965).

DODGE, O. G., LINSELL, C. A., DAVIES, J. N. P.: Circumcision and the incidence of carcinoma of the penis and cervix. A study in Kenya and Uganda Africans. E. Afr. med. J. 40, 440—444 (1963).

DODGE, O. G., LINSELL, M. D.: Carcinoma of the penis in Uganda and Kenya Africans. Cancer (Philad.) 16, 1255—1263 (1963).

DOLL, R.: Bronchial Carcinoma: Incidence and Aetiology. Brit. med. J. 2, 521—527 and 585—590 (1953).

DOLL, R., HILL, A. B.: The Mortality of Doctors in Relation to their smoking habits. A preliminary report. Brit. med. J. i, 1451—1455 (1954).

DOLL, R., MUIR, C. S., WATERHOUSE, J. A. H., eds.: Cancer Incidence in Five Continents, Vol. II. U.I.C.C. Geneva: Springer 1970.

DOLL, R., PAYNE, P., WATERHOUSE, J. A. H., eds.: Cancer Incidence in Five Continents, Vol. 1, U.I.C.C. Berlin: Springer 1966.

DONIACH, I.: In: Recent Advances in Pathology. Ed.: C. V. HARRISON. London: Butterworth 1960.

DORFMAN, R. F.: Follicular (nodular) lymphoma in South Africa. Symposium on Lymphoreticular Tumours in Africa, Paris, 1963. Ed.: F. C. ROULET. Basel-New York: Karger 1964, pp. 211—228.

DORN, H. F., CUTLER, S. J.: Morbidity from cancer in the United States. U.S. Public Health Monograph No. 29, 1955.

DOUGLAS, G. W.: Geographic variation in the occurrence of hydatidiform mole and choriocarcinoma. (By the joint project for study of choriocarcinoma and hydatidiform mole in Asia.) Ann. N. Y. Acad. Sci. 80, 195—196 (1959).

DREYFUSS, W., NEVILLE, W. E.: Buschke-Loewenstein Tumors (Giant Condylomata Acuminata). Amer. J. Surg. 90, 146—150 (1955).

DUNHAM, L. J., BAILAR, J. C.: World maps of cancer mortality rates and frequency ratios. J. nat. Cancer Inst. 41, 155—204 (1968).

DUTZ, W., STOUT, A. P.: Kaposi's sarcoma in infants and children. Cancer (Philad.) 13, 684—694 (1960).

EDINGTON, G. M.: Malignant disease in the Gold Coast. Brit. J. Cancer 10, 595—605 (1956).

EDINGTON, G. M., MACLEAN, C. M. U.: The relative incidence of tumours of the reticuloendothelial system in Ibadan, Nigeria. p. 54—66. In: Lymphoreticular Tumours in Africa. Ed.: ROULET, F. C. Basel: Karger 1964 a.

EDINGTON, G. M., MACLEAN, C. M. U.: Incidence of the Burkitt tumour in Ibadan, Western Nigeria. Brit. med. J. 1, 264 (1964 b).

EDINGTON, G. M., MACLEAN, C. M. U.: A cancer rate survey in Ibadan, Western Nigeria, 1960—63. Brit. J. Cancer **19**, 471—481 (1965).

EDMONDSON, H. A.: Tumors of the liver and intrahepatic bile ducts. In Atlas of Tumour Pathology. Armed Forces Institute of Pathology, Washington, D. C., Section 7, Fascicle 25, 1958.

EDMONDSON, H. A., STEINER, P. E.: Primary carcinoma of the liver: an autopsy study. Cancer (Philad.) **7**, 462—502 (1954).

EDWARDS, D. L., STERLING, L. N., KELLER, R. H., NOLAN, J. F.: Mixed heterologous mesenchymal sarcomas (mixed mesodermal sarcomas) of the uterus. Amer. J. Obstet. Gynec. **85**, 1002—1011 (1963).

EFRON, G.: Glomus Jugulare tumour. A case report. S. Afr. med. J. **31**, 164—168 (1957).

EISENBERG, H.: Cancer Incidence in Connecticut. In: U.I.C.C. Cancer Incidence in 5 Continents, Vol. I. Eds.: DOLL, R., PAYNE, P., WATERHOUSE, J. A. H. Geneva, U.I.C.C., 1966.

EL GAZAYERLI, M., KHARADLY, M., KHALIL, H., GALAL, R., RIAD, W., EL GAZAYERLI, M. M.: Primary tumours of lymph nodes. In: Lymphoreticular Tumours in Africa. Ed.: ROULET, F. C. Basel: Karger, p. 36—41, 1964.

EL HASSAN, A. M., MILOSEV, B., DAOUD, E. H., KASHAN, A.: Malignant disease of the upper respiratory tract in the Sudan. In: Cancer in Africa. p. 307—314, Eds.: CLIFFORD, P., LINSELL, C. A., TIMMS, G. L. Nairobi: East African Publishing House 1967.

ELIAS, H.: Multicentric carcinogenesis in the human liver. Acta hepato-splenol. (Stuttg.) **7**, 65—86 (1960).

ELLIOTT, R. I. K.: On the prevention of Carcinoma of the Cervix. Lancet **1**, 231—235 (1964).

ELLIS, M.: Chronic mastitis in the African native. Its relation to carcinoma of the breast. Brit. J. Surg. **25**, 39 (1937).

ELMES, B. G. T., BALDWIN, R. B. T.: Malignant Disease in Nigeria: An analysis of 1000 tumours. Ann. trop. Med. Parasit. **41**, 321—328 (1947).

EMIRU, V. P.: The Conjunctiva in Kwashiorkor. M. D. Thesis, Makerere University, 1970.

ENOS, W. F., HOLMES, R. H.: Malignant Melanoma in the Tropics. Amer. J. Path. **27**, 523—535 (1951).

ENZINGER, F. M.: Fibrous hamartoma of infancy. Cancer (Philad.) **18**, 241 (1965).

ENZINGER, F. M.: (In collaboration with R. LATTES, H. TORLONI and pathologists in 14 countries.) Histological Typing of Soft Tissue Tumours. Geneva, World Health Organization, 1969.

ENZINGER, F. M., SHIRAKI, M.: Alveolar Rhabdomyosarcoma (a review of 110 cases). Cancer (Philad.) **24**, 18—31 (1969).

EPSTEIN, M. A.: Long-term tissue culture of Burkitt Lymphoma cells Ch. 13 in "Burkitt's Lymphoma". Eds.: BURKITT, D., WRIGHT, D. H. Edinburgh and London: Livingstone 1970.

ERASMUS, J. F. P.: Carotid body tumour with invasion of the cerebello pontine angle. S. Afr. med. J. **21**, 225—227 (1947).

ESSIAN, E. M.: Leukemia in Nigerians: The Acute Leukemias. Afr. J. Med. Sci. **3** (1972) in press.

FALLS, H. F., NEEL, J. V.: Genetics of retinoblastoma. Arch. Ophthal. **46**, 367—389 (1951).

FARRER BROWN, G., BENNETT, M. H., HARRISON, C. V., MILLET, Y., JELLIFFE, A. M.: The pathological findings following Laparotomy in Hodgkin's disease. Brit. J. Cancer **25**, 449—457 (1971).

DE FAVIA, J. J., CUTIN, M., MORGANTE, A. P., FERRI, R. G.: Malignant granuloma of the face: contributions to its nosology. Arch. Otolaryng. **65**, 255—262 (1957).

FENTON, A. N., BURKE, L.: Sarcoma of the uterus: a record of 26 cases. Amer. J. Obstet. Gynec. **63**, 158—162 (1952).

FINN, W. F., JAVERT, C. T.: Primary and metastatic carcinoma of the Fallopian Tube. Cancer (Philad.) **2**, 803—814 (1949).

FISHER, E. R., REIBORD, H.: Electron microscope evidence suggesting the myxogenous derivation of the so-called Alveolar soft part Sarcoma. Cancer (Philad.) **27**, 150—159 (1971).

FOLLIS, R. H., CONNOR, D. H.: Some patterns of urinary iodine excretion in Uganda. E. Afr. med. J. **43**, 114—118 (1966).

FOSTER, W. D.: The early history of scientific medicine in Uganda. Nairobi: East African Literature Bureau 1970.

FRANKS, L. M.: Latent carcinoma of the prostate. J. Path. Bact **68**, 603—616 (1954).

FRAUMENI, J. F.: Stature and malignant tumors of bone in childhood and adolescence. Cancer (Philad.) **20**, 967—973 (1967).

FRAUMENI, J. F., Jr., EVERSON, R. B., DALAGER, N. A.: Declining Mortality from Wilms' Tumour in the United States. Lancet **1972 II**, 48.

FRAUMENI, J. F., GLASS, A. G.: Rarity of Ewing's sarcoma among U.S. Negro Children. Lancet **1970 I**, 366—367.

FRAUMENI, J. F., LI, F. P.: Hodgkin's disease in childhood: An epidemiologic study. J. nat. Cancer Inst. **42**, 681 (1969).

FRICK, H. C., JACOX, H. W., TAYLOR, H. C.: Primary carcinoma of the vagina. Amer. J. Obstet. Gynec. **101**, 695—703 (1968).

FRIEDMAN, N. B., ASH, J. E.: Tumours of the urinary bladder. Atlas of Tumour Pathology, Section VIII, Fasc. 31 a. Armed Forces Institute of Pathology, Washington, D. C., 1959.

FRIPP, P. F.: Bilharziasis and bladder cancer. Brit. J. Cancer **19**, 292—296 (1965).

GALL, E. A.: Primary and metastatic carcinoma of the liver. Relationship to hepatic cirrhosis. Arch. Path. **70**, 226—232 (1960).

GALL, E. A., MALLORY, T. B.: Malignant lymphoma. A clinico-pathologic survey of 618 cases. Amer. J. Path. **18**, 381—430 (1942).

GELFAND, M.: The Sick African. Cape Town: Juta 1957.

GIBSON, J. B.: Parasites, Liver Disease and Liver Cancer. In: Liver Cancer. I.A.R.C. Scientific Publications, No. 1, p. 42. Lyon 1971.

GILLMAN, J., PRATES, M. D.: Histological types and histogenesis of bladder cancer in the Portuguese East African with special reference to bilharzial cystitis. Acta Un. int. Cancr. **18**, 560 (1962).

GINSBERG, R., DAVIES, J. N. P.: Unpublished, 1972.

GLASS, A. G., FRAUMENI, J. F.: Epidemiology of bone cancer in children. J. nat. Cancer Inst. **44**, 187—199 (1970).

GOLDENBERG, D. M., FISHER, E. R.: Histogenetic relationship between carcinoid and mucin secreting carcinoma of the colon as revealed by heterotransplantation. Brit. J. Cancer **24**, 610—614 (1970).

GOUGH, J.: Hodgkin's disease: A correlation of histopathology with survival. Int. J. Canc. **5**, 273—281 (1970).

GRECH, E. S., LEWIS, M. G.: Ovarian Tumours in Ugandan Africans. E. Afr. med. J. **44**. 487—492 (1967).

GRIEVE, J. M., LINDER, A. M.: In: Cancer Incidence in Five Continents, II, p. 98. Ed.: DOLL, R., MUIR, C, WATERHOUSE, J. Berlin-Heidelberg-New York: Springer 1970.

GRIFFITH, H. B.: Gonorrhoea and fertility in Uganda. Eugen. Rev. **55**, 103—108 (1963).

GRIFFITHS, I. H., THACKRAY, A. C.: Parenchymal carcinoma of the kidney. Brit. J. Urol. **21**, 128—151 (1949).

HAENSZEL, W.: Variations in skin cancer incidence within the United States. In: Conference on Biology of Cutaneous Cancer (Ed.: URBACH, F.), p. 225. Nat. Cancer Inst. Monograph no. 10 ,N.I.H., Bethesda 1963.

HAENSZEL, W., CORREA, P.: Cancer of the Colon Rectum and Adenomatous Polyps. A review of epidemiological findings. Cancer (Philad.) **28**, 14—24 (1971).

HAGHIGHI, P., NABIZADEH, I., ASUADI, S., MOHALLATEE, E. A.: Cancer in Southern Iran. Cancer (Philad.) **27**, 965—977 (1971).

HAINES, M., TAYLOR, C. W.: Gynaecological Pathology, p. 238. London: J. & A. Churchill Ltd. 1962.

HALL, S. A., LANGLANDS, B. W. (Eds.): Uganda Atlas of Disease Distribution. Makerere University College, 1968.

HAMPERL, H., HELLWEG, G.: On Mucoepidermoid tumours of different sites. Cancer (Philad.) **10**, 1187—1192 (1957).

HANCOCK, P. E. T.: Malignant lymphoma: clinico-pathologic correlation, pp. 412—428. Cancer. Vol. 4. Ed.: RAVEN, R. W. London: Butterworth 1958.

HANDLEY, W. S.: The Genesis of Cancer, p. 25. London: Lewis 1931.

HARNETT, W. L.: A survey of cancer in London: Report of the Clinical Cancer research Committee, p. 576—588. British Empire Cancer Campaign. London: Sumfield & Day 1952.

HASEGAWA, K.: A case of Kaposi's sarcoma. Jap. J. Derm. **72**, 379 (1962).

HASHEM, M.: The aetiology and pathogenesis of the bilharzial bladder cancer. J. Egypt. med. Ass. **44**, 857 (1961).

HAZEN, H. H., FREEMAN, C. W.: Skin cancer in the American Negro. Arch. Derm. Syph. (Chic.) **62**, 622 (1950).

HEINS, H. C., DENNIS, E. J., PRATT-THOMAS, H. R., CHARLESTON, S. C.: The possible role of smegma in Carcinoma of the Cervix. Amer. J. Obstet. Gynec. **76**, 726—733 (1958).

HELLWIG, C. A.: Malignant lymphoma. Analysis of 202 cases. Amer. J. clin. Path. **16**, 564 —573 (1946).

HEMS, G.: Epidemiological characteristics of breast cancer in middle and late age. Brit. J. Cancer **24**, 226—233 (1970 a).

HEMS, G.: Aetiology of bone cancer, and some other cancers, in the young. Brit. J. Cancer **24**, 208—214 (1970 b).

HENLE, W., HENLE, G., HO, H. C., BURTIN, P., CACHIN, Y., CLIFFORD, P., DE SCHRYVER, A., DE THE, G., DIEHL, V., KLEIN, G.: Antibodies to Epstein-Barr virus in nasopharyngeal carcinoma, other head and neck neoplasms, and control groups. J. nat. Cancer Inst. **44**, 225—231 (1970).

HENNEBERT, P. N., SEGHERS, M. J.: Apercu de pathologie chirurgicale des machoires au Congo. Ann. soc. belge Méd. trop. **44**, 1081—1094 (1964).

HERTIG, A. T., GORE, H.: Atlas of tumor pathology. Washington. Fascicle **33**, Part 2 (1960) and Part 3 (1961). Armed Forces Institute of Pathology.

HESELSON, J.: Moles and Melanomas of the skin. S. Afr. med. J. **35**, 1113—1120 (1961).

HEWER, T. F.: Malignant Melanoma in Coloured Races; The Role of Trauma in its causation. J. Path. Bact. **41**, 473—477 (1935).

HIGGINSON, J., OETTLÉ, A. G.: Cancer Incidence in the Bantu and "Cape Colored" races of South Africa: Report of a cancer survey in the Transval (1953—55). J. nat. Cancer Inst. **24**, 589—671 (1960).

HIGGINSON, J., OETTLÉ, A. G.: Cancer of the bladder in the South African Bantu. Acta Un. int. Cancr. **18**, 579 (1962).

HILL, M. J., CROWTHER, J. S., DRASAR, B. S., HAWKSWORTH, G., ARIES, V., WILLIAMS, R. E. O.: Bacteria and Aetiology of Cancer of the Large Bowel. Lancet **1971** I, 95—100.

HILTON, G., SUTTON, P. M.: Malignant lymphomas: Classification prognosis and treatment. Lancet **1962** I, 283.

HOLLAND, J. F., HRESHCHYSHYN, M. M. (Eds.): Choriocarcinoma. U.I.C.C. Monograph Series, Vol. 3. Berlin: Springer 1967.

HORN, R. C.: Malignant Potential of Polypoid Lesions of the Colon and Rectum. Cancer (Philad.) **28**, 146—152 (1971).

HUBER, A.: Uteruskarzinom und Zirkumzision. Wien. med. Wschr. **110**, 571—574 (1960).

HUEPER, W. C.: Occupational and environmental cancers of the urinary system. New Haven and London: Yale Univ. Press 1969.

HUEPER, W. C., CONWAY, W. D.: Chemical Carcinogenesis and Cancers. Springfield (Ill.): Charles C Thomas 1964.

HUTT, M. S. R.: Epidemiology of human primary liver cancer. In: Liver Cancer. Lyon: I.A.R.C. Scientific Publications 1971 a, No. 1, p. 21.

HUTT, M. S. R.: Some aspects of liver disease in Ugandan Africans. Trans. roy. Soc. trop. Med. Hyg. **65**, 273 (1971 b).

HUTT, M. S. R., BURKITT, D.: Geographical distribution of cancer in East Africa: a new clinico-pathological approach. Brit. med. J. **2**, 719—722 (1965).

HUTT, M. S. R., BURKITT, D. P., SHEPHERD, J. J., WRIGHT, B., MATI, J. K. G., AUMA, S.: Malignant Tumors of the Gastrointestinal Tract in Ugandans, p. 41—47. In: Tumors of the Alimentary Tract in Africans. National Cancer Institute Monograph 25, 1967.

HUTT, M. S. R., MODY, N. J.: A malignant carotid body tumour in an African. J. Path. Bact. **86**, 534—535 (1963).

HUTT, M. S. R., TEMPLETON, A. C.: The geographical pathology of Bowel Cancer and some related diseases. Proc. roy. Soc. Med. **64**, 962—964 (1971).

IBRAHIM, H.: Bilharziasis and bilharzial cancer of the bladder. Ann. roy. Coll. Surg. Engl. **2**, 129 (1948).

IKONOPISOV, R. L., LEWIS, M. G., HUNTER-CRAIG, I. D., BODENHAM, D. C., PHILLIPS, T. M., ALEXANDER, P., COOLING, C. I., PROCTOR, J.: Autoimmunization with Irradiated Tumour Cells in Human Malignant Melanoma. Brit. med. J. 2, 752—754 (1970).

International Agency for Research on Cancer: Scientific Publications No. 1: Liver Cancer. Lyon, France 1971.

IRIBE, K.: (1969) quoted by GLASS and FRAUMENI. In: Epidemiology of bone cancer in children. J. nat. Cancer Inst. 44, 187—199 (1970).

JACKSON, H., Jr., PARKER, F., Jr.: Hodgkin's disease and allied disorders. London: Oxford University Press 1947.

JACKSON, J. G., REEVE, J. D.: Carcinoma of the thyroid in Africans. W. Afr. med. J. 10, 396—401 (1961).

JACKSON, S. M.: Ovarian dysgerminoma. Brit. J. Radiol. 40, 459—462 (1967).

JACOBS, A.: In: Encyclopedia of Urology. Ed. by: ALKEN, C. E., DIX, V. W., GOODWIN, W. E., WILDBOZ, E. Vol. 2. Berlin: Springer 1967.

JAMES, P. D., TEMPLETON, A. C.: Carcinoma of the Pancreas. E. Afr. med. J. 47, 699 (1972).

JANOTA, I.: Involvement of the nervous system in malignant lymphoma in Nigeria. Brit. J. Cancer 20, 47—61 (1966).

JANSSENS, P. G., QUERTINMONT, M. J., SIENIAWSKI, J., FATTI, F.: Necrotische tropenzweer en nieuwe mycobacteriele verwekkers (Myobacterium N. SP.). Verh. vlaam. Akad. Geneesk. Belg. 20, 420 (1958).

Joint Project for Study of Choriocarcinoma and Hydatidiform Mole in Asia. Geographic Variation in the Occurrence of Hydatidiform Mole and Choriocarcinoma: Ann. N. Y. Acad. Sci. 80, 178—196 (1959).

JONDAHL, W. H., DOCKERTY, M. B., RANDALL, L. M.: Brenner tumour of the ovary: a clinico-pathologic study of 31 cases. Amer. J. Obstet. Gynec. 60, 160—167 (1950).

JORGENSEN, E. O., DOCKERTY, M. B., WILSON, R. B., WELCH, J. S.: Clinico-pathologic study of 53 cases of Brenner's tumor of the ovary. Amer. J. Obstet. Gynec. 108, 122—127 (1970).

JUSSAWALLA, D. J.: Cancer Incidence in Bombay, 1970. See DOLL, MUIR and WATERHOUSE.

JUSSAWALLA, D. J., DESHPANDE, V. A., HAENSZEL, W. et al.: Differences observed in the site incidence of cancer, between the Parsi community and the total population of greater Bombay. Brit. J. Cancer 24, 56—66 (1970).

KADIN, M. E., BENSCH, K. G.: On the origin of Ewing's tumour. Cancer (Philad.) 27, 257—273 (1971).

KADIN, M. E., GLATSTEIN, E., DORFMAN, R. F.: Clinico-pathologic studies of 117 untreated patients subjected to Laparotomy for the staging of Hodgkin's disease. Cancer (Philad.) 27, 1277—1294 (1971).

KAFUKO, G. W., BAINGANA, N., KNIGHT, E. M., TIBEMANYA, J.: Association of Burkitt's tumour and holoendemic malaria in West Nile District, Uganda: Malaria as a possible aetiologic factor. E. Afr. med. J. 46, 414—436 (1969).

KAFUKO, G. W., BURKITT, D. P.: Burkitt's lymphoma and malaria. Int. J. Cancer 6, 1—9 (1970).

KASSEL, S. H., ECHEVARIA, R. A., GUZZO, F. P.: Midline malignant reticulosis (so-called lethal midline granuloma). Cancer (Philad.) 23, 922—935 (1969).

KAPOSI, M.: Idiopatisches multiples Pigmentsarkom der Haut. Arch. Derm. Syph. (Berl.) 4, 265 (1872).

KAYABUKI, D. W., GWATA, A. T., TEMPLETON, A. C.: Carcinoma of the Male Breast in Uganda Africans. Makerere Med. J. 12, 35—36 (1968).

KEELING, J. W.: Liver Tumours in infancy and childhood. J. Path. Bact. 103, 69—83 (1971).

KEEN, P.: Carcinoma of the Antrum in the South African Bantu. In: Cancer of the Nasopharynx. U.I.C.C. Monograph Series, Vol. 1, p. 95—100. Copenhagen: Munksgaard 1967.

KEEN, P., DE MOOR, N. G., SHAPIRO, M. A., COHEN, L.: The aetiology of respiratory tract cancer in the South African Bantu. Brit. J. Cancer 2, 528—538 (1955).

KENT, S. W., McKAY, D. G.: Primary cancer of the ovary. Amer. J. Obstet. Gynec. 80, 430—438 (1960).

KERR, W. K., BARKIN, M.: Aetiology and biochemistry of cancer of the bladder. In: Modern trends in Urology. Series 3. Ed. by: Sir ERIC RICHES. London: Butterworths 1970.

KERR, W. K., BARKIN, M., MENCZYK, Z.: Cancer of the bladder: biochemical factors in its etiology. Canad. J. Surg. **7**, 414—419 (1964).

KIBUKAMUSOKE, J. W.: Venereal Disease in East Africa. Trans. roy. Soc. trop. Med. Hyg. **59**, 642—648 (1965).

KING, H., BAILAR, J. C.: Epidemiology of urinary bladder cancer. A review of selected literature. J. chron. Dis. **19**, 735—769 (1966).

KING, H., DIAMOND, E., LILIENFELD, A. M.: Some epidemiological aspects of cancer of the prostate. J. chron. Dis. **16**, 117—153 (1963).

KING, M. H.: Medical care in developing countries. Nairobi and London: Oxford University Press 1965.

KIRYABWIRE, J. W. M., MUGERWA, J. W.: Teratoma of the liver in an African child. Brit. J. Surg. **54**, 585—587 (1967).

KOCSARD, E.: Kaposi's sarcoma in a Chinese boy (aged 16) with localisation on the left lower extremity and on the right caruncula lacrimalis. Dermatologica (Basel) **99**, 43—48 (1949).

KOLLER, O., GJONNAESS, H.: Dysgerminoma of the ovary. Acta obstet. gynec. scand. **43**, 268—278 (1964).

KOTTMEIER, H. L.: Carcinoma of the female genital tract. The Abraham Flexner Lecture Series, Number 11. Baltimore: Williams and Wilkins Co. 1953.

KOVI, J., LAING, W. N.: Tumours of mandible and maxilla in Accra, Ghana. Cancer (Philad.) **19**, 1301—1307 (1966).

KREMENTZ, E. T., SHAUER, J. O.: Behaviour and treatment of soft tissue sarcomas. Ann. Surg. **157**, 770—784 (1963).

KREYBERG, L., SAXEN, E.: A comparison of Lung tumour types in Finland and Norway. Brit. J. Cancer **15**, 211—214 (1961).

KRIBLER, D. M.: Hypertension and extra-adrenal phaeochromocytoma. S. Afr. med. J. **40**, 1130 (1966).

KRUGMAN, S., GILES, J. P.: Viral hepatitis. New light on an old disease. J. Amer. med. Ass. **212**, 1019—1029 (1970).

KUSNEZOW, W. N.: A case of sarcoma multiplex Idiopathicum (Kaposi) with fatal outcome. Urol. cutan. Rev. **37**, 230—235 (1933).

KYALWAZI, S. K.: Carcinoma of the penis: a review of 153 patients admitted to Mulago Hospital, Kla. Uganda. E. Afr. med. J. **43**, 415—425 (1966).

LAHEY, F. H., HARE, H. F., WARREN, S.: Carcinoma of the thyroid. Ann. Surg. **112**, 911—1005 (1940).

LAUREN, P.: The two histological main types of gastric carcinoma: diffuse and so-called intestinal type carcinoma. Acta path. microbiol. scand. **64**, 31—49 (1965).

LAWRENCE, A. W.: Adamantinoma. W. Indian med. J. **15**, 226—229 (1966).

LEDER, L. D.: Der Nachweis der Naphthol-AS-D-Chloroacetateesterase und seine Bedeutung für die histologische Diagnostik. Verh. dtsch. Ges. Path. **48**, 317—320 (1964).

LEE, F. D.: A comparative study of Kaposi's sarcoma and granuloma pyogenicum in Uganda. J. clin. Path. **21**, 119—128 (1968).

LEE, F. I.: Cirrhosis and hepatoma in alcoholics. Gut **7**, 77—85 (1966).

LEIGHTON, P. C., ZEIGLER, O., TRUSSELL, R. R., SHARMA, S. D.: Exfoliative Cervical Cytology in Uganda. In preparation 1972.

LENNOX, B.: The histopathology of tumours. Melanomata, p. 17—24, 7th. ed. Recent Adcances in Clinical Pathology. Ed.: HARRISON, C. V. London: Churchill 1960.

LEWIS, M. G.: Malignant melanoma in Uganda. (The relationship between pigmentation a malignant melanoma on the soles of the feet.) Brit. J. Cancer **21**, 483—495 (1967 a).

LEWIS, M. G.: Possible Immunological Host Factors in Human Malignant Melanoma. Lancet **1967 b II**, 921—922.

LEWIS, M. G.: Malignant Melanoma in Uganda. (A Dissertation presented for the Degree of Doctor of Medicine of the University of London. January, 1968.) M. D. Thesis, University of London, 1968.

LEWIS, M. G.: Melanoma and pigmentation of the leptomeninges in Ugandan Africans. J. clin. Path. **22**, 183—186 (1969).

Lewis, M. G., Ikonopisov, R. L., Nairn, R. C., Phillips, T. M., Hamilton-Fairly, G., Bodenham, D. C. Alexander P.: Tumour-Specific Antibodies in Human Malignant Melanoma and their Relationship to the extent of the Disease. Brit. med. J. 3, 547—552 (1969).

Lewis, M. G., Johnson, K.: The Incidence and Distribution of Pigmented Naevi in Ugandan Africans. Brit. J. Derm. 80, 362—366 (1968).

Lewis, M. G., Kiryabwire, J. W. M.: Aspects of behaviour and natural history of malignant melanoma in Uganda. Cancer (Philad.) 21, 816—881 (1968 a).

Lewis, M. G., Kiryabwire, J. W. M.: Differential Diagnosis of Malignant Melanoma of Feet in Uganda. Brit. J. Surg. 55, 207—211 (1968 b).

Lewis, M. G., Martin, J. A. M.: Malignant melanoma of the nasal cavity in Ugandan Africans. Relationship to ectopic pigmentation. Cancer (Philad.) 20, 1699—1705 (1967).

Lewis, T. L. T.: Progress in Clinical Obstetrics and Gynaecology 2nd edition. London: Churchill 1965.

Liang, P. C., Tung, C.: Morphologic study and etiology of primary liver carcinoma and its incidence in China. Chin. med. J. 79, 336—347 (1959).

Lichtiger, B., Mackay, B., Tessmer, C. F.: Spindle cell variant of squamous carcinoma. Cancer (Philad.) 26, 1311—1320 (1970).

Des Ligneris, M. J. A.: Tumours in Northern Transvaal. J. med. Ass. S. Afr. 1, 102 (1927).

Linden, G., Dunn, J. E., Jr., Arellano, M. G.: Cancer in Alameda County California. See Doll, Muir and Waterhouse 1970.

Linsell, C. A.: Nasopharyngeal cancer in Kenya (Pathology). Brit. J. Cancer 18, 49—51 (1966).

Linsell, C. A., Martyn, R.: The Kenya Cancer Registry. E. Afr. med. J. 39, 642—648 (1962).

Linsell, C. A., Peers, F. G.: Personal communication, 1972.

Livingstone, R. G.: Primary carcinoma of the vagina. Springfield: Charles C. Thomas 1950.

Lofgren, K. A., Dockerty, M. B.: Primary carcinoma of the Fallopian Tube. Surg. Gynec. Obstet. 82, 199—206 (1946).

Long, M. E., Taylor, H. C.: Endometrial carcinoma of the ovary. Amer. J. Obstet. Gynec. 90, 936—950 (1964).

Lopez, A., Crawford, M. A.: Aflatoxin content of groundnuts sold for human consumption in Uganda. Lancet 2, 1351 (1967).

Lothe, F.: Kaposi's Sarcoma in Uganda Africans. Acta path. microbiol. scand., Suppl. 161 (1963).

Lothe, F.: Leukaemia in Uganda. Trop. geogr. Med. 19, 163—171 (1967).

Low, G. C., Castellani, A.: Sleeping Sickness Commission Reports. No. 4. Royal Society. London 1903.

Lowe, C. R., MacMahon, B.: Breast cancer and reproductive history of women in South Wales. Lancet 1970 I, 153—156.

Lowenthal, M. N., Hutt, M. S. R.: Serial Liver Biopsies in Big Spleen Disease. E. Afr. med. J. 45, 100—111 (1968).

Lukes, R. J., Butler, J. J.: The pathology and nomenclature of Hodgkin's disease. Cancer Res. 26, 1063—1081 (1966).

Lumb, G., Newton, K. A.: Prognosis in tumours of lymphoid tissue. An analysis of 602 cases. Cancer (Philad.) 10, 976—993 (1960).

Lynch, J. B., Verzin, J. A., Hassan, A. M.: Cancer of the female genital tract amongst the Sudanese. J. Obstet. Gynaec. Brit. Cwlth. 70, 495—504 (1963).

Lyon, F. A., Senykin, M. B., Mickelvey, J. L.: Granulosa cell tumours of the ovary. Obstet. and Gynec. 21, 67—74 (1963).

MacDonald, E. J.: Malignant Melanoma among Negroes and Latin Americans in Texas. In: Pigment Cell Biology, p. 171—181. Ed.: Gordon, M. New York: Acad. Sci. Press 1959.

MacFarlane, K. T.: Sarcoma of the uterus: an analysis of 42 cases. Amer. J. Obstet. Gynec. 59, 1304—1316 (1950).

MacKenzie, A. R., Whitmore, W. F. J., Melamed, M. R.: Myosarcomas of the bladder and prostate. Cancer (Philad.) 22, 833—844 (1968).

MacMahon, B., Cole, P., Brown, J. B., Aoki, K.: Oestrogen profiles of Asian and North American Women. Lancet 1971 II, 900—902.

MacMahon, B., Cole, P., Lin, T. M., Lowe, C. R., Mirra, A. P.: Age at First Birth and Breast Cancer Risk. Bull. Wld. Hlth Org. **43**, 209—221 (1970).

McMaster, D. N.: A subsistence crop geography of Uganda. Bude (England): Geographical Publications Ltd. 1962.

Madden, S.: Chorioepithelioma of the Fallopian Tube. J. Obstet. Gynec. Brit. Emp. **57**, 68—70 (1950).

Magee, P. N.: Liver carcinogens in the human environment. In: Liver Cancer. I.A.R.C. Scientific Publications No. 1, p. 110, Lyon 1971.

Malhotra, S. L.: A study of carcinoma of the uterine cervix with special reference to causation and prevention. Brit. J. Cancer **15**, 62—71 (1971).

Malkasian, G. D., Dockerty, M. B., Symmonds, R. E.: Benign cystic teratomas. Obstet. and Gynec. **29**, 719—725 (1967).

Marneffe, J.: Tumours malignes O.R.L. et maxillo-faciales an Ruanda Urundi. Ann. Soc. belge Méd. trop. **38**, 681—696 (1958).

Marsden, H. B., Steward, J. K. (Eds.): Tumours in Children. Springer 1968, 347 pp.

Marsden, P. D., Hutt, M. S. R., Wilks, N. E., Voller, A., Blackman, V., Shah, K. K., Connor, D. H., Hamilton, P. J. S., Banwell, J. G., Lunn, H. F.: An investigation of tropical splenomegaly at Mulago Hospital, Kampala, Uganda. Brit. Med. J. **1**, 89—92 (1965).

Martin, J. A. M.: Cancer of the nose, throat and ear in Uganda. In: Cancer in Africa, 1967, pp. 287—293. Eds.: Clifford, P., Linsell, C. A., Timms, G. L. Nairobi: East African Publishing House.

Martinez, I.: Relationship of Squamous Cell Carcinoma of the Cervix Uteri to Squamous Cell Carcinoma of the Penis among Puerto Rican women married to men with penile carcinoma. Cancer (Philad.) **24**, 777—780 (1969).

Masseyeff, R., Sankale, M., Onde, M. et al.: Valeur de la recherche de l'alpha foetoproteine serique pour le diagnostic du cancer primitif du foie. Bull. Soc. méd. Afr. noire Langue franç. **13**, 537 (1969).

Matas, R.: Surgical Peculiarities in the Negro. Trans. Amer. surg. Ass. **14**, 483—610 (1896).

Maynard, E. P., Sadikali, F., Anthony, P. P., Barker, L. F.: Hepatitis-associated antigen and cirrhosis in Uganda. Lancet **1970 II**, 1326—1328.

McGlashan, N. D., Walters, C. L., McLean, A. E. M.: Nitrosamines in African alcoholic spirits and oesophageal cancer. Lancet **1968 II**, 1017.

McIntosh, J. F., Worley, G., Jr.: Adenocarcinoma arising in exstrophy of bladder: report of 2 cases and review of literature. J. Urol. (Baltimore) **73**, 820—829 (1955).

Medical Services Statistical Records: 1962—63 and 1968—69. Ministry of Health, Uganda.

Melamed, M. R., Koss, L. G., Flehinger, B. J., Kelisky, R. P., Dubrow, H.: Prevalence rates of uterine cervical carcinoma in situ for females using the diaphragm or contraceptive oral steroids. Brit. med. J. **3**, 195—200 (1969).

Middlebrook, L. F., Tennant, R.: Rhabdomyosarcoma of the uterine corpus. Obstet. and Gynec. **32**, 537—542 (1968).

Miller, R. W.: Relation Between Cancer and Congenital Defects: An Epidemiologic Evaluation. J. nat. Cancer Inst. **40**, 1079—1085 (1968).

Morris, G. C., Horn, R. C.: Malignant Melanoma in the Negro. Surgery **29**, 223—230 (1951).

Morrow, R. H., Pike, M. C., Smith, P. G., Ziegler, J. L., Kisuule, A.: Burkitt's Lymphoma: A time-space cluster of cases in Bwamba County of Uganda. Brit. med. J. **1**, 491—492 (1971).

Morrow, R. H., Smetana, H. F., Sai, F. T., Edgcomb, J. H.: Unusual features of viral hepatitis. Ann. intern. Med. **68**, 1250 (1968).

Morson, B. C.: The pathology and results of treatment of squamous cell carcinoma of the anal region. Ch. 7. In: Cancer of the Rectum. Ed.: Dukes, C. E. Edinburgh and London: Livingstone 1960.

Morson, B. C.: Precancerous conditions of the large bowel. Proc. roy. Soc. Med. **64**, 959—962 (1971).

Morson, B. C., Pang, L. S. C.: Rectal biopsy as an aid to cancer control in ulcerative colitis. Gut **8**, 423—434 (1967).

MORTON, D. G.: Ovarian Carcinoma. Amer. J. Obstet. Gynec. 95, 359—361 (1966).

MOSTOFI, F. K.: Pathological aspects and spread of carcinoma of the bladder. J. Amer. med. Ass. 206, 1764—1769 (1968).

MOVSAS, S.: Prostatic obstruction in the African and Asiatic. Brit. J. Surg. 53, 538—543 (1966).

MUELLER, C. W., TOPKINS, P., LAPP, W. A.: Dysgerminoma of the ovary. Amer. J. Obstet. Gynec. 60, 153—159 (1950).

MUELLING, R. J., JR., BURDETTE, W. J.: A Comparative Study of Malignant Melanoma among Negro and White Patients. Zoologica 35, 12—13 (1950).

MUIR GRIEVE, J.: Cancer Incidence in Cape Province. See DOLL, MUIR and WATERHOUSE (1970)

MUNOZ, N., ASVALL, J.: Time trends of Intestinal and diffuse types of gastric cancer in Norway. Int. J. Cancer 8, 144—157 (1971).

MUNOZ, N., CONNELLY, R.: Time trends of intestinal and diffuse types of gastric cancer in the United States. Int. J. Cancer 8, 158—164 (1971).

MUNOZ, N., CORREA, P., CUELLO, C., DUQUE, E.: Histologic types of gastric carcinoma in high-risk and low-risk areas. Int. J. Cancer 3, 809—818 (1968).

MURRAY, H. R.: Characteristics of human Schwann cells in vitro. Anat. Rec. 84, 275—285 (1942).

MURRAY, J. F.: Editor, Symposium on Tumors of the Alimentary Tract in Africans. Nat. Cancer Inst. Monogr. 25 (1967).

MUWAZI, E. M. K., TROWELL, H. C.: Neurological disease among African natives of Uganda. A review of 269 cases. E. Afr. med. J. 21, 2—19 (1944).

NASR, A. LOTFY ABOUL: Epidemiology of Cancer of the Gastrointestinal Tract in Egyptians. In: Tumours of the Alimentary Tract in Africans. Nat. Cancer Inst. Monogr. 25, 1—6 (1967).

NEFZGER, M. D., CHALMERS, T. C.: The treatment of acute infectious hepatitis. Amer. J. Med. 35, 299—309 (1963).

NEWBERNE, P. M., BUTLER, W. H.: Acute and chronic effects of aflatoxin on the liver of domestic and laboratory animals: a review. Cancer Res. 29, 236—250 (1969).

NOVAK, E., WOODRUFF, J. D.: Gynecologic and Obstetric Pathology, 5th ed. Philadelphia: Saunders 1962.

OBERLING, C., RIVIÈRE, M., HAGUENAU, F.: Ultrastructure of the clear cells in renal carcinomas and its importance for the demonstration of their renal origin. Nature (Lond.) 186, 402—403 (1960).

O'CONOR, G. T.: Malignant lymphoma in African children. 2. A pathological entity. Cancer (Philad.) 14, 270—283 (1961).

O'CONOR, G. T.: Persistent Immunologic Stimulations as a Factor in Oncogenesis, with special reference to Burkitt's tumor. Amer. J. Med. 48, 279—285 (1970).

O'CONOR, G. T., DAVIES, J. N. P.: Malignant tumors in African children: with special reference to malignant lymphoma. J. Pediat. 56, 526—535 (1960).

O'CONOR, G. T., TATARINOV, Y. S., ABELEV, G. I., URIEL, J.: A collaborative study for the evaluation of a serologic test for primary liver cancer. Cancer (Philad.) 25, 1091 (1970).

ODEKU, E. L., JANOTA, I.: Intracranial masses — Ibadan. W. Afr. med. J. 16, 31—42 (1967).

OETTLÉ, A. G.: Problems of research into diseases of the Bantu. S. Afr. J. Lab. clin. Med. 1, 57—79 (1955).

OETTLÉ, A. G.: Geographical and racial differences in the frequency of Kaposi's sarcoma as evidence of environmental or genetic causes. Acta Un. int. Cancr. 18, 330—363 (1962).

OETTLÉ, A. G.: Regional variations in the frequency of Bantu oesophageal cancer cases admitted to hospitals in South Africa. S. Afr. med. J. 37, 434—439 (1963 a).

OETTLÉ, A. G.: Skin cancer in Africa. In: Conference on Biology of Cutaneous Cancer (Ed.: URBACH, F.), p. 197. Nat. Cancer Inst. Monogr. 10, N.I.H., Bethesda (1963 b).

OETTLÉ, A. G.: Primary malignant neoplasms of the lymphoreticular tissues (200—203, 205): A histopathological series from white and Bantu races in the Transvaal, 1949—1953. Symposium on Lymphoreticular Tumours in Africa, Paris, 1963. Ed.: ROULET, F. C. Basel-New York: Karger 1964, pp. 24—35.

OETTLÉ, A. G.: Cancer in Africa, especially in regions south of the Sahara. J. nat. Cancer Inst. 33, 383—439 (1964 b).

OETTLÉ, A. G.: Primary Neoplasms of the Alimentary Canal in Whites and Bantu of the Transvaal, 1949—1953. A histopathological series. p. 97—109. In: Tumours of the Alimentary Tract in Africans. Nat. Cancer Inst. **25** (1967).

OJIAMBO, H. P.: Neurological disease at Kenyatta Hospital Nairobi. A retrospective study of 75 cases. E. Afr. med. J. **43**, 366—376 (1966).

OLWENY, C. L. M., ZIEGLER, J. L., BERARD, C. W., TEMPLETON, A. C.: Adult Hodgkin's disease in Uganda. Cancer (Philad.) **27**, 1295—1301 (1971).

OWOR, R.: Gallstones in Ugandan Africans. E. Afr. med. **41**, 251 (1964).

OWOR, R.: The pathology of chronic pancreatic disease. Thesis submitted for M. D. (E. A.), Makerere University Medical School, Kampala, 1970.

PACK, G. T.: Clinical Study of Pigmented Nevi and Melanomas. Biology of Melanomas. Ann. N. J. Acad. Sci. **4**, 52 (1948).

PACK, G. T., ARIEL, I. M.: Tumors of the Soft Somatic Tissues. London: Cassel & Co. Ltd. 1958.

PACK, G. T., MILLER, T. R.: Metastatic Melanoma with Indeterminate Primary Site (Report of two instances of long term survival). J. Amer. med. Ass. **176**, 55—56 (1961).

PALMER, J. P., SADUGOR, M. G., REINHARD, M. C.: Carcinoma of the vulva: a report of 313 cases. Surg. Gyn. Obstet. **88**, 435—440 (1949).

PARK, W. W.: In: Choriocarcinoma. See HOLLAND and HRESHCHYSHYN. The Pathology of Trophoblastic Tumours. 1967.

PARLICA, D., SAMUEL, I.: Primary carcinoma of the liver in Ethiopia. Brit. J. Cancer **24**, 22 —29 (1970).

PATEY, D. H., SCARFF, R. W.: The position of histology in the prognosis of carcinoma of the breast. Lancet **1928 I**, 801—804.

PAUTRIER, L. M., DISS, A.: Kaposi's idiopathic sarcoma is not a genuine sarcoma but a neuro-vascular dysgenesis. Brit. J. Derm. **41**, 93—105 (1929).

PAYET, M.: African cirrhosis in relation to primitive cancer of the liver. Acta Un. int. Cancr. **13**, 712. Primary cancer of the liver; statistical, anatomical and etiological considerations. Acta Un. int. Cancr. **13**, 860. Les orientations dans la recherche dans l'etude du cancer primitif du Foie. Acta Un. int. Cancr. **13**, 956 (1957).

PAYET, M.: Schistosomiasis and cancer of the urinary bladder in Senegal. 11. Mortality and morbidity from bladder cancer in West Africa. Acta Un. int. Cancr. **18**, 641 (1962).

PAYLING WRIGHT, G., SYMMERS, W. ST. C.: Systemic Pathology, Vol. I. 1st ed. London: Longmans 1966.

PELLAKALLIO, P., KALIMA, T. V.: Malignant tumours of the male breast in Finland. Brit. J. Cancer **23**, 480—487 (1969).

PELLER, S.: The function of circulatory organs in the genesis and distribution of primary cancers in man. Angiology **16**, 114—120 (1965).

PERSAUD, V., KNIGHT, L. P.: Carcinoma of the body of the uterus in Jamaica. W. Indian med. J. **14**, 42—51 (1968).

PETERSON, W. F., PREVOST, E. C., EDMUNDS, F. T., HUNDLEY, J. M., MORRIS, F. K.: Benign cystic teratomas of the ovary. Amer. J. Obstet. Gynec. **70**, 368—382 (1955).

PIKE, M. C., WILLIAMS, E. H., WRIGHT, BARBARA: Burkitt's tumour in the West Nile District of Uganda 1961—1965. Brit. med. J. **2**, 395—399 (1967).

POLTERA, A. A., TEMPLETON, A. C.: Intracranial tuberculosis in Uganda. A postmortem Survey. (Presented at the Pan African Symposium on Tumours of the Central Nervous System in the African, Nairobi, January 1972.) African J. med. Sci. (in press).

POPOV, L.: Medical study of goitre in Ethiopia. Ethiopian Med. J. **6**, 5—14 (1967).

PRATES, M. D.: Malignant neoplasms in Mozambique. A frequency ratio study from 1944—1957 and a comparison with other parts of Africa. Brit. J. Cancer **12**, 177—194 (1958).

PRATES, M. D.: The rates of cancer of the bladder in the Portuguese East African of Lourenço Marques. Acta Un. int. Cancr. **18**, 643—647 (1962).

PRATES, M. D., GILLMAN, J.: Carcinoma of the urinary bladder in the Portuguese East Africans with special ref. to bilharzial cystitis and preneoplastic reactions. S. Afr. J. med. Sci. **24**, 13—40 (1959).

PRATES, M. D., TORRES, F. O.: A cancer survey in Lourenço Marques, Portuguese East Africa. J. nat. Cancer Inst. **35**, 729—757 (1965).

PRINCE, A. M.: Relation of Australia and SH antigens. Lancet 1968 II, 462.

PRINCE, A. M.: Prevalence of serum-hepatitis-related antigen (SH) in different geographic regions. Amer. J. trop. Med. Hyg. 19, 872—879 (1970).

PRINCE, A. M.: Role of viruses in chronic liver disease in man and animals. In: Liver Cancer. I.A.R.C. Scientific Publications No. 1, p. 51, Lyon 1971.

PUGH, R.: In: Tumours of the bladder. Ed. WALLACE, D. M. Edinburgh and London: Livingstone 1959.

PURCHASE, I. F. H., VAN DER WATT, J. J.: Carcinogenicity of sterigmatocystin. Food Cosmet. Toxic. 6, 555 (1968).

PURVES, L. R., BERSOHN, I., GEDDES, E. W.: Serum alpha-feto-protein and primary cancer of the liver in man. Cancer (Philad.) 25, 1261—1270 (1970).

QUÉRÉ, M. A., BASSET, A., CAMAIN, R.: Les localisations oculaires de l'angioreticulosarcomatose de Kaposi. Ophthalmologica (Basel) 146, 23—33 (1963).

QUÉRÉ, M. A., CAMAIN, R., LAMBERT, D.: In: The pathology of orbito-ocular tumors in tropical African. Klin. Mbl. Augenheilk. 144, 829—840 (1964).

RAPER, A. B., ELMER, B. G. T., MUSOKE, L. K.: Cancer of the lung in Africans. A report of 6 autopsies. E. Afr. med. J. 29, 433—437 (1952).

RAPPAPORT, H.: The histologic aspects of malignant lymphoreticular neoplasms. Symposium on Lymphoreticular Tumours in Africa, Paris, 1963. Ed.: ROULET, F. C. Basel-New York: Karger 1964, pp. 174—210.

RAPPAPORT, H.: Tumors of the Hemato-poietic System. Washington, D. C. Armed Forces Institute of Pathology, 1966.

RAPPAPORT, H., WINTER, W. J., HICKS, E. B.: Follicular lymphoma: A re-evaluation of its position in the scheme of malignant lymphoma, based on a survey of 253 cases. Cancer (Philad.) 9, 792—821 (1956).

RAVEN, R. W.: Medical Progress. Brit. Encyclopaedia of Med. Practice. Ed.: Lord COHEN. London: Butterworth's press 1966.

RAWLS, W. E., TOMPKINS, W. A. F., MELNICK, J. L.: The Association of Herpes virus Type 2 and Carcinoma of the Uterine Cervix. Amer. J. Epidem. 89, 547—554 (1969).

REDDY, D. B., GANAPATHY, M. N., REDDY, D. J.: Malignant Melanoma and Allied Tumours. Indian J. Surg. 16, 308—323 (1954).

REESE, A. B.: Tumours of the Eye. New York: Paul B. Hoeber, 2nd ed. 1963.

REESE, A. J. M., WINSTANLEY, D. P.: The small tumour-like lesions of the kidney. Brit. J. Cancer 12, 507 (1958).

REYE, R. D. K.: A consideration of certain subdermal "fibromatous tumours" of infancy. J. Path. Bact. 72, 149—154 (1956).

REYNAUD, J., BEL, J., LY, B.: Les adamantinomes chez l'African. Bull. Soc. méd. Afr. noire Langue franç. 6, 352—359 (1961).

REYNAUD, J., LY, B.: "Tumeurs fibreuses" et fibromes osteogeniques des maxillaires. Bull. Soc. méd. Afr. noire Langue franç. 6, 466—470 (1961).

RICHARDSON, I. M.: Prostatic cancer and social class. Brit. J. prev. soc. Med. 19, 140—142 (1965).

RICHES, E. R.: Prostatic obstruction: the treatment of associated conditions. Proc. roy. Soc. Med. 55, 744—746 (1962).

RIOPELLE, J. L., THÉRIOULT, J. P.: Sur une forme méconnue de sarcome des parties molles: Le rhabdomyosarcome alvéolaire. Ann. Anat. path. 1, 88—111 (1956).

ROBB-SMITH, A. H. T.: Reticulosis and reticulosarcoma: Histological classification. J. Path. Bact. 47, 458—480 (1938).

ROBERTSON, M. A., HARINGTON, J. S., BRADSHAW, E.: The cancer pattern in Africans at Baragwanath Hospital, Johannesburg. Brit. J. Cancer 25, 377—384 (1971).

ROBSON, M. C.: Incidence of benign prostatic hyperplasia and prostatic carcinoma in cirrhosis of liver. J. Urol. (Baltimore) 92, 307—310 (1964).

ROMERO, L., METH, V.: Endonasal lymphoma of Weiss. Derm. ibero lat.-amer. 5, 61—79 (1970).

ROSE, R. J.: Cancer in New Zealand. See: DOLL et al., 1970.

ROSENBERG, S. A., DIAMOND, H. D., CRAVER, L. F.: Lymphosarcoma, survival and the effects of therapy. Amer. J. Roentgenol. 85, 521—532 (1961).

Ross, M. D.: Tumours in Mashonaland Africans. Cent. Afr. J. Med. **13**, 107—116 and 139—145 (1967).

Rouhani, A.: Kaposi's sarcoma. The first case observed in Afghanistan. Lyon. méd. **216**, 194—195 (1966).

Russell, W. O., Wynne, E. S., Loquvam, G. S.: Studies in bovine ocular squamous carcinoma (Cancer Eye). I. Pathological anatomy and his torical review. Cancer (Philad.) **9**, 1—52 (1956).

Sagoe, A. S.: Tropical splenomegaly syndrome. Long term Proguanil therapy correlated with spleen size, serum IgM and lymphocyte transformation. Brit. med. J. **3**, 378—382 (1970).

Sall, S., Sonnenblick, B., Stone, M. L.: Factors affecting survival of females with endometrial adenocarcinoma. Amer. J. Obstet Gynec. **107**, 116—123 (1970).

Saxen, E. A., Saxen, L. O.: Mortality from thyroid diseases in an endemic goitre area. Studies in Finland. Docum. Med. geogr. trop. (Amst.) **6**, 335—341 (1954).

Scheuer, P. J.: Pathogenesis and morbid anatomy of human primary liver cancer. In: Liver Cancer. I.A.R.C. Scientific Publications No. 1, p. 13, Lyon, 1971.

Schiffner, M. A., Mackles, A., Wolf, S. A.: Reappraisal of the diagnosis in Uterine Sarcoma. Amer. J. Obstet. Gynec. **70**, 521 (1955).

Schmauz, R., Jain, D. K.: Geographical variation of carcinoma of the Penis in Uganda. Brit. J. Cancer **25**, 25—32 (1971).

Schmauz, R., Templeton, A. C.: Nasopharyngeal carcinoma in Uganda. Cancer (Philad.) **29**, 610—621 (1972).

Schoental, R.: Toxicology and carcinogenic action of pyrrolizidine alkaloids. Canad. J. Res. E. **28**, 2237 (1968).

Schonland, M., Bradshaw, E.: Cancer in the Natal African and Indian, 1964—1966. Int. J. Cancer **3**, 304—316 (1968).

Schonland, M. M.: Cancer Incidence in Natal. See Doll et al., 1970.

Scott, J. S.: Choriocarcinoma. Observations on the etiology. Amer. J. Obstet. Gynec. **83**, 185—193 (1963).

Scoville, A. de: A propos des tumeurs maxillofacides dans la race noire. Ann. Soc. belge Méd. trop. **44**, 983—988 (1964).

Segi, M., Kurihara, M.: Cancer mortality for selected sites in 24 countries, 1960—1961. Tohoku Univ. Sch. Med., Sendai, Japan, 1964.

Segi, M., Kurihara, M.: Cancer mortality for selected sites in 24 countries, 1962—1963. Tohoku University School of Medicine, Sendai, Japan. 1966.

Sequeira, J. H., Vint, F. W.: Malignant Melanoma in Africans. Brit. J. Derm. **46**, 361—367 (1934).

Serck-Hanssen, A.: Aflatoxin induced fatal hepatitis? A case report from Uganda. Arch. environm. Hlth. **20**, 729 (1970).

Serck-Hanssen, A., Purohit, G. P.: Histiocytic medullary reticulosis. Report of 14 cases from Uganda. Brit. J. Cancer **22**, 506—516 (1968).

Shaper, A. G.: Cirrhosis and primary liver cell carcinoma in Uganda. J. trop. geogr. Med. **22**, 161 (1970).

Shaper, A. G., Patel, K. M.: Diseases of the biliary tract in Africans in Uganda. E. Afr. med. J. **41**, 246—250 (1964).

Shaper, A. G., Shaper, L. J.: Analysis of medical admissions to Mulago Hospital 1957. E. Afr. med. J. **35**, 648 (1958).

Shapiro, M. P., Keen, P., Cohen, L., de Moor, N. G.: Malignant disease in the Transvaal. II. Tumours of the musculo skeletal system; III. Cancer of the respiratory tract. S. Afr. med. J. **29**, 95—101 (1955).

Sharma, S. D., Zeigler, O., Trussell, R. R.: A cytologic study of *Dipetolenema perstans* in cervical smears. Acta cytol. (Philad.) **15**, 419—481 (1971).

Shedd, D. P., von Essen, C. F., Connelly, R. R., Eisenberg, H.: Cancer of the Buccal Mucosa, Palate and Gingiva in Connecticut, 1935—1959. Cancer (Philad.) **21**, 440—446 (1968).

Shedd, D. P., von Essen, C. F., Eisenberg, H.: Cancer of the Nasopharynx in Connecticut, 1935—1959. Cancer (Philad.) **20**, 508—511 (1967).

SHEPHERD, J. J.: Breast cancer in African women in Uganda. E. Afr. med. J. **41**, 467 (1964).

SHEPHERD, J. J.: Tribal variation in cutaneous tumours of the leg. E. Afr. med. J. **44**, 600—602 (1966).

SHEPHERD, J. J.: Volvulus. Chapter 25. In: Companion to Surgery in Africa by DAVEY, W. W. Edinburgh and London: Livingstone 1968.

SHEPHERD, J. J., MANTHY, I. A.: Thyroid carcinoma in Uganda. E. Afr. med. J. **40**, 445—447 (1963).

SHEPHERD, J. J., WRIGHT, D. H.: Burkitt's tumour presenting as bilateral swelling of the breast in women of childbearing age. Brit. J. Surg. **54**, 776—780 (1967).

SIMONS, J. N., BEAHRS, O. H., WOOLNER, L. B.: Tumors of the Submaxillary Gland. Amer. J. Surg. **108**, 485—494 (1964).

SIMONS, M. J., YU, M., CHEW, B. K., TAN, A. Y. O., YAP, Y. E. H., SEAH, C. S., FUNG, W. P., SHANMUGARATNAM, K.: Australia antigen in Singapore Chinese patients with hepato-cellular carcinoma. Lancet **1971 I**, 1149.

SINGH, P., COOK, J.: Tumours of the jaws. E. Afr. med. J. **33**, 383—390 (1956).

SINGH, S. P., MARTINSON, F. D.: Malignant Diseases of the Paranasal Sinuses in Nigeria. J. Laryng. **83**, 239—250 (1969).

SIRSAT, M. V.: Malignant Melanoma of the Skin in Indians. Indian J. med. Sci. **6**, 806—813 (1952).

SIRSAT, M. V.: Malignant Melanoma in Indians. A Review of 60 Cases. Indian J. med. Sci. **10**, 629—638 (1956).

SKINNER, M. E. G.: Malignant disease of the gastro-intestinal tract in the Rhodesian African. Nat. Cancer Inst. Monogr. **25**, 57—72 (1967).

SKINNER, M. E. G.: Cancer Incidence in Rhodesia. See DOLL et al., 1970.

SLAVIN, G., CAMERON, H. M.: Ameloblastomas in Africans from Tanzania and Uganda. A report of 56 cases. Brit. J. Cancer **23**, 31—38 (1969).

SLAVIN, G., CAMERON, H. M., FORBES, C., MORTON MITCHELL, R.: Kaposi's sarcoma in East African Children. A report of 51 cases. J. Path. Bact. **100**, 187—199 (1970).

SMALBRAAK, J.: Trophoblastic growths: a clinical, hormonal and histopathologic study of hydatidiform mole and chorioepithelioma. Amsterdam: Elsevier 1957.

SMITH, E. C., ELMES, B. G. T.: Malignant Disease in Natives of Nigeria: an analysis of 500 tumours. Ann. trop. Med. Parasit. **28**, 461—476 (1934).

SMITH, J. L., JR., STEHLIN, J. S., JR.: Spontaneous Regression of Primary Malignant Melanoma with Regional Metastases. Cancer (Philad.) **18**, 1399—1415 (1965).

SMITH, P.: Choriocarcinoma in Uganda. A case for active prophylaxis. Aust. N. Z. J. Obstet. Gynaec. **10**, 109—111 (1970).

SMITH, R., WOLFE, L. G.: Kaposi's sarcoma: electron microscopic and tissue culture studies. Abstr. 85, Amer. Ass. Pathologists and Bacteriologists, 67th Annual Meeting, St. Louis, Mo., March 7—10, 1970.

SOBIN, L. H.: Cancer in Afghanistan. Cancer (Philad.) **23**, 678—688 (1969).

SOEJOENOES, A., DJOJOPRANOTO, M., POEN, H. T.: Observation of some aspects of Hydatidi-form Mole and Choriocarcinoma in Indonesia, p. 58. In: Choriocarcinoma (see HOLLAND) 1967.

SOMMERS, S. C.: Endocrine changes with prostatic carcinoma. Cancer (Philad.) **10**, 345—358 (1957).

SOMMERS, S. C.: Pulmonary emphysema, healed myocardial infarcts and other disease correlations with male breast structure. Amer. J. med. Sci. **248**, 341—344 (1964).

SOOD, V., HULLEY, G., HUTT, M. S. R.: Viral hepatitis in Karamoja. Makerere med. J. **10**, 46 (1966).

SOULE, E. H., GEITZ, M., HENDERSON, E. D.: Embryonal rhabdomyosarcoma of the limbs and limb girdles. A clinicopathologic study of 61 cases. Cancer (Philad.) **23**, 1336—1346 (1968).

Statistical Abstract, 1969: Statistics Division, Ministry of Planning and Economic Development. Entebbe: Government Printer 1969.

STEINER, P. E.: Cancer, Race and Geography. Baltimore: Williams, Wilkins 1954.

STEINER, P. E.: Carcinoma of the liver in the United States. Acta Un. int. Cancr. **13**, 628 (1957).

STEINER, P. E.: Cancer of the liver and cirrhosis in Trans-Saharan Africa and the United States of America. Cancer (Philad.) **13**, 1085 (1960).

STEINITZ, R.: Cancer Incidence in Israel, 1970. See DOLL et al. (1970).

STERN, E., DIXON, W. J.: Cancer of the Cervix — A biometric approach to Etiology. Cancer (Philad.) **14**, 153—160 (1961).

STEVENSON, W. H. D.: Malignant Melanomata, especially those occurring on the Heel and the Sole of the Foot. Indian J. med. Res. **3**, 166—179 (1925).

STEWART, H. L.: In: Primary Hepatoma. Ed.: BURDETTE, W. J. Univ. of Utah Press 1965.

STEWART, H. L.: Experimental Alimentary Tract Cancer, p. 199—217. In: Tumors of the Alimentary Tract in Africans. Ed.: MURRAY, J. F. Nat. Cancer Inst. Monogr. **25** (1967).

STOLL, H. C., MARCHETTA, F. C., SCHOBINGER, R.: Malignant epithelial tumors of the mandible and maxilla. Arch. Path. **64**, 239—244 (1957).

STOUT, A. P.: Solitary cutaneous and subcutaneous leiomyomata. Amer. J. Cancer **29**, 435—469 (1937).

STOUT, A. P.: Bizarre smooth muscle tumours of the stomach. Cancer (Philad.) **15**, 400 (1962).

STOUT, A. P., HILL, W. T.: Leiomyosarcoma of the superficial soft tissues. Cancer (Philad.) **11**, 844 (1958).

SVOBODA, D. J., KIRCHNER, F. R., SHANMUGARATNAM, K.: The Fine Structure of Nasopharyngeal Carcinoma. In: Cancer of the Nasopharynx. Eds.: MUIR, C. S., SHANMUGARATNAM, K. Copenhagen: Munksgaard. Un. int. Cancr. Monogr. **1**, 163—171 (1967).

SYMINGTON, T.: Functional pathology of the human adrenal gland. Edinburgh: Livingstone 1969.

SYMMERS, W. ST. C.: Primary malignant diseases of the lymphoreticular system. Cancer. Ed.: RAVEN, R. W., Vol. 2. London: Butterworth 1958, pp. 448—483.

SYMMERS, W. ST. C.: Survey of the eventual diagnosis in 600 cases referred for a second histological opinion after an initial biopsy diagnosis of Hodgkin's disease. J. clin. Path. **21**, 650—653 (1968 a).

SYMMERS, W. ST. C.: Survey of the eventual diagnosis in 226 cases referred for a second histological opinion after an initial biopsy diagnosis of reticulum cell sarcoma. J. clin. Path. **21**, 654—655 (1968 b).

TATARINOV, Y. S.: Embryospecific beta globulin in liver cell carcinoma. Vop. med. Khim. **11**, 20 (1965).

TAYLOR, J. F., TEMPLETON, A. C., LUBEGA, A.: Kaposi's sarcoma in pregnancy. Brit. J. Surg. **58**, 577—579 (1971 b).

TAYLOR, J. F., TEMPLETON, A. C., VOGEL, C. L., ZIEGLER J. C., KYALWAZI, S. K.: Kaposi's sarcoma in Uganda: A clinico-pathological Study. Int. J. Cancer **8**, 122—135 (1971 a).

TEMPLETON, A. C.: Tumours of the Eye and Adnexa in Africans of Uganda. Cancer (Philad.) **20**, 1689—1698 (1967 a).

TEMPLETON, A. C.: Phaeochromocytoma in East Africa. E. Afr. Med. J. **44**, 271—277 (1967 b).

TEMPLETON, A. C.: Orbital Tumours in African Children. Brit. J. Ophthal. **55**, 254—261 (1971).

TEMPLETON, A. C.: Cutaneous leiomyoma, a neglected entity. E. Afr. med. J. **49**, 521 (1972 a).

TEMPLETON, A. C.: Superficial vascular tumours in Ugandan Africans, the relationship to Kaposi's sarcoma. In preparation (1972 b).

TEMPLETON, A. C.: Studies in Kaposi's sarcoma. I. Post-mortem observations. 2. Disease patterns in females. Cancer **30**, 854—867 (1972 c).

TEMPLETON, A. C.: Testicular tumours in Ugandan Africans. African Journal of Medical Sciences **3**, 157—161 (1972).

TEMPLETON, A. C.: Kaposi's sarcoma. In: Cancer of the Skin. Ed.: ANDRADE, G. New York: Saunders, in press (1973).

TEMPLETON, A. C., BIANCHI, A.: Bias in an African Cancer Registry. Int. J. Cancer **10**, 186—193 (1972 a).

TEMPLETON, A. C., BIANCHI, A.: How much Cancer is there in Uganda. E. Afr. med. J., in press (1972 b).

TEMPLETON, A. C., BUXTON, E., BIANCHI, A.: Cancer in Kyadondo County, Uganda 1968—
1970. J. nat. Cancer Inst. 48, 865—874 (1972).

TEMPLETON A. C., HUTT, M. S. R., DODGE, O. G.: Cryptogenic Metastases in Uganda Africans. J. Bone Jt Surg. 54 B, 125—129 (1972).

TEMPLETON, A. C., SCHMAUZ, R.: Cervical Lymphadenopathy in Ugandans. E. Afr. med. J.
47, 1—6 (1970).

TEMPLETON, A. C., VIEGAS, O. A. C.: Racial Variations in Tumour Incidence in Uganda.
Trop. geogr. Med. 22, 431—438 (1970).

TEN SELDAN, R. E. J.: Skin cancer in Australia. In: Conference on Biology of Cutaneous
Cancer. Ed.: URBACH, F. p. 153. Nat. Cancer Inst. Monogr. 10, N.I.H. Bethesda, 1963.

TESTU, J., RICHIR, C., GOUDOTE, E.: Un cas africain de tumeur d'Ewing. Bull. Soc. méd. Afr.
noire Langue franç. 8, 644—648 (1963).

THACKRAY, A. C.: Histological classification of rodent ulcers and its bearing on their prognosis. Brit. J. Cancer 5, 213—224 (1951).

THIJS, A.: L'angiosarcomatose de Kaposi au Congo belge et au Ruanda Urundi. Ann. Soc.
belge Méd. trop. 37, 295—307 (1957).

THORBJARNASON, B.: Sarcomata at New York Hospital. Arch. Surg. 82, 489—510 (1961).

THYS, A.: Considérations sur les tumeurs malignes des indigènes du Congo belge et du Ruanda-
Urundi Apropos de 2536 cas. Ann. Soc. belge Méd. trop. 37, 483—514 (1957).

TICHO, U., BEN SIRA, L.: Clinical and Pathologic correlation of non-pigmented tumors of the
conjunctiva and pingueculae among Africans. Amer. J. Ophthal. 70, 757—763 (1970).

TJALMA, R. A.: Canine bone sarcoma; estimation of relative risk as a function of body size.
J. nat. Cancer Inst. 36, 1137—1150 (1966).

TOKER, K.: Observations on the composition of certain colonic tumors. Cancer (Philad.) 24,
255—260 (1969).

TORPIN, R., PUND, E., PEEPLES, W. J.: The etiologic and pathologic factors in a series of 1241
fibromyomas of the uterus. Amer. J. Obstet. Gynec. 44, 569 (1942).

TORRES, F. O., PURCHASE, I. F. H., VAN DER WATT, J. J.: The aetiology of primary liver
cancer in the Bantu. J. Path. Bact. 102, 163 (1970).

TOUGH, I. C. K., CARTER, D. C., FRASER, J., BRUCE, J.: Histological grading in breast cancer.
Brit. J. Cancer 23, 294—301 (1969).

TROWELL, H. C.: Non-Infective Disease in Africa. London: Arnold 1960, p. 437.

TRUSSELL, R. R.: The treatment of carcinoma of the cervix by continuous intra-arterial metho-
trexate and by intermittent intramuscular leucovorin. Proc. roy. Soc. Med. 55, 759—760
(1962).

TRUSSELL, R. R.: Pelvic Inflammatory Disease. Proc. roy. Soc. Med. 61, 365—368 (1968).

TRUSSELL, R. R., GRECH, E. S., GALEA, J.: Maternal Mortality. In: Uganda Atlas of Disease
Distribution, p. 144—152. Eds.: HALL, S. A., LANGLANDS, B. W. Makerere University
College, Kampala 1968.

TULINIUS, H.: Frequency of some morphological types of neoplasm of five sites. In: Cancer
Incidence in Five Continents, Vol. II. Eds.: DOLL, R., MUIR, C. S., WATERHOUSE, J. A. H.
Geneva: Springer U.I.C.C., 1970.

UDEKWU, F. A. O., PULVERTAFT, J. V.: Studies of an aveolar soft tissue sarcoma. Brit. J.
Cancer 19, 744—748 (1965).

Uganda Atlas: Department of Lands and Survey, Kampala 1967.

Uganda Census, 1959: Statistics Branch, Ministry of Economic Affairs, Uganda. Entebbe:
Government Printer.

Uganda Census, 1969: Statistics Division, Ministry of Planning and Economic Development.
Entebbe: Government Printer.

United States Public Health Service: Smoking and Health. Public Health Service Publication 1103. Washington, D. C.: U.S. Government Printing Office 1964.

URIEL, J.: Transitory liver antigens and primary hepatoma in man and rat. In: Liver Cancer.
I.A.R.C. Scientific Publications. No. 1, p. 58. Lyon 1971.

URIEL, J., NESCHAUD, B. DE, STANISLAWSKI-BIRENSWAJG, M.: Le diagnostic du cancer primaire
du foie par des méthodes immunologiques. Presse méd. 76, 1415 (1968).

VAITHIANATHAN, T., FISHKIN, S., GRUHN, J. G.: Histiocytic medullary reticulosis. Amer. J.
clin. Path. 47, 160—166 (1967).

VANIER, T. M., PIKE, M. C.: Leukaemia incidence in tropical Africa (Letter). Lancet **1967 I**, 512—513.

VAN ZYL, J. J. W., DU TOIT, F. D., WICHT, C. L.: Phaeochromocytoma of the organ of Zucker-kandl. S. Afr. J. Surg. **4**, 43—49 (1966).

VINT, F. W.: Malignant disease in the natives of Kenya. Lancet **1935 II**, 628.

VOGEL, C. L., ANTHONY, P. P., MODY, N., BARKER, L. F.: Hepatitis-associated antigen in Ugandan patients with hepatocellular carcinoma. Lancet **1970 II**, 621.

VOGEL, C. L., ANTHONY, P. P., SADIKALI, F., BARKER, L. F., PETERSON, M. R.: Hepatitis-associated antigen and antibody in hepatocellular carcinoma. J. nat. Cancer Inst. **48**, 1583—1588 (1972 b).

VOGEL, C. L., ANTHONY, P. P., SADIKALI, F., BARKER, L. F., PETERSON, M. R.: Alpha-feto-protein and hepatocellular carcinoma in Uganda (in press 1972 a).

VOGEL, C. L., TEMPLETON, C. J., TEMPLETON, A. C., TAYLOR, J. F., KYALWAZI, S. K.: Treatment of Kaposi's sarcoma with Actinomycin D and cyclo-phosphamide. Results of a randomised clinical trial. Int. J. Cancer **8**, 136—143 (1971).

WAHNER, H. W., CUELLO, C., CORREA, P., URIBE, L. F., GAITAN, E.: Thyroid carcinoma in an endemic goitre area. Cali, Colombia. Amer. J. Med. **40**, 58—66 (1966).

WANG, D. Y., BULBROOK, R. D., CLIFFORD, P.: Plasma-testosterone levels in Kenyan men in relation to cancer of the nasopharynx. Lancet **1966 II**, 1342—1344.

WATERHOUSE, J. A. H.: Cancer Incidence in Birmingham, 1970. See DOLL et al. (1970).

WEBSTER, J. P., STEVENSON, T. W., STOUT, A. P.: The surgical treatment of malignancy of the skin. Surg. Clin. N. Amer. **24**, 319—339 (1944).

WHEELOCK, M. C., WARREN, S.: Leiomyosarcoma of the uterus. Ann. Surg. **116**, 882 (1942).

WILLIAMS, E. H.: Variations in Tumour Distribution in the West Nile District of Uganda, p. 37—42. In: Cancer in Africa. Eds.: CLIFFORD, P., LINSELL, C. A., TIMMS, G. L.: Nairobi: East African Publishing House 1967.

WILLIAMS, E. H. Personal Communication, 1972.

WILLIAMS, E. H., SPIT, P., PIKE, M. C.: Further Evidence of Space-Time Clustering of Bur-kitt's lymphoma patients in the West Nile district of Uganda. Brit. J. Cancer **23**, 235—246 (1969).

WILLIAMS, E. H., WILLIAMS, P. H.: A note on the apparent similarity in distribution of oncho-cerciasis, femoral hernia and Kaposi's sarcoma in the West Nile District of Uganda. E. Afr. med. J. **43**, 208—209 (1966).

WILLIAMS, H. M., DIAMOND, H. D., CRAVER, L. F., PARSONS, H.: Neurological complications of lymphomas and leukemias. Springfield (Ill.): Charles C Thomas 1959.

WILLIS, R. A.: Pathology of Tumours. 4th edition. London: Butterworth 1967.

WINSHIP, T.: Malignant tumours of the thyroid gland. In: Ch. 20. Vol. 2. Pt 2. Cancer. Ed.: RAVEN, R. W. London: Butterworth 1958.

WOGAN, G. N.: Chemical nature and biological effects of the aflatoxins. Bact. Rev. **30**, 460 —470 (1966).

WOGAN, G. N.: Aflatoxin risks and control measures. Fed. Proc. **27**, 932 (1968).

WOODMAN, H.: Endemic goitre in Central Africa. E. Afr. med. J. **29**, 217—228 (1952).

WOODRUFF, J. D., JULIAN, C. G., NOVAK, E. R.: Diverse patterns of endometrial malignancy. Amer. J. Obstet. Gynec. **108**, 34—40 (1970).

WOODRUFF, J. D., PROTOS, P., PETERSON, W. F.: Ovarian Teratomas. Amer. J. Obstet. Gynec. **102**, 702—714 (1968).

World Health Organization: Manual of the International Statistical Classification of Diseases, Injuries, and Causes of Death, Vol. I. (Based on the recommendations of the Seventh Revision Conference, 1955.) World Health Organization, Geneva 1957.

WRIGHT, D. H.: Cytology and histochemistry of the Burkitt Lymphoma. Brit. J. Cancer **17**, 50—55 (1963).

WRIGHT, D. H.: Microscopic features, histochemistry, histogenesis and diagnosis. In: Burkitt's Lymphoma. Ed.: BURKITT, D. P., WRIGHT, D. H. Edinburgh and London: Livingstone 1970 a, pp. 82—102.

WRIGHT, D. H.: Gross distribution and haematology. In: Burkitt's Lymphoma. Ed.: BURKITT, D. P., WRIGHT, D. H. Edinburgh and London: Livingstone 1970 b, pp. 64—81.

Wright, D. H.: Burkitt's Lymphoma: A review of the pathology immunology and possible etiologic factors. Pathology Annual, 1971: Ed.: Sommers, S. C. New York: Appleton-Century-Crofts 1971.

Wright, D. H., Roberts, M.: The geographical distribution of Burkitt's tumour compared with the geographical distribution of other types of malignant lymphoma in Uganda. Brit. J. Cancer 20, 469—474 (1966).

Wright, R., McCollum, R. W., Klatskin, G.: Australia antigen in acute and chronic liver disease. Lancet 1969 II, 117—121.

Wynder, E. L., Bross, I. J., Feldman, R. M.: Etiological factors in Cancer of the Mouth. Cancer (Philad.) 10, 1300—1323 (1957).

Wynder, E. L., Dodo, H., Barber, H. R. K.: Epidemiology of cancer of the ovary. Cancer (Philad.) 23, 352—370 (1969).

Wynder, E. L., Hultberg, S., Jacobsson, F., Bross, I. J.: Environmental factors in cancer of upper alimentary tract. Swedish study with special reference to Plummer-Vinson (Paterson-Kelly) syndrome. Cancer (Philad.) 10, 470—487 (1957).

Wynder, E. L., Kajitani, T., Ishikawa, S., Dodo, H., Takano, A.: Environmental factors of cancer of the colon and rectum. II — Japanese epidemiological data. Cancer (Philad.) 23, 1210—1220 (1969).

Wynder E. L., Mabuchi, K., Whilmore, W. F.: Epidemiology of Cancer of the Prostate. Cancer (Philad.) 28, 344—360 (1971).

Yahia, G., Benirschke, K., Sturgis, S. H.: Carcinoma of endometrium. Progr. Gynaecology IV, 410—425 (1963).

Yeh, S.: A histological classification of carcinomas of the nasopharynx with a critical review as to the existence of lymphoepitheliomas. Cancer (Philad.) 15, 895—920 (1962).

Yeh, S.: Histology of Nasopharyngeal Cancer. In: Cancer of the Nasopharynx. Eds.: Muir, C. S., Shanmugaratnam, K. U.I.C.C. Monogr. Series, Vol. 1, p. 147—152. Copenhagen: Munksgaard 1967.

Yesudian, P.: A case of Kaposi's Sarcoma. Indian J. Derm. 14, 121 (1969).

Yoshida, Y.: Malignant Melanoma in Japan. Indian J. Ven. Dis. 21, 59—64 (1955).

Ziegler, J. L., Bluming, A. Z., Morrow, R. H., Cohen, M. H., Fife, E. H., Finerty, J. F., Woods, R.: Burkitt's Lymphoma and Malaria. Trans. roy. Soc. trop. Med. Hyg. 66, 285—292 (1972).

Ziegler, J. L., Bluming, A. Z., Morrow, R. H., Fass, L., Carbone, P. P.: Central Nervous System Involvement in Burkitt's Lymphoma. Blood 36, 718—728 (1970).

Ziegler, J. L., Morrow, R. H., Bluming, A. Z., Fass, L., Templeton, A. C., Templeton, C., Kyalwazi, S. K.: Clinical Features and Treatment of Childhood Lymphoma in Uganda. Int. J. Cancer 5, 415—425 (1970).

Ziegler, J. L., Morrow, R. H., Fass, L., Kyalwazi, S. K.: Childhood Hodgkin's disease in Uganda. E. Afr. med. J. 47, 191 (1970).

Ziegler, J. L., Wright, D. H., Kyalwazi, S. K.: The differential diagnosis of Burkitt's lymphoma of the face and jaws. Cancer (Philad.) 27, 503—514 (1971).

Zimmerman, L. M., Wagner, D. H.: Relation of Nodular Goiter to Thyroid Carcinoma. In: Clinical Endocrinology. Ed.: Astwood, E. B. Vol. I, p. 160. New York-London: Grune and Stratton 1960.

Subject Index

Recent Results
in Cancer Research

Sponsored by the Swiss League against Cancer
Editor in chief: P. Rentchnick, Genève

In Production

In Preparation

* Distribution rights for U. K., Commonwealth and the Traditional British Market (excluding Canada): W. Heinemann, Medical Books Ltd., London.